HERBS

AGAINST

CANCER

— Important Note to Reader —

ALL HEALTH BOOKS CARRY DISCLAIMERS AND WARNINGS. THIS ONE HAS TO BE TAKEN QUITE LITERALLY. *HERBS AGAINST CANCER* IS intended as a work of historical and critical analysis. It is not a book of instructions for cancer patients on how to treat themselves. Given the nature of the subject, it necessarily discusses some herbs and related compounds of extreme, even deadly, toxicity. These include but are not limited to poison hemlock, deadly nightshade, oleander, etc.

It would be tragic if any reader were to misunderstand the author's or the publisher's intentions and attempt to use such information to self-medicate for any indication or condition. Readers with cancer should seek out the help of skilled oncologists, other physicians and trained herbalists. In this context, I can do no better than to repeat the words that appeared in bold type on the back of Jonathan Hartwell's book, *Plants Used Against Cancer:*

WARNING: Neither the author nor the publisher makes any medical claims for any herb. This information is compiled from the published literature. Some plants contain deadly poisons and some mentioned herein are extremely dangerous.

This book contains general information about cancer. Neither the author nor the publisher makes warranties, expressed or implied, that this information is complete, nor do we warrant the fitness of this information for any particular purpose. This information is not intended as medical advice, and we disclaim any liability resulting from its use. Neither the author nor the publisher advocates any treatment modality. Each reader is strongly urged to consult qualified professional help for medical problems, especially those involving cancer.

HERBS
AGAINST
CANCER

HISTORY AND
CONTROVERSY

RALPH W. MOSS PHD

EQUINOX PRESS, INC.
Brooklyn, New York

Copyright © 1998 by Ralph W. Moss
Manufactured in the United States of America
by Equinox Press, Incorporated
144 St. John's Place, Brooklyn, New York
718-636-4433

Cover Art
Botanical Frame, Tempera on Gold Leaf by Enrique Moreiro
Botanical Illustrations
The Plant Kingdom Compendium and *Henning Anthon*
Typography and Design
Movable Type, Inc., Brooklyn, New York
(Monotype Bembo Text)
Digital Photography of Cover Art
Jellybean Photographics, Inc., New York, New York
Printing
Malloy Lithographing, Inc., Ann Arbor, Michigan

Library of Congress Cataloging-in-Publication Data

Moss, Ralph W.
    Herbs against Cancer : history and controversy / Ralph W. Moss.
        p.   cm.
    Includes bibliographical references and index.
    ISBN 1-881025-40-3 (trade paper)
    1. Cancer -- Alternative treatment.   2. Herbs -- Therapeutic use.
    I. Title
    RC291.A62.M67   1998
616.99′406 -- dc21   98-26261
                                                                      CIP

3   5   7   9   10   8   6   4   2

HERBS AGAINST CANCER

TABLE OF CONTENTS

DEDICATION

To the scientists
who have investigated and validated
folk treatments for cancer

especially

JONATHAN L. HARTWELL, PhD (1906–1991)
National Cancer Institute

and

JAMES A. DUKE, PhD
US Department of Agriculture (ret.)

"Oh mickle is the powerful grace that lies
In herbs, plants, stones, and their true qualities....
Within the infant rind of this small flower
Poison hath residence, and medicine power."
—Shakespeare, Romeo and Juliet, Act II Scene III

❧ Preface

THIS IS THE FIRST OF TWO BOOKS ON THE TOPIC OF BOTANICALS AND CANCER. IN THIS VOLUME I TRACE SOME OF THE HISTORY AND particularly the controversies that have erupted around the use of herbs to treat cancer in the Western world. I focus on what economic botanist James A. Duke, PhD, has called "herbs of contention." My main focus has been on the perennial conflict of regular doctors versus advocates of natural agents that are used to prevent, treat, diagnose, or mitigate the Dread Disease.

Choosing the topics for extended discussion from a list of more than 3,000 such herbs has been difficult. In making my selection, I have had to set several limitations:

● I deal exclusively with herbs in the Western tradition, which emerged in the ancient civilizations of Mesopotamia and Egypt, was transmitted to the Greeks and Romans, preserved throughout the Middle Ages and then transformed by science in modern times. It also includes other streams that have fed this river, particularly the Native American.

I felt it would be fruitless to discuss Chinese, Japanese, Indian or other Eastern herbs outside the context of their respective philosophical systems. An understanding of Traditional Chinese Medicine (TCM), Kampo, and Ayurveda was clearly beyond the scope of this book. I should acknowledge, however, that in doing so, I have given up a lot. There are those who believe that TCM in particular holds greater promise for cancer patients than the European-American tradition. Perhaps. But I believe that Western herbs are important in their own right and deserve a more lucid exposition

5

than they have received so far.

• In two instances, I have stretched some peoples' definition of "herb" by including fruits and fruit juices. These are "The Grape Cure," an historically interesting and important controversy, and noni juice.

• I have chosen not to write about the use of mushrooms, fungi, or their byproducts in the treatment of cancer. Although their inclusion would have bolstered my argument that botanicals are an effective but largely neglected aspect of cancer care, I was uncomfortable with the notion of mushrooms as "herbs." Also, most medicinal mushrooms emerge from Chinese and Japanese medicine and should not be wrenched out of their cultural contexts.

• Similarly, I have decided not to write, in this book, about sea vegetables, mosses, or various one-celled organisms, such as green or blue-green algae. A discussion of Chlorella and Spirulina might also have bolstered my argument, but to include such items stretched the definition of "herbs" past the point that I was willing to go.

• With a few exceptions, I have avoided a discussion of homoeopathic preparations entirely. (My main exception is HANSI and, as I explain, this cannot be considered a classical homoeopathic formulation.) Many homoeopathic drugs are indeed of vegetable origin and some are used against cancer. In the past, some herbalists have mingled homoeopathic with allopathic uses. However, this seems pointless. The method by which homoeopathic preparations are made, their indications for use, and their proposed mechanism of action put them in a class apart from the usual botanical medicines.

• I have also chosen to exclude one botanical product that otherwise might have figured prominently. That is amygdalin, or laetrile, which is a plant constituent found in the bitter almond, the kernels of peaches and apricots, and hundreds of other plants of the Prunus genus. My primary reason is that I have written extensively about this controversy in two books that are still in print: *The Cancer Industry* (rev. 1996) and *Cancer Therapy* (1992). Interested readers can consult those volumes.

This book does not pretend to completeness, since many of the 3,000 traditional anticancer herbs have been objects of their own fascinating controversies. What I have attempted to do is present about two dozen items that have been the object of struggle in a wide variety of countries and eras.

A note on abbreviations:

Throughout the text, sources are identified by a number, in parentheses, pertaining to the References. There are instances in which a few commonly cited works are referred to without such footnotes.

Unless otherwise noted, the following abbreviations are used:

AHPA refers to the *Botanical Safety Handbook of the American Herbal Products Association;*

ASCO to the American Society of Clinical Oncology;

CAM to complementary and alternative medicine;

EB to the *Encyclopedia Britannica,* 15th Edition;

Hartwell to Jonathan Hartwell's *Plants Used Against Cancer;*

Medline to the US National Library of Medicine's database; this indispensible online resource gives titles, and often abstracts, of over nine million peer-reviewed medical journal articles (www4.ncbi.nlm.nih.gov/PubMed/).

A note on terminology:

In this work, I have tried to keep technical terms to a minimum. However, the use of the following terms was unavoidable.

1. *Anticancer* refers to ability of a compound to destroy cancer in humans.
2. *Antineoplastic* is a broad term that refers to any agent that fights against cancer in any way.
3. *Antitumor* refers to the ability of a compound to destroy cancer in experimental animals.
4. *Apoptosis* is a process by which a cell engages in programmed cell death or cellular suicide; a more refined way of killing a cell than cytotoxicity.
5. *Biopsy* is a surgical operation to determine whether or not a particular tissue is malignant or benign.
6. *Cancer* is a general term for a group of more than 100 diseases characterized by uncontrolled and abnormal growth of cells in different parts of the body. Solid cancers are corrosive, invasive, and metastatic (can colonize other parts of the body).
7. *Conventional treatments* refers to those that are routinely taught in medical schools, discussed in textbooks, and practiced in accredited hospitals. Primary treatments are surgery, radiation therapy, and chemotherapy, with hormones, cytokines and a few immunostimulants.
8. *Cytotoxicity* refers to the ability of a substance to kill or harm cells. It can refer to the action of drugs on healthy cells but in this book more usually refers to the action of drugs or herbs on cancer cells.
9. *Host-mediated responses* refers to antitumor or anticancer effects that result not from cytotoxicity (*q.v.*) but from an effect on the patient's inherent defense systems, particularly immunity.
10. *Induration* refers to a lump or hardening, which may or may not be malignant, depending on the results of a biopsy.
11. *Lesion* refers to any localized abnormal change in the structure of an organ or tissue. Usually, it is applied to cancerous changes in such structures.

Chapter 1 ❧ Introduction

*"There is a wonderful science in Nature, in trees, herbs, roots,
and flowers, which man has never yet fathomed."* —Jethro Kloss, Back to Eden

*"The great deluge of modern chemotherapy is about to wash away
the plant and vegetable debris."* —Morris Fishbein, MD (1927)

THE WORLD IS CHANGING. MEDICAL TREATMENTS THAT WERE CONSIDERED SHEER QUACKERY A FEW YEARS AGO ARE NOW BEING given serious consideration by government researchers. In the developing world, herbal medicine has attained new prestige, thanks mainly to the sponsorship of the World Health Organization (WHO). In the developed world, the public, by the tens of millions, is demanding an integration of conventional Western medicine and the once-scorned approaches of complementary and alternative medicine (CAM).

Cancer is one of the diseases whose treatment is being re-evaluated around the world. There is widespread dissatisfaction with surgery, radiotherapy, and especially chemotherapy. Even oncologists (cancer specialists) are being caught up in that trend. You will notice that the latest cancer "breakthroughs" mainly involve innovative and less toxic agents, such as hormonal drugs (tamoxifen), angiogenesis inhibitors (Angiostatin and Endostatin), and monoclonal antibodies (Herceptin).

More and more, doctors (prodded by outspoken and well-informed patients) are realizing that they need to do more than just kill cells. They must also foster wellness, by supporting the body's defense mechanisms and utilizing the biochemical peculiarities of the tumor against itself.

One possible "new" avenue of treatment is herbal medicine, with "new" in quotes because, as you shall see, it is one of the oldest ways of treating illness.

First of all, what do we mean by herbs and herbal medicine? We all have a commonsensical definition of herbs, which is basically "anything that grows and is useful." More technically, the *Concise Oxford Dictionary* defines an herb as (a) any non-woody seed-bearing plant which dies down to the ground after flowering, or (b) any plant with leaves, seeds, or flowers used for flavoring, food, medicine, scent, etc.

The World Health Organization (WHO), which has done much to promote the use of herbs, defines "herbal medicines" as "finished, labeled medicinal products that contain as active ingredients aerial or underground parts of plants, or other plant material, or combinations thereof, whether in the crude state or as plant preparations." Such plant materials can include juices, gums, fatty oils, essential oils, and any other substances of this nature.

Herbal medicines may also contain not just excipients (such as binders that help in the preparation of pills and capsules) but also, by tradition, natural organic or inorganic active ingredients, which are not of plant origin. In other words, the fact that an herbal remedy also contains potassium iodide, zinc chloride, or even bat dung does not invalidate it as an "herbal medicine," in the eyes of the World Health Organization (415).

Herbal medicine is regarded, in the United States at least, as an offshoot of complementary and alternative medicine (CAM). It has been called "hippy medicine"—or worse. However, although my own focus is on events in the English-speaking world, it is important from the start to put the use of herbal medicine in a worldwide context. Much of the resurgence of herbs in America, England, Canada, and Australia has to do with the acceptance of cultural pluralism in those countries. In many other countries, including the European Continent, the use of herbal medicine never entirely died out, and in some instances has been officially sanctioned and fostered. At the very least, there has been greater tolerance. It is mainly in the English-speaking countries, especially the USA, that such treatments were for a long time stigmatized as "health fraud" and "quackery."

One reason for the profound change in climate has been the activities of the World Health Organization, and its many affiliated agencies and congresses. The prestige of the WHO and the United Nations has done much to dissolve the atmosphere of hostility that surrounded traditional medicines.

For example, the Declaration of Alma-Ata in 1978 called for the accommodation of proven traditional remedies within national drug policies and regulatory measures. The World Health Assembly, a branch of the United

Nations (in resolution WHA 22.54), dealing with pharmaceutical production in developing countries, called on the Director-General to provide assistance to health authorities of member states to ensure that the drugs used were those most appropriate to local circumstances, that they were rationally used, and that the requirements for their use were assessed as accurately as possible.

Another 1989 resolution (WHA 42.43) explicitly supported national traditional medicine programs and drew attention to herbal medicine as being of "great importance" to the health of individuals and communities. These, and many other proclamations, led to a new validation of traditional health practices in a great many countries and to programs for their preservation and investigation. It is estimated that 80 percent of the world's population relies on traditional herbal medicines for a significant part of their healthcare. Although this is often by necessity, it is also frequently by choice.

Meanwhile, in the developed countries, we have seen a "preference of many consumers for products of natural origin" (415). This trend is reinforced by the desire of many immigrants to incorporate the traditional remedies of their former homes into the context of Western scientific medicine. A significant and related development has been the entry of many excellent scientists, especially Asians, into the research establishment. The reader will notice how many of the finest scientists in this field are of Chinese, Japanese or East Indian origin. A large percentage of the members of the American Society of Clinical Oncology (ASCO) are now either non-Americans or Americans of recent immigrant stock. This, too, is bound to have a profound impact on the future of cancer research.

At the same time, it is universally recognized that, in both developed and developing countries, the status of information on herbal medicine is often deficient. WHO has stated that "consumers and health care providers need to be supplied with up-to-date and authoritative information on the beneficial properties, and possible harmful effects, of all herbal medicines" (415).

To that end, several world conferences of drug regulatory authorities have been held by United Nations agencies. The US Food and Drug Administration (FDA) and the National Institutes of Health's Office of Alternative Medicine (OAM) jointly sponsored a similar groundbreaking conference called: "A Symposium on Botanicals: a Role in US Health Care?" at the Omni-Shoreham Hotel in Washington, DC from December 14-16, 1994. At that time the issues of safety and efficacy of medicinal herbs were intensively discussed.

It is my hope that this book, and its forthcoming companion volume, will help provide "up-to-date and authoritative information" on the benefits and deficits of using herbs in the treatment of cancer.

In America, there is no question that medical herbalism is undergoing an astonishing resurgence. The signs of vital growth are everywhere. In 1993, when David Eisenberg, MD of Harvard Medical School conducted his groundbreaking survey on the use of complementary and alternative medicine (CAM), a mere three percent of Americans were using therapeutic herbs. (The survey actually studied patient use in 1990.) In 1994, the FDA conducted its own survey and estimated that eight percent of Americans were now using herbal products. One year later, and the Gallup Poll showed that the number had leaped to 17 percent. By 1997, according to a Website called *MarketFacts,* it appeared that an astonishing 40 percent of the American public were using herbs regularly (www.marketfacts.com).

Because of this growing popularity, herbs are starting to wield clout in the medical marketplace. Annual sales, which were $1.0 billion in 1991, had jumped to $3.24 billion by 1997 (109).

"The interest in medicinal herbs has exploded in the last two or three years," said Kathleen Halloran, editor of the magazine *Herb Companion.* "Many people are amazed at the many uses of the herbs growing in their gardens." And not just their gardens. Presently in America there are around 1,600 different herbal products on the market. Some of these have become household words, and are advertised in mainstream media. Those of us who grew up thinking of herbs as "guerrilla medicine" did neck-wrenching doubletakes when we saw packages of St. John's Wort and *Ginkgo biloba* piled high at Wal-Mart.

The majority of consumers (79 percent in one survey) feel that herbs are safe and probably effective for many conditions currently treated with pharmaceuticals or over-the-counter drugs. And there is not yet an end in sight. A 1998 *MarketFacts* survey showed that many more Americans would take medicinal herbs if they knew more about them. In this respect Americans are merely catching up with the Germans, Indians, Chinese and many other people who rely on herbs for a good part of their health care. They are also returning to the health habits that dominated our country's history from the time the Pilgrims landed until well into the 20th century. Our exclusive reliance on pharmaceuticals is beginning to look just like a brief hiatus in a long history in which herbs held an important place in the national consciousness.

But what about cancer? Are cancer patients also turning to herbs? And, if they are, should they be encouraged in this trend?

Cancer is the second most common cause of death in America. Over 1.2 million Americans (nine million people worldwide) develop some form of internal cancer each year. Over half a million Americans per year die of the disease. Given the overall statistics, it is inevitable that many cancer patients, especially those already familiar with the use of herbs for minor ailments, will start to explore the possibility of using herbs to assist them with this most serious of health crises.

And in fact this is already happening. A 1998 study of women with breast cancer revealed that 80.9 percent were using dietary supplements of some sort in the course of their illness. This included some herb-derived products such as evening primrose oil. Researchers at the University of California–San Diego found that such women were better educated, slimmer, etc. than their non-herb-using counterparts. In California at least, herbalism is chic (300).

Yet most people frankly admit that they are poorly educated on the topic of herbs. In the above study, only 19 percent of those taking supplements said they knew "quite a bit" about herbs, and only two percent said they knew "a great deal." When it comes to herbs, people generally don't consult their medical doctors. Their attitude is "Why bother?," since most people assume that MDs were never trained in the subject and are prejudiced against it. In fact, rather than consulting their doctors about herbs, five times as many people turn to popular books, according to *MarketFacts*.

But what is the quality of the information they receive? I have attempted to read every book on the topic of herbs and cancer, even tracking down the rare and out-of-print ones. Generally speaking, I have not been impressed. With some notable exceptions, many are biased, one-sided, and gullible about the virtues of herbs. Sometimes, they "puff" products of dubious value. They may ignore the possibility of adverse effects, contraindications, or common drug interactions.

I must warn you that some seemingly objective health information on herbs is crypto-advertising. Some of the sincere-sounding "patient testimonials" come from people who are themselves integrated into multi-level or network marketing schemes.

There are some "scientific papers" that never have and never will see the light of day in any medical journal; journalistic reports in magazines that are "sponsored" by herbal product manufacturers. In fact, new herbal products are the subject of entire "newsletters," which turn out to be simply advertising gimmicks, ready to be sent out by the hundreds of thousands. Some of these products (but not all) are worthless and dangerous. This is the seamy side of the herb and cancer business.

Yet other books and articles err in the opposite direction. They sneeringly denigrate any possible use of herbs for cancer, while managing to insult the reader's intelligence. These are the pronouncements of professional detractors of CAM and herbal treatments. There is a group of individuals whose careers revolve around lurid exposés of alternative approaches—the so-called "quackbusters." They are the mirror image of the herbal promoters.

Quackbusters are motivated by a reflexive hostility towards anything smacking of deviance in medicine. They are quick to apply the words "quack," "scam," or "fraud" to treatments and individuals they disapprove of. In the words of Larry Dossey, MD, they are victims of the "right men syndrome," and cannot tolerate having their rigid views contradicted. The term "right man" describes "an individual, almost always male, who has a dynamic yet fragile personality and always possesses a manic need to feel that his actions are perfectly justified and correct at all times" (111).

A typical product of "right" thinking is the Website *QuackWatch,* edited by a leading crusader against "quackery," Stephen Barrett, MD.

Dr. Barrett issues this warning to cancer patients: "Be wary of herbal remedies." He offers no differentiation between treatments that are seeking scientific validation, and arrant fraud. According to his site, "herbs are promoted primarily through literature based on hearsay, folklore and tradition." This ignores the decades of work by such genuine experts as Jonathan Hartwell and James Duke in verifying such claims, filtering them through the sieve of scientific inquiry.

"As medical science developed," says Dr. Barrett, "it became apparent that most herbs did not deserve good reputations...." What an odd statement, when in fact the traditional uses of many herbs have now been confirmed, in part or in whole, by medical science.

"Most that did," Barrett continues, "were replaced by synthetic compounds that are more effective." This is only partially true. Synthetic compounds can never fully replace herbs, because herbs are extremely complex things, which can have multiple physiological or psychological effects in the body. And many of the best herbs have never been synthesized. Even Dr. Barrett concedes that "many herbs contain hundreds or even thousands of chemicals that have not been completely cataloged." However, he draws a negative conclusion from that fact. Barrett contends that certain chemicals in herbs could "well prove toxic."

This is obviously true, although most herbs are safe when used as recommended. Oftentimes, critics point to a particular chemical in plants and claim that it is toxic or even carcinogenic. However, one must be cautious about such claims and take every instance on a case-by-case basis. As Paracelsus said centuries ago, everything, even water, is toxic if taken in sufficient doses. For example, I will enjoy some beets this afternoon. Yet beets contain, among other toxic chemicals, arsenic! Am I engaging in reckless behavior by eating them? Of course not, since the arsenic is present in 0.01 to 0.08 parts per million, a homoeopathic dose. Similarly, some of the scares about "toxic" ingredients in herbs are exaggerated by die-hard critics of CAM who have an ideological ax to grind. (Occasionally, however, common herbs do prove to have unexpected toxicities.)

Finally, Barrett concludes that "with safe and effective treatment available, treatment with herbs rarely makes sense." This is a specious argument. While I agree with Dr. Barrett that cancer patients should never forego surgery, radiation therapy, or chemotherapy when these treatments have been proven to be effective and reasonably safe, even this leaves a wide area for herbal treatments.

Cancer treatments in general are not always very safe. And ultimately they are not effective for about 40 to 50 percent of the patients. For the 564,800 Americans expected to die in 1998 of cancer, there are neither safe nor effective conventional treatments. There are also about eight million people who have been treated for cancer and who might want to do something besides worry about the recurrence of their disease.

While I deplore the activity of the "quackbusters," I want to make clear that I think there are also reasonable critics of herbal treatment who have studied the question and come up with less optimistic assessments than I have.

They have their reasons. Some are skeptical of the power of herbs to possibly affect a deep-seated condition such as cancer. Others are afraid that patients will be deterred from taking proper treatments by the illusory promise of herbal cures.

In recent years, researcher John Boik has issued a sober and rather pessimistic judgment on the potential of using herbs against cancer. He believes that the efficacy of complementary treatments is "largely unknown" (47). In an unpublished article he has written:

"In the end, two things are clear to me. First, no alternative/complementary therapy has as yet been proven to cure or significantly affect cancer in humans. And, second, few, if any, individual natural agents appear to have the potential to produce dramatic clinical effects...."

But he adds, "That natural anticancer therapies are unproven is a direct consequence of the lack of research on these agents. It is not that they are proven useless, it is that proof is lacking either way" (48).

Boik further believes that when used alone, relatively high doses of natural agents would be required to influence specific processes and he worries that these doses could cause severely adverse side effects. However, he also believes that combinations of agents (such as is traditional in Chinese and some Western medicine) might have effects over a longer period of time without the deleterious side effects.

Richard Grossman, author of *The Other Medicines,* holds a similarly negative view. Grossman is a psychotherapist who incorporates herbs into his regimens for people with cancer. But he does not believe that these regimens are curative for any cancers. He does feel, however, that they can be of great value in alleviating some of the side effects of toxic mainstream therapies and for their general health-enhancing effects.

Michael Lerner and his colleagues at Commonweal take an even more negative stance. In a recent addition to *Choices in Healing,* they write:

"But there are also many herbal remedies for cancer sold in health food stores and by mail order that have no long empirical tradition of ethical use, or have been taken out of the context in which they were used properly, or are adulterated, or are not what they are represented to be, or are sold for unethical markups. Like pharmacological treatments for cancer, herbal remedies can be an area where quackery is a very real concern. They have no intrinsic health promoting benefits..." (133).

While sharing their concern over potential health fraud, I think this is phrased too negatively. I remain more optimistic about the role of herbs and feel that herbs have great potential as treatment and can play a more positive role for cancer patients. I would not rule out the possibility of a curative role in some cases.

However, my point is that there are skeptics and there are Skeptics. I am excited by the prospect of using herbs against cancer. But it is possible to make an honest appraisal of this field and come away disappointed. Such genuine critics are clearly not motivated by any ingrained hostility towards alternative medicine, or freedom of choice, but by a sincere desire to guide patients in the most useful directions. I respect and have learned from their approach.

I have tried to look at herbs used in the treatment of cancer in an even-handed way. In a field that has been marred by outrageous exaggeration on both sides, I have tried to offer accurate and dispassionate information.

My viewpoint is essentially that of "friendly skepticism." I am neither promoter nor denigrator of such usage. Certainly, I am rooting for the roots. But I demand proof for any claims. If this proof is deficient (as is too often the case) I clearly say so. Unlike some authors in this field, I have no economic interest in any of the treatments I write about.

In these pages I have avoided the more ethereal regions and tried to stick to the facts as they are revealed by history and the scientific record. I am neither by inclination or training inclined to explicate on phenomena that cannot be measured or observed through the senses.

Historically, we know that herbalism evolved in close proximity with magic (black and white) as well as religious rites. It has also been intertwined with astrology and alchemy. (But, then again, so was chemistry.)

Many old herbalists mixed charms and magic with their potions. They often subscribed to a "Doctrine of Signatures," which meant that healing plants resembled the parts of the human body they most influenced. By such *a priori* reasoning, walnuts were considered good for the brain. As odd as it may seem, there are still a few prominent herbalists who promulgate such views. I consider this a fallacy and will point it out where it occurs.

Astrology continues to have adherents in herbal circles. There is an ancient pedigree to such beliefs. Nicholas Culpeper (1616-1654), who wrote one of the first English herbals, was an inveterate astrologer. "He who would know the reason of the operation of the Herbs, must look up as high as the stars," he said (90). One modern student of this topic considers herself primarily a "medical astrologer."

Even alchemy has its modern adherents. A highly regarded herbalist in New Jersey titled his company Herbalist & Alchemist. He claims to use alchemical methods, combined with modern science, to transform common substances into their vital essences. "Alchemical preparations have a synergistic principle that gives them a unique vitality and activity," he writes (412).

Many other writers believe that there is a religious component to herbalism, and that a beneficent Deity put herbs in a locale in order to cure the human illnesses found there. It simply a matter of matching up the symptoms with the cure. This approach is epitomized by a bestselling book, *God's Pharmacy,* which appeared originally in Germany. Other writers have put forward fanciful ideas of direct or subtle communication between plants and humans.

I enjoy reading such theories. Nevertheless, I have approached the question of herbs in a very materialistic way, without recruiting any higher powers onto my side. It is not my intention to insult anyone's beliefs, and I respect the enormous efforts that some herbalists have made in trying to understand and apply ancient and esoteric healing traditions. However, fundamentally, I am trying interpret herbalism through the prism of science, not religion. For that reason, in this book you will find no explanations of herbs based on any mystical concepts (251). My motto is the same as the one often heard at the US National Institutes of Health: "In God we trust. All others show data."

By using the tools of the appropriate sciences, I believe we can arrive at valuable knowledge about plants and how they can be used to fight malignant diseases. I also want to share this fascinating history, and to impart knowledge that patients can use in making decisions, if they so choose.

Surveying the scene, I am amazed that none of the scholars in medical botany thought to write a book like this before. One reason has to be that more practical authors have avoided a topic that is so obviously fraught with peril.

First of all, many people seem to want sensational accounts of miracle cures, or nothing at all. They have had enough "reality" from their oncologists. Stories of fantastic cures stimulate the imaginative side of the brain. The popular book market seems to demand either the word "miracle" or the word "cure" in the title—and preferably both. Just scanning my book shelf I see such recent titles as *Cancer Cure, Curing Cancer, The Man Who Cures Cancer* and *The Cure for All Cancers*. I am awaiting delivery of a new title that deals in part with cancer. It is called *Miracle Herbs*.

Second, John Heinerman (who himself wrote a now out-of-print book on herbs and cancer) explained the economic dilemma this way:

"Publishers of health books generally like authors to include information that is safe, simple, and for everyday aches and pains. Few of them venture into areas such as cancer, believing that they are potential mine fields of explosive consequences" (174).

Why a Mine Field?

You are bound to anger many conservative doctors if you say anything positive about herbal cancer treatments. No matter how cautiously one writes, some people seem intent on misunderstanding the message. Desperate or distracted patients may read a book such as this and then decide to use herbs in unwise fashion.

So let's get the issue of toxicity on the table. I recently saw a magazine article that blared, "If it's natural, it can't do you any harm." What pernicious nonsense! I think of the patient in Michigan who died when his doctor injected an anticancer tea into his veins (*The Holland Sentinel*, 4/18/97). In another well-publicized instance, numerous patients were injected with a concentrated form of aloe vera juice and some died immediately afterwards (209). There are instances in which cancer patients seem to have damaged their livers by taking herbal tea. Some "cancer remedies" contain cancer-promoting substances. So not everything natural is safe or good for you. In fact, some of the herbs discussed in this book are deadly poisons.

A writer's nightmare is the desperate patient who misunderstands all the warnings and caveats and decides to brew up a little *Conium maculatum* (hemlock) to treat his malignancy. Gentle reader, I have two words for you. Please. Don't.

In this book I will not sweep potentially unpleasant or dangerous facts about herbs under the rug. If I know about them, so will you. However, that said, it is emphatically true that herbs in general are much safer than pharmaceuticals. A March, 1998, article in the *Journal of the American Medical Association (JAMA)* revealed that more than 100,000 people a year die in American hospitals from adverse reactions to properly prescribed medication. Prof. Bruce Pomeranz of the University of Toronto calculated that this makes drug reactions themselves between the fourth and sixth leading cause of death (249). (And understand that this does not even include drug accidents.)

Herbs may very well represent a gentler way to accomplish some of the same therapeutic aims as drugs, with less adverse effects. The number of deaths that occur because of the deliberate intake of medicinal herbs is very small. However, shocking revelations about pharmaceuticals do not give herbalists a free ride. They, too, have to take responsibility for any adverse effects from their products.

Remember too that untoward or idiosyncratic reactions can and do occur and cause considerable suffering. I remember the sight of a good friend of mine—an ardent advocate of alternative medicine—who smeared tea tree oil on his feet to kill athlete's foot. Instead of being cured, his feet blew up like balloons and he had to leave the meeting we were attending and take allopathic medicine to relieve his suffering.

More tragically, I can't get out of my mind the sight of a young girl who bought a salve on the Internet and seriously disfigured herself (see Chapter 6). The "good news" in her case was that the offshore manufacturer offered her her money back. Unfortunately, they couldn't offer her her face back.

These are, to be sure, uncommon occurrences. Nevertheless, they demonstrate why one must be careful to detail the potential toxicities of herbs, even in situations in which they are unlikely to occur.

Although I have tried to be very careful, I also must caution you not to rely on this book, or any other single book, as a guide to herb toxicity. Cross check the safety of plants with various other up-to-date authorities and never rely on any single source for such information. Bear in mind that a celebrated old reference book, Sturtevant's *Edible Plants of the World,* states that the seeds of the "love pea" (*Abrus precatorius*) have nourishing qualities. In fact, they are extremely poisonous and need prolonged special preparation to destroy the poison. At least eight other plants are similarly mislabeled in this "classic" work (229). As Mark Twain once said, "Be careful about reading health books. You may die of a misprint."

Another danger is that patients may enthusiastically turn to an herbal (or other non-conventional) treatment when a conventional treatment is more appropriate. This is the old shibboleth of conventional medicine. Like many such arguments, the problem is often exaggerated for its propagandistic value—nevertheless there is a grain of truth in it.

Surgery, radiation and chemotherapy all have their place in the treatment of cancer. Surgery for small tumors can be lifesaving in many situations. Radiation and chemotherapy can also extend life, improve quality of life, and even cure in other situations. Frequently, the three methods are used in conjunction. I hope you will share my boundless enthusiasm for herbs. However, please don't neglect treatments that are well proven to increase overall survival.

In rare instances, foolish or desperate people refuse or delay surgery to take herbs and then may have to deal with disseminated cancers. While propagandists routinely exaggerate the extent of such problems, that does not make them non-existent. In the course of dealing with thousands of cancer patients over a period of 25 years, I have personally seen this happen only two or three times. But each time was a tragedy.

Also, please remember that advanced cancer is not properly a self-help disease. The person with cancer should try to assemble a team. This could include surgeons, radiotherapists, oncologists, nurses, psychological and spiritual counselors, and should include the best herbalists and complementary practitioners available as well. It may not be easy to find oncologists willing to work with herbalists. However, there is an increasing willingness on the part of some to do so.

Finally, we should always keep an eye on the bottom line. Cancer can involve punishing expenses. Alternative treatments have increased in cost along with conventional ones, and they have the further disadvantage of not being covered by standard health insurance. One of the potentially great things about botanicals is how inexpensive they often can be. Think about garlic, turmeric, soy, broccoli—each of these has health-promoting powers and can be purchased for very little. Even most herbs in the health food store or pharmacy are inexpensive.

Then again, some of the herbal products discussed in this book are inordinately expensive. The worst involve some secret remedy that has allegedly been suppressed by the cancer establishment. An individual who died from some irresponsible injections of herbs gave her "alternative" doctor $16,000 in three weeks for the privilege (209).

Occasionally, suppression of competitive treatments by the medical establishment does take place. I have detailed some instances of such suppression in my book, *The Cancer Industry*. The problem is that the historical occasions of persecution do not in any way exonerate the shady practices of some hustlers in the herbal field. All too often, unscrupulous operators try to whip up patient paranoia as a cover for money-making operations. They shout "Persecution!" to avoid their own responsibilities to the patient and to charge a lot of money. These same people do an absolute minimum of research to validate their therapies.

The historical background of cure mongering, and the deep divisions within the medical profession, have made the evaluation of cancer treatments difficult. Clearly, herbal cancer treatments could not develop along lines entirely free of charlatanism. There is no reason to deny that health fraud has always been a feature of the alternative cancer field. On the other hand, there were some authentic folk traditions that, even in America, managed to survive the patent medicine era.

In general, I avoid the words quack and quackery in my discussion. Athough we all have a commonsensical notion of quackery, the word lacks scientific precision. It is usually used as an ugly pejorative to denigrate those with whom one violently disagrees.

I say this not in order to shield anyone from deserved criticism. But unless we can accommodate nuances, we shall miss the most important part of this story. As we shall show in the case of Harry Hoxsey, various elements, positive and negative, are bound up in the phenomenon usually called quackery (see Chapter 5).

The classic definition of a quack is "one who pretends to medical skill he does not possess" (25). One thinks of the slick but uncredentialed layperson who breezes into town and hangs out his shingle as a physician. Such things occur. But today such an opportunist is most likely to adhere as closely as possible to conventional practices in order to escape detection.

I believe that anyone who claims to administer a sure-fire cure for cancer, based on methods that have not been proven through the regular avenues of science, will almost certainly be unmasked as a fraud. There is usually a good dose of secrecy and paranoia thrown in.

For example, consider this Website for an herbal cancer "cure":

"In my worldly travels I have come to know the underlying causes of many diseases including cancer. I would like to point out that I don't believe in treating or masking symptoms—I CURE!! I work with a money back guarantee: If the Level 1 program and it fails [sic], you pay nothing. If you think this is putting my money where my mouth is you are right. All of my programs are non-medical and so are not toxic" (www.telusplanet.net/public/herbrem1/).

Interestingly, the author has posted Webster's definition of "quack" and "quackery" at the site, in support of his belief that "western allopathic medicine is no less than 75 percent very well organized quackery." Talk about beating your opponent to the punch!

Most "cancer quacks" do not pretend to the skills of surgery, radiotherapy or chemotherapy. Their claims are based on treatments not utilized by conventional doctors. So the question of "quackery" inevitably moves from the training and education of the individual practitioner to the methods he or she advocates.

Unfortunately, the efficacy of any new method cannot be known *a priori*. We also must be circumspect in making charges, since many excellent ideas in medicine were initially rejected as worthless quackery. If we are to have progress in medicine, we must foster an atmosphere of friendly skepticism.

Quackbusting further obscured the nuggets that existed in the ancient traditions. Certainly, we can criticize the methods and presentation of herbal advocates. But to attain true knowledge about safety and efficacy requires serious scientific testing. And, as you shall see, such testing, for a variety of reasons, has rarely been carried out by either side in this debate.

A related question is that of secrecy. At the aforementioned Website there are repeated claims of "cure" for all the common types of cancer, but not one word on the nature of the treatment itself. While most of us have a gut feeling that secrecy and quackery are intimately related, this is not always the case. Many of the most controversial methods (such as the Eli

Jones formula) were public. And occasionally, valid methods were kept secret for prolonged periods of time. The obstetrical forceps, for instance, was kept as the private possession of a single English family of doctors (the Chamberlens) for almost 100 years. Even when they were thrown in jail they refused to talk. "They kept their instrument a close secret," one historian has written, "and they went to extraordinary lengths to mislead observers," literally attached bells and whistles to the instrument's cart in order to fool would-be competitors (272).

There is often an aura of strict secrecy around pharmaceuticals leading up to the time they are patented. I well remember the persistence of Wall Street analysts who tried to sweet talk news of cytokine development out of me when I was at Memorial Sloan-Kettering. (Little did I realize what a huge business this was about to become.) After a drug is patented, of course, the company may be reasonably open about its nature. But by then it has secured a legal monopoly for seventeen years. Looked at from an economic, rather than an idealistic or humanitarian, perspective, secrecy is a weapon in the fierce economic competition that often characterizes the health field.

There are so many pitfalls in the evaluation of these products that one can well ask: Should people who are fighting cancer use herbs at all? Is it ethical to produce, sell, or even write favorably about this topic? I am painfully aware of the lack of really good studies to prove the value of herbs, especially as treatment. But I think we know enough about both safety and effectiveness to answer with a qualified yes.

There are a number of situations in which herbs could profitably be used in the fight against malignancy:

● *When the immune system is deficient.* Many scientists believe that a weakened immune system contributes to the growth of cancer. Some herbs have been demonstrated to improve, or modulate, various aspects of immunity.

● *To counteract the side effects of conventional treatments.* Conventional treatments are directed at killing or removing cancer cells. However, they are not specific and many normal cells get destroyed in the process. The immune system is often devastated in the fight. Herbs (and other non-conventional approaches) can help build up the body's defenses. Even the American Cancer Society now concedes that herbs can be useful as adjuncts. (They continue to caution patients against using herbs as anticancer agents.)

● *Primary prevention.* There is evidence that herbs (or special "designer" foods) may actually be able to help prevent cancer from occurring. Wouldn't that be wonderful! Really fine scientists are deep at work isolating compounds from soy, broccoli, grapes, etc. that have powerful cancer-preventing effects.

● *Secondary prevention.* Herbs may help prevent a recurrence of disease, once a tumor has been removed and the treatment period is over.

- *Watchful waiting.* In some situations (such as prostate cancer), many doctors urge watchful waiting. This involves intensive and repeated diagnostic procedures, but no treatment. But one can just as easily take some herbs as wait passively for the cancer to spread.

- *Primary treatments.* This of course is most controversial, but if cancer has recurred, or if it is discovered at a stage where no life-extending treatment is available, herbs can be used as part of cancer treatment. Many scientists would dispute this, and they are right that the evidence for such usage is thin. But, my feeling is "What exactly do you have to lose?" The main consideration of using herbs in this situation are (a) safety; (b) cost; and (c) psychological impact.

- *Psychological benefit.* Herbs can provide a psychological boost through the feeling that something worthwhile is being done.

Remember that alternative medicine is more than just herbs. It can include the use of food supplements, modulators of the immune system (vaccines, etc.) and mind-body techniques, such as meditation and guided visualization. All of these can be powerful and of great benefit to cancer patients. Thus, while I have isolated the herbal contribution for the sake of exposition, I do not believe it should be so isolated in actual practice. This is part of what we mean by "holistic" or "complementary" medicine. Hopefully, more and more physicians are becoming educated in the use and value of such techniques, and are willing to work with non-conventional practitioners in a cooperative fashion. We hope that the 21st century will usher in a new era of integrative oncology rather than the competition between different medical paradigms that marked the 19th and 20th centuries.

It is my hope that this book will play a role in bringing about this integration and will help introduce the use of non-toxic and less-toxic herbs into the practice of scientific oncology.

Finally, I want to address some words to the cancer patient who has picked up this book. If you are fighting cancer now, I wish you success in your struggle. I know that cancer is a formidable foe. But in the course of my career I have also known individuals with extremely advanced cancers who have turned the tide in the most unpromising of situations. Of course, we both know that this is more than just a matter of taking a few herbs. There has to be a skillful application of a number of approaches, orthodox, experimental and unconventional, and of faith—not just in a higher power, but in one's healers and their methods.

If you are battling cancer, I hope that this book will contribute to your knowledge and lift your spirits. I strongly urge you and your caregivers not to despair, but to keep searching, struggling and hoping. It is my firm belief that there are answers, if we use our intelligence, energy, and intuition to seek them out.

Chapter 2 🌸 Early Treatments

"The idea that the American Indians, or this person or that person...would accidentally stumble upon some herb that would cure [cancer] is rather far-fetched. It's like the idea that if you put three billion monkeys in a room, one of them might write a Shakespearean sonnet."—William Grigg
       Public Information Officer
       Food and Drug Administration (25)

"It is easy to make fun of medieval recipes; it is more difficult and may be wiser to investigate them. Instead of assuming that the medieval pharmacist was a benighted fool, we might wonder whether there was not sometimes a justification for his strange procedure."—Jonathan Hartwell
       National Cancer Institute scientist (165)

THE USE OF HERBS AGAINST CANCER IS A VERY ANCIENT PRACTICE, FOUND IN EVERY CULTURE AND REGION OF THE WORLD. THERE are even reasons to believe that animals may also use herbs to combat cancer.

Cancer is a disease of great antiquity. Some people have called cancer a "disease of civilization" and attribute its rise to industrialization and pollution. This definitely has something to do with it. However, there is evidence that animals, even in the wild, also develop cancer. Bone cancer was detected in a dinosaur bone discovered in Wyoming in 1992. There may even be a form of cancer in plants.

How prevalent is cancer in animals? A survey found cancer in 2.75 percent of all the mammals at the San Diego Zoo (118). Some wild animals also get cancer. For example, certain strains of wild Asian mice developed breast cancer with alarming frequency, 80 to 90 percent of the individuals

23

(199). Malignant melanoma has been found in the eye of a wild penguin and a red-tailed hawk (241). Wild kangaroos have been found with cancer in their livers (62). Chondrosarcoma was discovered in the eye of a great white heron (362). And as for wild skunks....well, you get the point.

I believe it will one day be proven that non-human species also have the ability to choose herbs that have some activity against cancer. The evidence for this is circumstantial, but intriguing.

Animals have long been known, anecdotally at least, to seek out healing herbs. "The dog taken by a fever seeks rest in a quiet corner, but is found eating herbs when his stomach is upset," wrote the great medical historian, Henry Sigerist, MD. "Nobody taught him what herbs to eat, but he will instinctively seek those that made him vomit or improve his condition in some other way" (355). (As we shall see, the greatest American herb controversy centered on exactly such claims—that an ailing stallion discovered a complicated herbal remedy known as the Hoxsey formula.)

Primates, such as the Japanese macaques, eat mineral-rich earths, luxuriously bathe in hot springs on snowy winter days, and smear a honey-like substance on their wounds. They perform simple "surgery" on cuts and bruises using sticks (334). Crude toothpicks have been found dating back 1.84 million years and, believe it or not, chimpanzees have been seen employing a kind of dental floss. A zoopharmacognosist (who studies such behavior professionally) humorously called this type of behavior "practicing medicine without a license."

But most intriguing of all is the primate use of "pharmaceuticals." Primatologist Karen Strier of the University of Wisconsin at Madison discovered that during their nonreproductive periods, muriqui monkeys in Brazil eat large amounts of plants containing fertility-reducing plant estrogens (isoflavonoids). When they are ready to mate, however, they switch to plants with steroid compounds that promote fertility. (Indigenous tribes in that part of South America employ identical compounds for their own birth control.)

In the mid-1980s, Harvard anthropologist Richard Wrangham observed chimpanzees in the Gombe National Park in Tanzania making special trips to find a type of sunflower called Aspilia. This is a virtually inedible plant, yet sometimes chimps chewed or even swallowed its leaves whole. Astonishingly, Aspilia was found to contain an oil called thiarubrine-A, which has the ability to kill many types of bacteria, fungi, and parasitic worms. This same leaf is also used by the local human population for many therapeutic purposes.

But that's not all. This combination of animal and human use led scientists to further explore the nature of thiarubrine-A. They found that it has "significant anticancer activity as well" (334). Coincidence? Could a monkey, primate or primitive human know on some level that it has cancer and instinctively seek out an anticancer herb? It's an intriguing possibility.

And this is not the only instance. *Vernonia amygdalina* is another plant eaten by wild chimpanzees. Certain bitter chemicals in the leaf (called sesquiterpene lactones) are now being investigated as both antimicrobial and antitumor agents (206). A related species, *Vernonia cinerea,* called purple flea-bane, happens to be a folk remedy for cancer in India. *Angelica sinensis,* the famous Dong Quai, has a strong reputation in China as a treatment for cancer of the cervix, esophagus, lung and nose (34). And it also contains sesquiterpene lactones.

It's a good guess that the use of plants with antitumor activity predates modern civilization by eons and may even indicate one way we could discover useful plants in the future.

There is also cancer as far back in human history as we can look. British scientists reported signs of a similar kind of cancer (osteochondroma) in a Neolithic human skeleton (72). Utah scientists found the telltale signs of a metastatic nasopharyngeal cancer in a prehistoric Great Basin hominid skeleton. Five cases of malignant bone cancer have been identified among prehistoric skeletons in Japan. The oldest case, from the "Jomon" period (5th or 4th millennium BC to around 250 BC) on Honshu Island, showed clear signs of a metastatic malignant bone tumor in the skull (382).

In 1983, archeologists found an isolated, calcified tumor among a group of human remains—a calcified uterine leiomyoma. They dated it as 5,000 years old (235). Signs of metastatic prostate cancer were found in a cremated pelvis dating from the 1st century AD (151). Roman antiquity, medieval Canterbury, pre-Columbian Chile, "precontact" Hawaii—wherever you look you find signs of ancient cancer. Most of these are bone cancers or bone metastases, for the simple reason that skeletons are all that usually remain of prehistoric corpses. They speak to us eloquently about human suffering (6, 339).

We can also assume that our distant ancestors were seeking cures among the herbs, just as we are. "The empirical search for agents to cure disease," wrote Dean Varro E. Tyler, "probably began with the earliest stirrings of thought and reason in the brains of humanoid creatures—the forerunners of *Homo sapiens*" (390). Discoveries made at Shanidar in the Zagros mountains give a strong indication that even Neanderthal man practiced some form of herbal medicine (371).

Humans turned to plants initially for food, of course, but while some of these were rejected as unpalatable, they "were found nevertheless to exert interesting physiological effects on those who consumed them," says Tyler (390).

Some of the obvious plants of this sort were coffee beans (*Coffea spp.*)

and tea leaves *(Camellia sinensis)*, which could stimulate the senses or cause insomnia; opium poppy latex *(Papaver somniferum)*, which could dull painful sensations; cinchona bark *(Cinchona spp.)*, which could cure the intermittent fever of malaria; ergot *(Claviceps purpurea)* which could cause abortions; nightshade *(Atropa belladonna)* which, if it didn't kill the intrepid Neolithic, could stop intestinal spasms; or digitalis *(Digitalis purpurea)*, which could cure dropsy (cardiac edema).

Here we are on shaky ground, of course, but it is likely that some plants were similarly found which seemed to suppress the growth of tumors, or at least reduce the pain or swelling. Others, like bloodroot, when smeared on a strange skin growth, were probably found to eat away and destroy it.

It might have taken centuries, millennia, eons before such crude observations were systematized into the powerful oral traditions of folk medicine. About 4,000 years ago this folk tradition began to be written down, in China and Egypt at first, and later in Babylonia, Israel, Africa, Greece and Rome. Shamans, the magic workers who still exist in many cultures, gradually

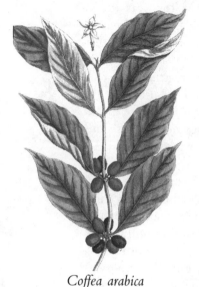

Coffea arabica (coffee)

evolved into medical herbalists. In the last few hundred years these herbalists have evolved into medical botanists, pharmacognosists, and molecular biologists.

Cancer in Early History

As far back as we go in the written medical records as well, we find mentions of cancer and cancer-like diseases. Indeed, as Dr. Jonathan Hartwell wrote, to study the history of cancer is to study not just the history of medicine but of humanity itself. Every ancient culture (except, for inexplicable reasons, the Mesopotamians and Hebrews) knew cancer well and devised elaborate ways to treat it.

We often speak glibly of "Western medicine," but this type of medicine has its roots in Western Asia and Africa, especially among the ancient Sumerians, Assyrians, and Egyptians. E.A. Wallis Budge (1857-1934), the great Egyptologist, has said that an official School of Herbalists probably existed in Egypt as early as 3,000 BC.

"There may have been, and probably were, many physicians and herbalists who studied plants and anatomy in a scientific manner," he wrote, and "the actual effect of the herbal medicines which they prescribed for their patients" (59).

Twelve centuries later, around 1800 BC, certain medical papyri were finally written down. These include what are now called the Ebers, Berlin, British Museum, Hearst, and Edwin Smith Papyri. These are among the oldest and most important historical documents in the world. They reveal that the ancient Egyptians had an advanced medical system as well as a *Materia Medica,* or descriptive list of healing substances.

About five-sixths of the ingredients in their formulas were of herbal origin. Nevertheless, popular attention has focused on some of the more "disgusting" elements. These included the dung of asses, dogs, pigs, gazelles, and crocodiles, as well as other evil-smelling and evil-tasting stuff (59). The same type of ingredients have been found in Babylon, Greek, Syrian, and even some more modern European Herbals. You can even find bat dung and equally strange ingredients in some Chinese formulas that have been sold on the American market. (Such "weirdness" has been used to smear herbal medicine in general.)

We also know that cancer existed in ancient Egypt. There is a possible histiocytoma in the skin of the heel and a squamous papilloma of the hand of an Egyptian mummy (423, 377). In fact, the Ebers Papyrus discusses cancer and makes a number of recommendations for its treatment. This included precursors of most of today's methods, including surgery, cautery, minerals, and herbs. The Egyptians even knew about photosensitizing agents, 3,500 years before the Food and Drug Administration approved Sanofi's Photofrin® for the treatment of stage I diffuse lung cancer.

Some of the diagnoses in the Ebers Papyrus have been proven right over the years—they are "surprisingly accurate," according to the *Encyclopedia Britannica* (4:342). I am particularly intrigued by a recent development that confirms how astute the Egyptians could be. In cancer, the Egyptians relied upon an ointment made up of arsenic trioxide and vinegar. In fact this became known as *Unguentum Aegypticum,* or the Egyptian ointment. It remained in use until the 16th century AD (413, 296).

The Renaissance surgeon Fabricius Hildanus (1560-1634) is said to have been the first to reject the use of this treatment. But Benjamin Rush, MD, signer of the Declaration of Independence and first US Army surgeon general, was still using an arsenic paste for external cancers and it remained in use throughout the 19th century. The Eclectic physicians used arsenic iodide internally (in the form of Fowler's solution) to treat the burning pain of stomach cancer, three drops once every three hours (289).

So prevalent was the use of arsenic that in 1916 a historian stated that ancient cancer remedies "have invariably been found to consist of arsenic, zinc or the alkaline caustics" (374). Even pathologist James Ewing, MD, stated in 1942 that in cases of Kaposi's sarcoma "arsenic is believed to be of some value" (125). Coming from him that was high praise indeed. But after the emergence of cytotoxic chemotherapy, the use of arsenic in cancer largely died out and was considered a sign of quackery. Arsenic-containing Fowler's solution was still being used to treat cancer at Memorial Sloan-Kettering Cancer Center in the 1950s.

Fast forward to 1997. Leading scientists in Shanghai, China announce that they have discovered a startling new cure for a form of leukemia—arsenic. It turned out that this historic treatment never died out in rural China. In 1996, Chinese scientist Z.X. Shen and colleagues at the Shanghai Institute of Hematology, Rui-Jin Hospital, published a groundbreaking article on the use of arsenic trioxide (As_2O_3) in the treatment of acute promyelocytic leukemia (APL). Fifteen APL patients who had relapsed after standard treatment were given arsenic intravenously. There was a complete response in nine out of ten of the patients treated with arsenic alone. The remaining five had complete responses with a combination of arsenic and standard chemotherapy. Dr. Raymond Warrell is now pursuing this treatment at Memorial Sloan-Kettering Cancer Center in New York. Essentially, this is the same prescription an Egyptian doctor would have made 5,000 years ago.

Of course, it needs to be stated that herbs were never the totality of any cancer doctor's repertoire. In ancient times they also believed in a multi-modality approach, including magic, witchcraft, and astrology. The Egyptians were a highly religious people and they held definite views about the religious or what we would term the psychosomatic origin of illnesses. They thought that sickness was brought about by the intervention of evil spirits. Knowledge of healing herbs (and of medicine in general) was believed to come from the intervention of powerful and beneficent gods.

In fact, the intertwined serpents that eventually became the Caduceus, symbol of the medical profession, had its origin as the emblem of the Sumerian god Ningishzida, son of Ninazu, Master-physician.

The pharmacopoeia of the Greeks and Romans consisted mainly of plants. But starting in the Greco-Roman world there was a struggle between herbal and mineral treatments. In general, botanical treatment was seen as democratic, since herbs are available to all for the picking. Mineral or chemical treatments required more specialized skills and usually involved more side effects. It was thus seen as elitist.

Greco-Roman physicians knew a great deal about cancer. Many of the names we now apply to the disease (such as carcinoma, cancer, edema, etc.) were coined by them. Hippocrates, Galen (whose book about cancer has come down to us), Dioscorides, the first Western herbalist, Pliny the Elder, etc. all wrote about this disease. We shall have reason to refer to many of them at various points in this text (325).

During the Middle Ages, treatment consisted mainly of semi-magical practices. For example, because cancer means crab, crayfish were eaten and the ashes of a crab were sprinkled on external tumors. However, as the economy revived, so too did the quality of medical care (mainly under the influence of Arabic and Jewish physicians).

We know of at least three medical thinkers of the Middle Ages who employed herbs in the treatment of cancer. Oddly, all three of these treatments are still alive, in some form or other, in various parts of the world. Isidore of Seville used *Chelidonium majus* (greater celandine) to treat the disease. *C. majus* is the main ingredient in a formula called Ukrain, which is used by some non-conventional doctors in the United States and Europe (see Chapter 22).

A medieval doctor named Odo of Meuse (who lived in Lorraine) advocated the use of *Rumex acetosella* (sheep sorrel) as a cancer treatment. Centuries later, this became a key ingredient in the popular Canadian remedy called Essiac tea (see Chapter 7).

But the most important medieval herbalist to write about cancer was Saint Hildegard of Bingen (1098-1179), the so-called Sibyl of the Rhine. Hildegard was one of the most accomplished women of her day. She had mystical visions and, at the age of 43, reported these to her Archbishop. He appointed a committee of theologians to investigate. They declared these visions authentic and assigned a monk to help her record them. This became her work, *Scivias,* which is still in print and still fascinating to read. In 1147, Hildegard founded a convent and continued to put her visions onto parchment. At her death she was sanctified by popular acclaim.

To give an idea of the scope of Hildegard's genius, she also wrote a *Lives of the Saints;* carried on an extensive correspondence with the leading intellectual figures of her day; wrote abstruse allegorical treatises, and for the amusement of her teeming brain even contrived her own language. Today, she is best known as the author of a surprise best-selling compact disc of her music. But in her spare time she also wrote two treatises on medicine and natural history, "reflecting a quality of scientific observation rare in that period," according to the *Encyclopedia Britannica* (5:924).

Although Hildegard certainly had access to a large array of herbal lore (in the fashion of the fictional "Brother Cadfael"), her own prescriptions apparently stemmed from visions. "In all creation," she wrote, "trees, plants, animals, and gem stones, there are hidden secret powers which no person can know unless they are revealed by God" (375).

According to a modern student of her work, "Hildegard is the first historic figure whose cancer salve has been studied in modern times" (296). Her salve formula (used for external cancers) is as follows:

"Take violets, press out their juice, and strain it through a cloth. Add olive oil one-third weight of the juice and take just as much billy goat fat as violet juice. Boil everything in a pot and prepare a salve" (375).

This "violet cure" for cancer has engendered controversy for a millennium. Recently, when the Food and Drug Administration asked for the removal of another popular herb, chaparral, from health food stores, many manufacturers simply replaced it with violets. (We shall deal more fully with this question in the companion volume.)

Equally astonishing, Hildegard was probably the first person to put forward the theory that cancer was caused by a "virus." She used the word "vermes," literally worms, although it seems from the context that she meant invisible corrupting agents, not wriggly invertebrates. She predicted that these "vermes" would die when they tasted her salve. Since worms are not normally seen in cancers it is interesting to speculate on whether she also had a vision of such creatures invisible to the naked eye.

Hildegard also prescribed a complex internal medicine, or elixir, that was based on the aquatic duckweed (*Lemna spp.*), the smallest known flowering plants, which were used to protect against cancer. She also prescribed beverages made with yarrow (*Achillea millefolium*) to prevent against what we now know as metastases.

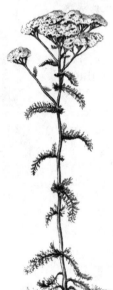

Achillea millefolium
(yarrow)

Her modern-day followers, and she has them, recommend three pinches of yarrow powder in fennel tea for three days prior to cancer surgery (375).

It is interesting that according to Hartwell, yarrow is a traditional cancer treatment in Germany, as well as in the US and UK.

When I visited the Lukas Klinik in Switzerland recently, external packs of yarrow were being placed over the livers of cancer patients. In fact, in 1994, Japanese scientists isolated three chemicals from the plant, achimillic acids A, B, and C, that were active against mouse P-388 leukemia (387). Violets have a long history as a cancer remedy as well, although most tests have not shown any activity in experimental systems.

Another famous Hildegardian formula was called anguillan, the "vulture remedy." This contained eel gall, ginger, long pepper, basil, ivory powder, and the pulverized beak of a vulture. How she coaxed the gall out of an eel I can only imagine. Since both elephants and vultures are on the endangered species list, modern-day Hildegardians are faced with a dilemma. Ingeniously, they have substituted a "homoeopathic" dose of this medicine, so that one vulture beak can service the entire world. Patients are being told to take ten drops of this mixture six times per day.

Why vulture beak? Probably because cancer tears like a vulture. And so, according to the medieval "Doctrine of Signatures" one should prescribe a real vulture's beak as treatment. Hildegard continues to have her followers. According to one writer, she "and her mystic brothers in Tibet apparently shared a kind of clairvoyance that has never been replaced by the microscope" (296). Two German admirers state: "This medicine comes from God's wisdom and is on the highest level of perception and needs no human justification" (375). To each his own.

The herbal traditions of Europe were dealt a tremendous blow by the Inquisition, which began in 1231 and didn't peter out until 1834. The Inquisition was established by the Holy Office to root out heresy wherever it could be found. Oftentimes, its victims turned out to be women, especially those who used herbs and salves to heal their neighbors. Had Hildegard been born a hundred years later, she might have been burned as a witch.

According to Ingrid Naiman, "Though women and homosexuals were the main target...it was midwives who were most severely attacked." The textbook of the medieval "quackbusters" was the *Malleus Maleficarum*. It stated that "midwives cause the greatest damage, either killing children or sacrilegiously offering them to devils...The greatest injury to the Faith is done by midwives, and this is made clearer than daylight itself by the confessions of some who were afterwards burned" (296).

It is said that as many as nine million people were burned at the stake during this nightmare. As one example, Jacoba Felicie was brought to trial by the Faculty of Medicine of the University of Paris in 1322, accused of curing her patients of internal illnesses and visiting the sick. Witnesses testified that after their University-trained physicians failed to cure them, they had been healed by Jacoba. She was convicted, and executed, because the *Malleus Maleficarum* taught that any knowledge of herbal healing reduced one's dependence on God. As Naiman has written, "European herbal traditions were nearly eradicated by the Inquisition" (296).

When the revival of interest in botanicals came, it came under the stimulus of the New World, and particularly from North American settlers and their Native American tutors.

American Treatments

The American settlers found themselves a long way from home, with no dependable supply of their familiar medicines, and a host of new diseases. They therefore had little choice but to turn to the native plants and, more importantly, the native healers, who generously shared their profound knowledge with the colonists. Within decades, native American folk remedies began to show up in books, and were being exported back to the mother country. Medical books and magazines of the 18th and 19th century were filled with enthusiastic accounts of such remedies as bloodroot, goldenseal and American ginseng.

The lack of trained physicians in America, and the distance of many of the pioneers from established cities, also led to a particular need for effective indigenous treatments. Although cancer had yet to become a statistically important problem, it was well known and tremendously feared.

Most of the regular doctors practiced in a few relatively wealthy coastal cities, like Boston, New York, and Philadelphia. But if you looked at colonial society as a whole, overwhelmingly the main responsibility for health care fell on the colonists themselves, and particularly the womenfolk. It was they who were responsible for diagnosing and treating common illnesses. More often than not, their first line of defense was herbal. Each household had its herb garden and a stock of remedies, some common, some private family recipes, stored away for various purposes. Medicinal herbs were generally gathered in the fall, along with the other crops. In addition, there was usually a wise woman or two in the community who had the "healing tetch," and who specialized in treating difficult cases.

Initially, the colonists found themselves surrounded by a baffling array of unfamiliar flora and fauna, and an equally baffling set of diseases. The Indians knew the peculiarities of plants, and also had a well-deserved reputation for excellent looks and health. Compared to the white men, they were striking in their appearance, tall and graceful with remarkably strong teeth and bones. The Noble Savage wasn't entirely a myth.

The Indians had had millennia to master the art of empirical medicine in the American terrain. Early settlers also drew upon the contributions of African-American slaves as well as other minority groups. From the start, America was a pluralistic society, even if it thought of itself as a New England or a New Amsterdam.

Every Man His Own Doctor

We are fortunate to have a book written nearly half a century before the American Revolution that gives us an intimate portrait of the state of popular healthcare. This was *Every Man His Own Doctor,* subtitled *The Poor Planter's Physician* (1732). Its goal was to describe "plain and easy means for persons to cure themselves of all, or most of the distempers, incident to this Climate, and with very little charge, the medicines being chiefly of the growth and production of this country."

When *Every Man* was first published, Americans still relied to a great degree on the sporadic arrival of trunks of medicine from the old country. But trunks and ships didn't always arrive in time, and some of the baffling illnesses encountered were unknown in the Old World. Clearly, there was a crying need for an economical and effective way to deal with them. *Every Man* tried to fill that void.

Although published at first anonymously, it soon became known that the author was Dr. John Tennent. Dr. Tennent has earned a very small footnote in orthodox medical history for his introduction of "snakeroot" (*Aristolochia serpentaria*) into regular medical practice. However, in its day, *Every Man* was a best seller, and editions came out regularly every year or two. One of its first publishers was Benjamin Franklin.

"Every Man" is unique in many ways. It can be seen as the beginning of American "alternative medicine," since it introduced the familiar and lucrative theme of "doctor-bashing" into our literature. Given the resentment that many people felt towards "elitist" doctors, it was fast tracked to best-seller status (384). The fact that Tennent himself was a medical school graduate did not preclude him from making scathing attacks on his own colleagues.

The cancer recommendations are at the end of the book, and from the scantiness of the remarks, one gets the impression that while known and dreaded, cancer was still a relatively rare affliction.

"Another woeful case," he writes, "is a cancer, which some despairingly imagine to be incurable." Cancer, he writes, begins with little hard lumps, or swellings in the breast, lip, or other glandulous parts of the body. "These afterwards break into painful Sores, which eat farther and farther, till at last they reach some large [blood] vessel or mortal part" (384).

Tennent claimed that "blessed by God, there have been some instances of success by the methods hereafter mentioned....In this case, the patient must submit, in the first place, to have the lump cut clean out, so soon as he is convinced it is cancer." To help heal the surgical wound, he recommended the following "balsam": boil six ounces of sassafras (*Sassafras albidum*) root and six ounces of dogwood (*Cornus spp.*) root in a gallon of water until it is reduced to a pint. Then after straining it, "drench a pledget therein" and apply it warm to the sore, renewing it every day. (A pledget is a small wad of lint or cotton used as a bandage or compress.) If the patient continues this on a daily basis, "I can assure him that he will not be the first that has been blest with Success."

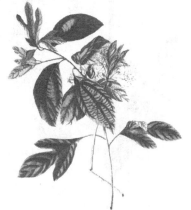

Sassafras albidum
(sassafras)

Hartwell tells us that a salve as well as a fluid extract of sassafras has been taken orally for general cancer in Georgia and California. However, there have been far more articles about the potential carcinogenicity of sassafras than its use as a cancer remedy (219, 348).

In addition, Tennent urged his cancer patients to drink sassafras tea every morning, live temperately, upon light and innocent food, and abstain entire-

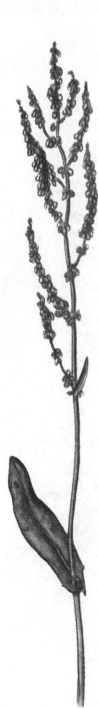

ly from strong liquor." He adds that "the way to prevent this calamity is to be very sparing in the eating of pork, to forbear all salt and high-seasoned meats, and live chiefly upon the Garden, the Orchard, and the Hen-house" (384, 289).

The strictures against eating pork and high-seasoned meats sounds modern, but actually hark back to Galen. The suggestion to "live chiefly upon the Garden, the Orchard, and the Hen-house" has its parallels in Galen as well (325).

Tennent believed that by using his poultice on the wound, his internal tea, and his mostly vegetarian diet, that people could decrease mortality from this disease. It was a humane suggestion and in some ways far ahead of its time.

Mrs. Johnson's Receipt

A few decades later there was an early attempt to find and evaluate an effective treatment for cancer. In Virginia, mid-century, the House of Burgesses of the General Assembly of Virginia offered the munificent sum of £100 for the discovery of a valid cure for cancer (60).

The committee took evidence over a period of six or seven years. They heard testimony from many practitioners and allegedly cured patients. One of those submitting a treatment was Mary Johnson, who offered her own family "receipt" for the judges' consideration. Little is known about her, but she is sometimes said to have been an herbal practitioner with a reputation for curing cancer. In the end, the House of Burgesses awarded Mrs. Johnson the £100 for her efforts. Apparently, in their view, the cancer puzzle had been solved.

Mrs. Johnson's formula is no secret. "Take a peck of garden sorrel (*Rumex acetosa*), and better than half as much celandine (*Chelidonium majus*); beat them in a mortar and express the juice through a fine cloth into a pewter basin. Take a large handful of persimmon (*Diospyros virginiana*) from the south side of the tree; beat it as firm as can be; pour a little spring water into it." Both sorrel and celandine are well known folk cancer remedies, whose use persists to the present day.

Other distinguished figures in America proposed herbal cancer cures from time to time. One of these was Cadwalader Colden who stood at the opposite end of the social scale from the obscure Mrs. Johnson. Colden was lieutenant governor of New York, a founder of the American Philosophical Association, and an

Rumex acetosa (garden sorrel)

intimate friend of Benjamin Franklin. He wrote an article for the *Gentleman's Magazine* in 1752 extolling the virtues of poke root (*Phytolacca americana*) as a cancer treatment. (*Penthouse* was therefore not the first men's magazine to publish stories on sensational cancer cures.) There is also a letter in the possession of the New York Historical Society to Benjamin Franklin expounding on this same theory. Poke root became a well regarded cancer treatment at that time, "known to all Europe" according to Carl Linnaeus.

Cadwalader Colden

Around the same time, Dr. Hugh Martin called sorrel a "sovereign specific" for cancer and reputedly cured 14 people in Philadelphia with this, as well as many others. One of his famous beneficiaries was Caesar Rodney (1728-1784), president of Delaware and signer of the Declaration of Independence (*EB* 10:132).

In the early 19th century, all sorts of adventurers and explorers were drawn to the new country. Constantine Rafinesque (1784-1840) was such a fascinating individual. He came from Turkey and made himself into a naturalist, traveler, and writer who "made major and controversial contributions to botany..."(*EB* 9:899). Rafinesque's name is now engraved in stone at the Brooklyn Botanic Gardens. But he was no stuffy academic. He traveled the world and at one time was a Levantine trader in Sicily. But he was consumed by scientific curiosity and spent his spare moments studying the natural history of plants and fish. In 1815, he returned to the United States and eventually became a professor at Transylvania University in Lexington, Kentucky. He was considered a "brilliant teacher" who also founded a botanical garden. Rafinesque "anticipated, to some extent, part of Charles Darwin's theory of evolution" (*EB* 9:899).

He was also the author of more than 950 works, including a two-volume medical botany (324). In it, Rafinesque extolled the virtue of many plants that were subsequently used against cancer. He gave a detailed description of goldenseal (*Hydrastis canadensis*), which was and is included in many cancer formulas.

Less scholarly but more influential was Samuel Thomson (1769-1843), who led the mass movement that bears his name. Early in the 19th century, Thomson, a layperson, joined an ardent faith in herbs to a Jacksonian-style rebellion against the elitist medical profession. Thomson's system was patented and he sold the rights to would-be practitioners. Thomsonianism grew enormously in popularity throughout the first half of the century. At one time it was used by one fifth of the inhabitants of the United States (86).

Thomson himself was obsessed with the action of a limited number of herbs, particularly Indian tobacco (*Lobelia inflata*). This herb mimicked the action of mercurous chloride, or calomel. Lobelia has many interesting biological effects and was used by the Iroquois as a treatment for uterine cancer (129). Lobeline, a constituent of Lobelia, causes regressions of liver carcinoma of Albino mice (175). Thomson also had formulas that included goldenseal and comfrey.

Thomson's influence was far-reaching. In the 1930s, Jethro Kloss urged the use of Lobelia in cancer as an herb that "loosens disease and opens the way for its elimination from the body....Its action is quick and more effective than radium, and Lobelia leaves no bad effects, while radium does" (232). Thomson developed a large following for his Botanical rebellion against regular medicine. Among other things, he developed a plaster for external cancers made of red clover blossoms. It is believed that he learned this treatment from the Penobscot Indians of Maine. The Penobscots also discovered the use of mayapple as a cancer remedy hundreds of years before scientists realized they were the source of chemotherapeutic drugs Etoposide and Teniposide (see Chapter 10).

At first, the discovery of authentic Indian remedies such as pokeroot, bloodroot, clover, or mayapple was fairly straightforward. A trader, settler, explorer, or scholar would make contact with the native Americans. Sometimes the white man himself had a personal problem and sought advice. Knowledge of the local flora was conveyed in a non-commercial and non-secretive atmosphere.

But this valuable medical legacy of the Native Americans was soon exploited for commercial gain, at the same time that the Indians themselves were being driven to extinction. As early as 1858, an "Indian Medical Institute" in Boston advertised a secret herbal cure. They claimed that "hundreds and thousands of men and women" formerly afflicted with cancer "are now rejoicing in health..." (345). After the Civil War, this exploitation of an Indian provenance for patent medicines became almost obligatory.

"From the older and much larger Kickapoo Indian Medicine Company, down to the smallest pitch doctor working Indian herbs," wrote popular historian Stewart Holbrook, "the factory and operating headquarters were all east of the Mississippi and commonly east of the Hudson; but the ingredients must of necessity be credited to some region or other in what was still thought of as genuine Indian country" (188).

Many fortunes were made in the Indian nostrum business. There was Trapper's Indian Oil, Indian Salve, Indian Worm Killer, Indian Cough Cure, and of course Kickapoo Indian Sagwa, which was composed of roots, herbs, barks and leaves, and "cured" dyspepsia, neuralgia, headache, constipation, kidney disease, etc. It cost a formidable $1.00 per bottle (21).

Although the promoters claimed that Kickapoo Sagwa was "at all times under the Indians' personal supervision," it is doubtful if these medicines had anything to do with Kickapoos. "Anything with the word 'Indian' was a sure winner," wrote two commentators on that era (21).

At first, merchandise was moved via the traveling medicine show, which was a colorful blend of circus-style entertainment and sales pitches. By 1906, the Healy and Bigelow company was sending out scores of troupes to rural America to sell Kickapoo Indian Sagwa. Doc Hamlin's Wizard Oil fronted many other shows. Many of the lesser shows featured actors posing as Quakers, such as Hal the Healer, Brother John, and Brother Benjamin, "all of whom used Thee and Thou most of the time and never failed to open with a strong pitch about the inherent honesty of the Friends and their remedies." In 1880, a successful show could expect to make about four thousand dollars in a three-week tour (188).

Such shows remained popular in rural America up to the 1940s (21). But eventually print advertising was found to be a more economical way to reach an expanding audience. This took the form of posters in shop win-

dows, trade cards and brochures left on drugstore counters, paintings on the sides of barns and rocks, and ads in almanacs, religious and country weeklies, on the back pages of popular novels and, primarily through ads in the daily newspapers.

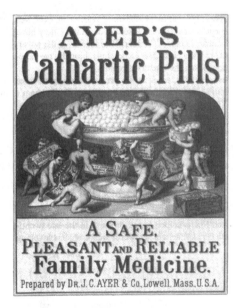

Along with cure-alls for every imaginable human ill, there were advertisements for cancer cures. "We remove Cancer without Pain, no Caustics or Knife used," read one ad. "The Cure is Perfect." Rupert Wells advertised his Radiatized Fluid for Cancer: "It will cure you at home without pain, plaster or operation."

In this climate, charlatanism flourished and it became impossible to distinguish valuable medicinal herbs from cynical frauds. This makes all evaluations from the post-Civil War era very difficult.

As Varro Tyler has said, "Medicine and quackery have always been close, if not compatible, partners. At times, they may appear to have separated, but sooner or later, in one place or another, they wind up united" (392).

Intellectual Beverages

Some of these patent medicines had big futures. One of the most popular, Dr. Miles' Compound Extract of Tomato, became catsup. Dr. John Pemberton's Coca-Cola was originally a "brain tonic and intellectual beverage" which contained a small amount of cocaine. Maine was one state where patent medicines thrived, since it was "dry" and most remedies contained considerable amounts of alcohol. The Giant Oxie Company of Augusta, manufactured an "improved Moxie nerve food." But as the American Medical Association (AMA) complained, "printer's ink is the very life blood of quackery." Eventually the Giant Oxie fortune was poured directly into the newspaper business. This eventually became the Gannett Company, publishers of USA Today.

For example, when Ulysses S. Grant was dying of cancer of the mouth, a vendor of patent medicines marched boldly onto the steps of his front porch and placed in his lap a package of chewing gum, with alleged medical properties (312). On the day that Grant died, the newspapers were filled not just with stories of his tragic demise, but ads for patent cancer remedies. One of these was for "Swift's Specific." The ad featured a testimonial from one Mrs. Mary Comer, who said that this nostrum had cured her of an awful cancer of the mouth which had proved resistant to the efforts of "six or seven of the best physicians of the country" (312). The oblique reference to Grant was clear to all readers.

During this time, medicine as a whole polarized between "regular" and "sectarian" practitioners. The regulars were then, as now, centered around the AMA. From 1880 until 1906, they allowed advertisements for patent medicine in their journal (much as they later allowed cigarette advertising). They opposed arrant quackery, which was of course good, but also attacked virtually all "botanical" practitioners, thus throwing out the baby with the bath water.

The "botanicals" were either non-credentialed lay healers or trained doctors who belonged to the schools of Homoeopathy or Eclecticism.

Eclecticism initially grew out of the activities of Jacob Tidd, a New Jersey practitioner who, like Samuel Thomson, also had a botanical system based on Indian lore. He passed this knowledge to Wooster Beach (1794–1868), who established a Reformed Medical School in New York City. Later, a more influential Eclectic medical school was founded in Cincinnati. It lasted until 1939. Today, the Eclectic flame is kept lit by the Lloyd Library of Cincinnati, which has preserved most of the papers and formulas of the Eclectic school.

Historian Harris Coulter, PhD, has called Eclecticism "a more sophisticated system of practice drawing on the same intellectual and philosophical sources" as Thomsonianism (86). However, they had no systematic theory of diagnostics or pharmacology, and basically accepted allopathic medicine's systems, substituting their own vegetable cures.

Regular and Eclectic physicians competed for the same clients and generally despised each other. *JAMA* editor Morris Fishbein, MD, called Eclecticism "the apotheosis of the old grandmother and witch-doctor systems of treatment" (132). He championed chemotherapy and denied any utility to herbs, whatsoever. For their part, the Eclectics tenaciously held to some absurd positions, e.g., rejecting the necessity of biopsies in the diagnosis of cancer or surgery in its treatment.

Secret Remedies

In the colonies, secret cancer cures appeared early. In the mid-18th century, one Francis Torres, described as an itinerant mountebank, wandered into Philadelphia with "Chinese Stones," which reputably cured cancer as well as toothaches and rattlesnake bites (420). What were they?

A Revolutionary War doctor, Hugh Martin, wrote a *Narrative of a Discovery of a Sovereign Specific for the Cure of Cancers* (1784). No one knows what was in it, as "nothing of great significance was disclosed beyond a bold claim of an efficient cancer remedy" (289). In New York in 1858, T.T. Blake, MD, issued a book, called *Cancers Cured Without the Use of the Knife,* which put forward a salve or ointment applied externally. Again, the author was careful to hide the nature of his remedy.

Most such remedies were never disclosed to the public. Invariably, "a cancer cure," as author Nat Morris remarked, "was a closely guarded secret and was regarded as valuable property" (289). Throughout history this issue of secrecy has dogged many developers of herbal treatments. Since herbs cannot generally be patented or otherwise monopolized, secrecy is the only way to protect one's economic interests. The regular medical profession abhors secrecy, however, and therefore this issue has long been herbal medicine's Achilles' heel.

John King

The history of Eclecticism is tied up with a plant familiar to students of cancer therapy, namely the mayapple (*Podophyllum peltatum*). In 1835, a young Eclectic physician, John King, MD (1813-1893) was preparing a water-alcohol extract of a mayapple root. Leaving the preparation unfinished, the next morning he and his colleagues discovered fragments of dark, brittle stuff floating in the mix.

Foolheartedly, this 22-year-old doctor administered it to a young girl who happened to be nearby and was feeling unwell. The rationale was that "podophyllum was especially prized by the Eclectics as a remedy for biliousness and other liver complaints," according to historian Barbara Griggs. It almost killed her. What Dr. King had discovered was the concentrated resin of the plant.

"To say that I was greatly alarmed," he later wrote, "would but feebly describe my mental condition." But this accidental discovery opened the floodgates to what became known as the "Concentrated Principles" of American plants. It set in motion a craze for ever more potent, concentrated and better defined extracts.

This story is especially germane since it was an extract of this same plant that was later, serendipitously, discovered by the NCI's Jonathan Hartwell to contain an antitumor principle. By a circuitous route these became two anticancer agents, the semisynthetic drugs etoposide and teniposide. In 1983, etoposide was approved by the FDA for the treatment of refractory testicular tumors and small cell lung cancer. It is also used in "front-line combination therapy" for many other kinds of cancer (104; see Chapter 10).

Incidentally, it was Hartwell's discovery that the Penobscot Indians had already "discovered" mayapple as a cancer treatment that led him to write *Plants Used Against Cancer.* A picture of the mayapple graced the front cover of Hartwell's book.

John Milton Scudder

Not everyone liked the idea of abandoning simple plant preparations however, and of isolating increasingly powerful fractions. One of those especially critical of this tendency was John Milton Scudder, MD (1829-1894). Scudder himself had graduated from the Eclectic Institute in 1856 and became the Professor of Materia Medica there. All writers agree he was "a man of passionate integrity." At a time when almost all Eclectics were carried away with enthusiasm for so-called "concentrated medicines" he successfully fought for the reintroduction of simple herbal remedies, formulas and teas (154).

Scudder was the author of *Specific Diagnosis, Specific Medication,* and many other medical textbooks. He was a well-known figure in American medicine for decades, and played a progressive role in medicine's development by arguing vigorously for an end to the use of violent cathartics, emetics and blisters. Instead, he advocated a gentler form of medicine.

"I look back on the old methods of drugging, with the same feelings of disgust and horror that I look back upon the thumb-screw, the cat, the rack," he once wrote (154).

Scudder wrote that "much of Eclectic Medicine was an unmitigated humbug. It was the day of so-called concentrated medicines and anything ending with the suffix '-in' was lauded to the skies."

Because of this internal squabbling, Eclecticism reached a low ebb in 1861. It was Scudder who saved the day. Ms. Griggs describes him as "a warm and attractive person who was adored by all his students, and a man of passionate integrity..." (154).

Scudder was particularly interested in cancer. Not a secretive man, Scudder's Alterative was widely published:

Botanical name	Common Name	Source
Scrophularia nodosa	Knotted Figwort	Fresh herb
Alnus serruleta	Tag alder	Bark
Rumex crispus	Yellow dock	Fresh root
Corydalis spp.	Chinese Corydalis	Tuber
Podophyllum peltatum	Mayapple	Water extract

Note: This formula should only be used under a physician's direction. Please see the warning in the front of the book.

Each of these will be discussed in full in this book's companion volume. What jumps out of course is the presence of mayapple. In a sense, the Eclectics were using epipodophyllotoxins, the precursors of Etoposide and Teniposide, at a time when their orthodox counterparts were mired in therapeutic nihilism.

Cancer and Syphilis

Some of the other herbs may also have anticancer activity as well. Figwort (Scrophularia marilandica) was an old treatment for syphilis. The "fathers of the Eclectic School of Medicine" believed that there was a relationship between syphilis and cancer (in part because they accepted without questioning the existence of an undefined cancer "germ"). It seems to be a harmless plant, but use is restricted in people who have a heart condition called ventricular tachycardia (278).

Eli Jones

An even more important chapter in the history of herbal medicine and cancer centered around the treatments of Eli Jones, MD.

The consensus of opinion in medicine in the 19th century was that neither drugs nor herbs could possibly cure cancer. For over 200 years cancer was thought to be basically a local disease, which could only be controlled through radical surgery. The only physicians in America and England who thought otherwise were the Homoeopaths and Eclectics. The Eclectics in particular had a virtual monopoly on the treatment of advanced cancer. They saw tens of thousands of such cases and claimed success. Naturally, they were hated for this by the "regular" physicians, who had usually given up on the same patients.

In 1865, Dr. John Skelton, the father of Eclecticism in England, published a book titled *Practice*. In it, he claimed that cancer was a constitutional—or blood—disease and that it could be cured by medicine alone. The august founders of American Eclecticism—Drs. Newton, Hill, Jones, Sherwood and Paine—all wrote that cancer was constitutional and could be cured by natural medicine. In fact, because of their positive attitude, the Eclectics became identified as "cancer doctors." Where else could one turn? To the back pages of the newspaper?

It is said that up to the time of his death, Dr. Robert S. Newton of New York City had treated more cases of breast cancer than any other doctor in the country (210). A prominent homoeopath, Edwin M. Hale, left behind several treatments for cancer. In 1878, Dr. J. Compton Burnett (father of the British novelist Dame Ivy Compton Burnett) published a book titled *Tumors of the Breast*. It included a record of 132 cases which he claimed were permanently cured through medical treatment (210).

As part of this vibrant Eclectic trend, in 1869, a young man named Eli Grellert Jones, MD (1850-1933) began treating cancer by medical means in the United States. Although today he is almost completely forgotten, Jones was as close as the Eclectic movement came to producing a true cancer specialist. He was an 1870 graduate of the Eclectic Medical College of Pennsylvania and of Dartmouth Medical College in 1871. Not only was he well trained but he did not share the penchant for secrecy that surrounded many herbal treatments.

Together with J. Weldon Fell and John Pattison (see Chapter 3), "he tore the veil of secrecy that had historically surrounded the use of salves and other botanical remedies used to treat cancer," wrote a modern commentator (296). In 1911, he published a 301-page book called *Cancer: Its Causes, Symptoms and Treatment*. This was subtitled, "the results of over forty years' experience in the medical treatment of this disease" (210). In it, Jones summarized his experience dealing with this disease as well as many concomitant problems. (It is still in print in India, where it is cherished as part of the homoeopathic tradition.)

Jones justifiably claimed that "the Eclectic School of Medicine were the pioneers in America in the successful treatment of cancer." While some might dispute his use of the word "successful," there is no doubt that the Eclectics initiated the first serious study of the medical (as opposed to the surgical) treatment of this disease. Not only did Jones himself publish a textbook summarizing his treatment of thousands of patients, but other Eclectics wrote optimistically about the possibilities of curing the disease with botanical medicines (210).

It will strike a modern day observer as curious that Jones has to argue not just for particular formulas but for the legitimacy of the medical treatment of cancer as a whole. This was the era in which "therapeutic nihilism" held sway. Typical was the opinion of one prominent Philadelphia surgeon

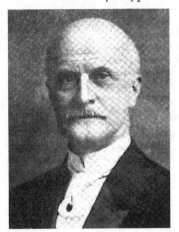

Eli Jones, MD

who declared about cancer, "All we know, with any degree of certainty, is that we know nothing." There was virtually no American cancer research. When the *Boston Medical and Surgical Journal* offered a prize of one thousand dollars in 1882 for the best essay on a "Cure for Malignant Disease," they did not receive a single credible entry! This fact alone, they complained, testified to the "comparative barrenness of American researchers in the field of medical science" (312).

At the same time, orthodox medicine was given to episodes of wild enthusiasm, invariably followed by dark despair. In the 1870s, "regulars" publicized a purported cancer "specific" from the bark of an obscure South American vine, Condurango. This was dropped when it turned out that it did not indeed cure all cancers in predictable fashion. "It has become obsolete," Jones remarked, "like one hundred other so-called 'cures' for cancer that the regular school has claimed as a cure for cancer." When the regulars were done with it, Condurango was picked up by the Eclectics, who assigned it a minor role as a remedial agent for certain cases of breast cancer.

During this period, the few people who attempted to research or treat cancer medically were frequently anathematized. The story of immunology pioneer William B. Coley, MD, is well known and has been summarized in Stephen S. Hall's 1997 book, *A Commotion in the Blood* (161). Dr. Kanematsu Sugiura, DSc, once told me that when he began his own research into this topic in 1912 (the year that Jones published his *Cancer* book), all medical treatments were regarded as virtual quackery (292). As late as 1940, Memorial Hospital pathologist James Ewing, MD, had hardly a word to say about the medical treatment of the disease in his 1,160 page magnum opus, *Neoplastic Diseases*. Orthodox treatment consisted of surgery, radiation and radium—and almost nothing else.

As odd as it may seem, during this period it was "quacks" such as Harry Hoxsey (see Chapter 5), who took up the banner of what they called "chemotherapy" against their surgical or nihilistic opponents. "Chemotherapy is the only true effective way to deal with this deadliest of all diseases afflicting modern mankind," Hoxsey wrote defiantly (194). Of course, the word "chemotherapy" had a different connotation in those days, and was often based on mild botanical medicines.

Unlike a host of cancer-treating charlatans, however, the Eclectics were real physicians, the equals in education, training, and ethics, of the regular physicians of their day. Jones insisted that "the medical treatment of cancer, in all its forms, is a specialty as much as surgery, otolaryngology, or gynecology, and that a doctor must prepare himself for such work in the same manner that he would for any special line of work in his profession." This was revolutionary.

Such a doctor "should endeavor...in every sense of the word to be a Specialist in Cancer. There is a great demand for good men [sic], men who will master this special work, as cancer is increasing, cases are dying every day, somewhere, for lack of proper treatment" (210). From 1894 on, Jones taught postgraduate courses to physicians from all over the country in the medical treatment of cancer.

"I do not ask what a physician's medical politics are," he said. "I only ask that he will carry out the plan of treatment, agreed upon, faithfully and conscientiously." At one time he had 15 physicians, from Maine to California, following his cancer regimens.

Jones also differed from the great mass of non-conventional practitioners in that he was entirely open about his methods, and even published formulas for them in his books *Definite Medication, Rational Treatment of Cancer,* and *Cancer: Its Causes, Symptoms and Treatment.*

Unlike the advertising quacks, he did not believe there was or could be a single remedy for all cancers. "I have never claimed to have a 'specific' for anything from an ingrown toenail to a cancer," he wrote, defiantly. "I do claim...that there are remedies which do have a curative effect upon cancer, as we find it in different portions of the body....No remedy...will cure all forms of cancer. Such a thing is impossible for the simple reason that the disease as it appears in different parts of the body, has a different anatomical structure."

He also said that "the day is past when a physician with an escharotic paste or bottle of herb syrup or some kind of 'injection dope' can start out to cure all kinds of cancer," he optimistically wrote.

"That is the worst form of Quackery," he continued. "Such men will always find their level." Jones believed that he had raised the medical treatment of cancer to the level of a science. "It has taken me many years to lift this business of treating cancer, in all its forms, out of the mire of quackery and raise it up to the dignity of a specialty." (One wonders what he would make of the Internet.)

It was a sign of the sectarian times, however, that Jones also engaged in intemperate attacks on conventional methods, just as they did upon him.

"Four-fifths of the cases of cancer I have seen in the past forty years," he wrote, "had been operated on and the cancer returned worse than before. Other cases have tried the x-ray, Radium, Escharotics, Hypodermic treatment, etc., etc., before I saw them, with the same results" (210).

Eli Jones is actually one of the founders of medical oncology in the United States. But because he was on the losing side in the sectarian wars, his contribution goes unrecognized to this day.

He is unmentioned in the official or academic histories of cancer. In that sense, the legacy of those bitterly sectarian days are still with us, a century later.

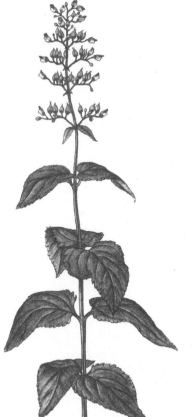

Scrophularia nodosa
(figwort)

Jones's Treatments

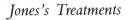

Jones had many cancer remedies, both herbal and homoeopathic, which he considered effective. But he is most remembered for his advocacy of poke root and for "compound syrup Scrophularia," or so-called "cancer syrup."

"After many years of testing different remedies for the internal treatment of cancer to form a combination which could be dignified with the name 'Cancer Syrup'—a remedy that could be depended on in the more advanced stages of cancer when the system has become saturated with the germs of cancer—I have devised the following formula," he wrote.

"I have utmost faith in the curative power of this combination," he said. "I have never mentioned this remedy to any one and would not until I had thoroughly tested it in many difficult cases of genuine cancer so that I could conscientiously recommend it in my book on cancer."

The Eli Jones Formula (★ = also included in Scudder's formula)

Scientific name	Common name	Part used	AHPA
Scrophularia nodosa★	Figwort	leaves/roots	2d
Phytolacca americana	Poke root		3
Rumex crispus★	Yellow dock	root	2d
Celastrus scandens	False bittersweet	bark/root	—
Corydalis formosa★	Chinese Corydalis	root	2b
Podophyllum peltatum★	Mayapple	root	2b
Juniperus communis	Juniper berries	(fruit)	2b
Zanthoxylum spp.	Prickly ash	berries (fruit)	2b
Guaiacum officinale	Guaiacum wood	—	

Note: This formula should only be used under a physician's direction. Please see the warning in the front of the book.

Also Note: AHPA Ratings are as follows: 1 = generally safe; 2a = for external use only; 2b = not to be used during pregnancy; 2d = other specific use indications; 3 = use with caution; 4 = insufficient data.

Great care should be taken to procure fresh herbs, Jones cautioned. The ingredients should be mixed and coarsely bruised. Then they are moistened with dilute alcohol and left to stand for two to three days. They are then put in a steam displacement apparatus and passed through the vapor of three pints of alcohol. This displacement is continued with the steam of water until the strength is exhausted. One sets aside the three pints of tincture which passed first and evaporates the remainder to two pints. These are mixed together with syrup. Oil of sassafras is added for flavor. The dose is one tablespoonful, three times a day, or sufficient to keep the bowels regular every day.

There is no mistaking Jones's debt to Scudder and the other Eclectics, nor would he have denied it. His personal motto was "What man has done, man may do." Each of these herbs will be discussed in detail in this book's companion volume.

The FDA and the Sherley Amendment

The Eclectics vanished from the scene in the decades that followed the famous Flexner Report (1910) on the state of medical education. However, we should note that they left their mark on the legal and regulatory aspect of herbal cancer treatments. In the early years of the new century, a Kansas City Eclectic doctor marketed a mixture of liquids and pills as "Dr. Johnson's Mild Combination Treatment for Cancer." His advertisements took a swipe at conventional treatments, as well.

Prof. James Harvey Young says Johnson was "vending an assortment of tablets and liquids." He remarks, "For this purpose, of course, the concoctions were worthless" (420). Young's language is loaded and his conclusion unsubstantiated. Without knowing what was in the treatments it is difficult to say what its effect on cancer might have been.

This case was a test, however, of the power of the new Food and Drug Administration (FDA). Even though Johnson had described the ingredients on the label, the FDA sought an injunction based on the "false claims." The case went all the way to the Supreme Court, which sided in Johnson's favor. Oliver Wendell Holmes, Jr., delivered the majority decision, writing that Congress had stipulated that labels must accurately reflect the contents, and not that all therapeutic claims be deemed true by some outside agency. The government should stay out of the business of scientific controversy. This "would distort the uses of its constitutional power to establish criteria in regions where opinions were far apart" (420).

Opponents of "quackery" considered this ruling "first aid to fraud and murder." They had President Taft and much of the Congress on their side. There were 150 such cases pending, and Taft said that they involved "some of the rankest frauds by which the American people were ever deceived."

The Supreme Court had made clear that "any attempt to legislate against mere expression of opinion would be abortive." But a new law was passed which supposedly got around this difficulty. It stated that the FDA act proscribed "knowingly false misstatements of fact as to the effect of the preparations." This was introduced by Rep. Swagar Sherley of Kentucky and passed easily. It thus entered history as the Sherley Amendment.

The focus of anti-fraud legislation became the motives and intentions of the proponents and led to a tremendous upsurge in ad hominem arguments. Since you had to prove that someone "knowingly" made false statements, this focused the debate on the motives of the promoter rather than the effectiveness of the remedies themselves.

The campaign against quackery inevitably netted not just many charlatans but quite a few legitimate practitioners of an alternative persuasion. Second, it willy-nilly got the government into the business of passing on what was "fact" in not just the preparation but the effects of various complex preparations.

Although the civil libertarian dangers of this Sherley Amendment were glossed over at the time, it also did exactly what Justice Hughes had warned about: it established a canon of orthodox opinion about cancer treatment. This is ironic, since at the time next to nothing was known about the causes, prevention, detection, treatment, or control of cancer. Thus, the battle between orthodoxy and "quackery" in cancer had the appearance of a battle between two ignorant armies clashing by night.

Through the first decades of the 20th century, however, orthodox medicine was increasingly recognized as the sole legitimate form of scientific medicine in the United States. All other philosophies were marginalized, tarred with the brush of quackery. This included the naturopaths (heirs of Eclecticism as well as Fr. Sebastian Kneipp's nature cure), the chiropractors, faith healers, and so forth.

"In America," wrote medical historian Fielding H. Garrison, "under existing legislation, every species of medical sect—osteopathy, chiropraxis, Christian Science, eclecticism, botanic medicine, etc.—has been permitted to flourish" (132).

In 1912, 1921 and 1936, the AMA issued three volumes called *Nostrums and Quackery*. These described the "evils" of patent medicines, which a few years before had been a mainstay of the *Journal of the American Medical Association's* revenue. In 1927, Morris Fishbein, MD, the editor of *JAMA*, issued a popular book that included an "Encyclopedia of Cults and Quackery." Fishbein saw "cults" everywhere. It is amusing that he even considered beauty parlors to be part of the medical cult phenomenon. And he filled page after page with descriptions of cults from Aero- to Zonotherapy.

"The appeal of the bizarre is strong even to enlightened men," wrote the enlightened Fishbein. "To a public educated to a belief in the black art, magic, alchemy, and the miracles of the saints, the unusual necessarily has an absolute fascination. Medicine in this way became inordinately complex and chaotic" (132).

Fishbein and his colleagues set out to make medicine simple and well organized, by centralizing everything under the control of the AMA. They especially aimed at the destruction of Eclecticism and its heirs. This set the stage for the great battle of the 20th century concerning herbs and cancer, the Hoxsey saga (see Chapter 5).

Back to Eden

Despite the AMA's opposition throughout the 20th century, medical herbalists were busy proposing and using cancer formulas. It is impossible to describe them all. One prominent exemplar was Jethro Kloss, whose book *Back to Eden* is arguably the best-selling herbal of modern times. (His family claimed that by 1975 the book had sold over one million copies.)

Born in Wisconsin on April 27, 1863, Kloss received training at the famous Battle Creek Sanitarium in Michigan (which is described in the book and movie, *The Road to Wellville*). From 1900 to 1905, he and his first wife operated a branch of "the San" in Rose Lawn, Wisconsin. With his second wife he operated the "Home Sanitarium" in St. Peter, Minnesota. This contained a small hospital and treated cancer patients extensively, using the popular electromagnetic therapies of the days. Some years later he opened a large health food manufacturing operation in Amqui, Tennessee, from which he shipped his health food throughout North America. He created many new food products and herbal combinations. With Kloss, as with many of his type, the philosophy of health food was indistinguishable from missionary Protestantism. "He believed that God had placed in the earth remedies for human ills and aids to human health," wrote his daughter. "He took a keen, almost evangelical interest in [the] effort to improve the general health of the public" (232, 139).

Kloss later founded health food cafeterias, health schools, and still other factories and stores. In the early 1930s, he moved to Washington, DC and became a prominent figure on what was called the health food circuit. He presented "Demonstration Dinners" for Washington notables and lectured in Constitution Hall "in promotion of the natural life." In 1946, he died peacefully in his eighty-fourth year.

He was representative of a number of prominent "health food" and physical fitness evangelists. John Harvey Kellogg, Bernarr Macfadden, Edgar Cayce, Charles Atlas, and many others were variations on this theme.

Kloss stands out because his lone book, *Back to Eden,* endures as a summary of the holistic-naturopathic approach of those days, Unlike the quacks that AMA described, Kloss is entirely open about his approach to cancer, which occupies 26 pages of his text; more if you include the discussion under particular herbs.

Kloss wrote at a time in which cancer appeared to be increasing "at an alarming rate" (139). (This rise, incidentally, was generally denied by orthodox medicine.) In his view, cancer was preventable. Its cause, he said, was essentially "chronic auto-intoxication." By this he meant constipation and the sluggishness of all the organs of elimination—the lungs, liver, kidneys, skin, and bowels. The system becomes "poisoned," and these poisons accumulate in the weakest organ, which usually had been injured by a blow, fall, or bruise. The use of "improper foods," such as tea, coffee, cola drinks, and alcohol all predisposed to cancer.

Although this philosophy of auto-intoxication sounds hopelessly outdated, we must remember that at the time it was generally believed in English-speaking countries. "Ninety-five percent of the human race suffer from chronic blood-poisoning," declaimed Dr. Walpole in George Bernard Shaw's *Doctor's Dilemma.*

"It's as simple as ABC. Your nuciform sac is full of decaying matter—undigested food and waste product—rank ptomaines....I tell you this: in an intelligently governed country people wouldn't be allowed to go about with nuciform sacs, making themselves centres of infection." Writer Lynn Payer sees a direct line from Shaw's Dr. Walpole to the famous oncologist Sir Denis Burkitt, who believes that intestinal statis leads to colon cancer. High-fiber diets, commented the *British Medical Journal,* seem "to arouse the same passions as teetotalism did in our Victorian ancestors" (313).

This was the essential philosophy of Kloss. Like many "health nuts" before and since, he abjured meat of all kinds, and especially pork; cane sugar products; white flour and white rice; and all "denatured" and "devitalized" foods. "The life-giving properties keep the blood stream pure," he wrote, "and cancer will not develop where there is a pure bloodstream." Probably unconsciously, he echoed some of the same dietary strictures about cancer of the Greco-Roman physician, Galen.

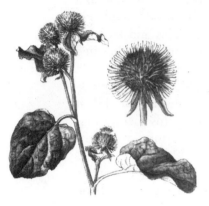

Before treatment with herbs could have an effect, patients had to "cleanse the blood stream" by thoroughly relieving constipation and making all the eliminative organs active. He urged people to take herbal laxatives and High Enemas. Well-ripened fruit, he claimed, was particularly beneficial.

"Tomatoes should be eaten by themselves—not with other foods. Make a meal of them." Again, he repeats, "Tomatoes are high in vitamin content. Use fresh ripe tomatoes or the best canned ones, but fresh, vine-ripened ones are better."

Eli Jones also extolled the tomato, almost a century before the discovery of lycopenes, phytochemicals with antitumor activity.

Arctium lappa
(burdock)

For the first ten days of treatment, Kloss said, "it is advisable to take nothing but unsweetened fruit juices, preferably orange, grapefruit, pineapple, lemon or grape. Do not mix the juices, but take different ones at different times." Vegetables juices are also very helpful, he said, especially carrot juice, again recalling recent work on beta-carotene.

Kloss's Primary Anticancer Herbs:

Scientific name	Common name	Part	AHPA
Trifolium pratense	Red clover	Blossoms	2b
Arctium lappa	Burdock	Root	1
Rumex crispus	Yellow dock	Root	2d
Viola spp.	Blue violet	Whole plant	1
Hydrastis canadensis	Goldenseal	Root	2b
Taraxicum officinale	Dandelion	Root	1
Helianthemum canadense	Rock rose	Leaves/plant	—

Note: Plants on this list should only be used under a physician's direction. Please see the warning in the front of the book.

These seven are to be combined in equal amounts, he says. As the reader can see, they are relatively safe herbs. He also recommends the following ten items, although he puts somewhat less stress on them than on the main combination:

Kloss's Secondary Anticancer Herbs:

Scientific name	Common name	Part Used	AHPA
Commiphora myrrha	Myrrh	Gum	2b
Echinacea purpurea	Echinacea	Flowers	1
Aloe vera	Aloe	Leaves	1
Iris versicolor	Blue flag	Root	2b,2d
Eupatorium purpureum	Joe Pye	Leaves, root	2a,b,c,d
Sanguinaria canadensis	Bloodroot	Root	2b,2d
Capsicum annuum	African cayenne	Pod	1
Stellaria media	Chickweed	Whole plant	1
Agrimonia eupatoria	Agrimony	Whole plant	1
Mahonia acquifolium	Oregon grape	Root	2b

Note: Plants on this list should only be used under a physician's direction. Please see the warning in the front of the book.

Kloss's descriptions of these various herbs are always interesting. One senses his vast experience as an irregular practitioner in his comments and judgments. In particular, he waxes rhapsodic over red clover, a plant that in summer is available fresh and free to almost everyone in the world.

This was based in part on what he learned from one of his mentors, the now forgotten Mrs. E. G. White. But it was also based on a personal experience he had growing up on a farm in Manitowoc, Wisconsin, on Lake Michigan. "When I was a boy," he wrote, "my parents had me gather it for their postmaster, who had a serious cancer. He lived to be an old man, without an operation.

"Every family should have a good supply of red clover blossoms," he added. "Gather them in the summer when in full bloom. Dry in the shade on papers. Put in paper bags when dry and hang in a dry place. Use this tea in place of tea and coffee and you will have splendid results. Use it freely. It can be taken in place of water" (232).

Used alone, he said, red clover tea was excellent for gastric cancer, four or more cups per day on an empty stomach. It is also good for cancer in other parts of the body. If the disease is in the throat, "make a strong tea and gargle four or five times a day, swallowing some of the tea. Open cancerous sores can be bathed freely with the tea....If in the rectum," he added, "inject with syringe [enema], five or six times a day. If in the uterus, inject with bulb syringe, holding the vagina closed after the syringe is inserted so the tea will be forced well around the head of the womb.

"Red clover is one of God's greatest blessings to man," he exulted. "Very pleasant to take and a wonderful blood purifier." Kloss offers no scientific evidence for his herbs' effectiveness. He is pre-scientific, as many healers were in those days. As naive as he seems, he may have been right on the anticancer value of these herbs.

Red clover has a long history of use in cancer all over the world. It contains a phenomenal array of anticancer and cancer preventive compounds. Like soy, it contains genestein, which is the subject of intense scientific work for its anticancer effects. The same is true of some of the other herbs on his list. In fact, many of these herbs—burdock, yellow dock, blue violet, Oregon grape—occur again and again in the story of herbalism. They weave in and out of various formulas, both secret and open, formulas which occur over the last 2000 years as treatments for cancer.

Out of thousands of possible candidates, these few have often been the standbys of herbalists of all eras. Is this just coincidence? Conscious or unconscious borrowing? Or are they used because they work, and are empirically discovered and rediscovered to have beneficial effects for cancer patients? Only scientific tests can answer that question.

Alternative practitioners are often accused of being secretive. However, in his book Kloss appears to be open and honest, to the point of naiveté. In March, 1939, he wrote to the newly formed National Cancer Institute, offering his treatment for cancer for testing. "I absolutely have a cancer cure that will cure any cancer which has not gone too far," he wrote. "I know the cause, prevention, and cure of cancer, also of heart diseases, pneumonia, asthma, infantile paralysis, gonorrhea, syphilis, and tuberculosis." We can only imagine the reaction of NCI scientists to these wild claims!

But Kloss persisted: "Will you permit one or more of your research doctors who know of a cancer patient who has not been treated by radium or X ray to let me treat this patient under their special observation by the methods which I have found successful? Thus they will see everything done for this patient and will know that a cure really can be effected by the means which I use."

The NCI scientist who answered his letter said they were not in a position to accept his offer. But they suggested that he go "to some hospital which takes cancer patients or to some regular practitioner." There is no record that any conventional doctor ever actually tested Kloss's method. It was not the first nor last time that naive laymen have attempted to get cancer scientists to test some formula and gotten the brush-off. In fact, one of the sources that Jonathan Hartwell drew on for his book, *Plants Used Against Cancer,* were dusty file drawers at the NCI filled with the similar hopes and dreams of many a bygone healer.

Chapter 3 ❀ Hemlock and Cancer

C ONIUM MACULATUM IS THE FAMOUS "POISON HEMLOCK," WHICH THE GREEK PHILOSOPHER SOCRATES WAS GIVEN TO DRINK AS A MEANS of execution. Poison hemlock is a tall, willowy, white-flowered plant indigenous to Europe and Asia, which has been widely naturalized in the United States and Canada. It dominates waste places in summer and particularly likes river banks. As an Umbellifera, it is in the same family as carrots, parsley, parsnip, and fennel.

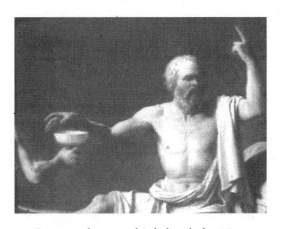

Socrates about to drink hemlock poison

Scientists tell of two healthy young men who were killed when they burned some incense that was contaminated with hemlock. What makes this case unusual is that it took place in the middle of the 13th century BC! (97) Hemlock poisoning is still fairly common in some parts of the world (such as rural Turkey), where enthusiasm for medicinal herbs sometimes outruns knowledge (309). I have heard of such accidents in Maine in recent years.

Socrates and Hemlock

There is some dispute over the identification of the "pharmakon" which killed Socrates. Most scholars believe it is Conium maculatum, *since like the Athenian potion it too kills without convulsions. Millspaugh, a famous American herbalist wrote, "From the careful observations of many pharmacographists and historians, there seems little doubt that the Grecian State potion…was principally, if not wholly, composed of the fresh juice of the leaves and green seeds of this plant" (277) But Plato never specified hemlock. A "pharmakon" is any strong drug, and not necessarily a poisonous one (hence our word "pharmacology"). Plato's description of Socrates' death is vivid. He suffered a slow paralysis that crept from his feet to his heart. Hemlock also causes a creeping muscular paralysis, with a slight trembling, but no spasm.*

That is why it is generally identified as the Athenian poison. The other major contender is Cicuta virosa, *or "water hemlock," also a member of the Umbelliferae family. But this is one of the most violently poisonous plants, when eaten (30). Cicuta causes convulsions, which neither Socrates nor other prisoners experienced. So Conium is still the most logical choice for the world's most celebrated poisonous plant.*

Conium and Cancer

There is fine line between poison and medicine. For example, most forms of chemotherapy could be classified as poisons. It was Paracelsus (1493-1541) who said that "all substances are poisons; there is none which is not a poison. The right dose differentiates a poison from a remedy."

Thus it is not surprising that Conium entered medicine as early as Dioscorides, who recommended its external use in herpes infections and erysipelas. Pliny the Elder made the first mention in writing of its use as a cancer treatment: its leaves keep down all tumors, he said (319). The Arabian physician Avicenna also praised it as a drug that could cure tumors of the breast (166).

In 1760, hemlock's use in cancer was reintroduced by a young professor at the Vienna Medical School, Baron Anton Storck (1731-1803). Storck wrote that Conium cured not just ulcers and other chronic diseases, such as schirrus (i.e., hard tumors) and cancer (342, 87).

Hemlock was not the first or only poison recommended for cancer.

Other such drugs of the time included aconite (*Aconitum napellus*), deadly nightshade (*Atropa belladonna*), and henbane (*Hyoscyamus niger*). Storck's advocacy of hemlock was not a departure from standard medicine, but an extension of the thinking of his age.

A coterie of like-minded doctors formed around Storck. Another celebrated physician of the day, Gaspard Laurent Bayle (1774-1816), collected 46 cases of cancer that were allegedly cured and 26 that were benefited by the use of this drug (86).

Dr. Storck also had some dietary recommendations. He urged patients to "avoid farinaceous substances not fermented, and too acrid aromatics." He adds that good wine will not be hurtful to those who are accustomed to it, but adds that "the patient should live in a pure free air, and keep his mind as quiet and cheerful as possible"—still excellent advice.

But a competing school of doctors was unable to achieve anticancer effects from this drug and pointed to its dangers and failures. "So frequent were the failures," said the American homoeopath Millspaugh, "that most careful and protracted experiments in gathering, curing, preserving, and preparing the drug were resorted to, analyses were made, essays written, and finally serious doubts expressed as to Baron Storck's cases" (277).

There were even suggestions of, if not fraud, then biased interpretations of the data. "It never succeeded so well as when under his own direction or confined to the neighborhood in which he resided," wrote one medical critic, "and to the practice of those physicians with whom he lived in habits of intimacy and friendship." It was suggested that the hemlock in the vicinity of Vienna was somehow more cytotoxic than that in other places, such as Britain or America. Baron Storck obligingly sent a supply of his medicine to England, but skeptical physicians there still could not get favorable results.

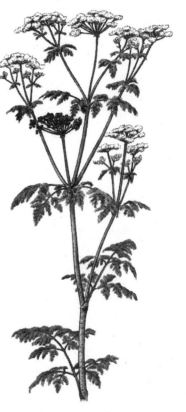

Conium maculatum
(poison hemlock)

Oddly enough, hemlock got caught up in the celebrated struggle between the British surgeon Richard Guy and Thomas Gataker, surgeon to the Royal Family (see Chapter 6). Because Guy had his own secret external remedy he tended to denigrate all other contenders. Thomas Gataker challenged him to reveal his formula and methods. Wishing to contrast his own successful treatment with the ineffective ones espoused by his competitors, Guy claimed that he had treated 100 patients with hemlock at the Manchester Infirmary, without any success. He had merely stupefied some and brought blindness to others, he said. To his *Practical Observations on Cancers* he appended "some remarks on the effects of hemlock, shewing the inefficacy of that medicine in cancerous complaints" (289).

He cited the case of one Jane Franklin of Knightsbridge who was afflicted with a schirrus (hardened) gland about the size of a walnut in the bend of her elbow. She "took the Hemlock for a long time under the direction of an experienced surgeon: She found not the least benefit from it," says Guy. "The gland became adherent and immovable, attended with acute pains that struck up to the axillary glands."

Guy goes on: "The above cases may shew, that the hemlock was possessed of no special virtue, either toward curing or abating the progress of cancers....nor does it appear that its effects are so innocent to the constitution, as Dr. Storck seems to insist upon" (289).

Buchan on Cancer

But Guy himself lost face in England after he was criticized for promoting a secret escharotic cure. Perhaps because of this, his criticism had little effect and the hemlock treatment proceeded. Its use was popularized by a Scottish physician, William Buchan, MD. In 1769, Dr. Buchan published the first edition of his *Domestic Medicine*. This was one of the most influential and popular medical books of all time. Buchan was a fellow of the Royal College of Physicians of Edinburgh, the most prestigious medical society in the English-speaking world. Like the American Dr. Tennent, Dr. Buchan's overarching purpose in writing his book was to advise patients how to avoid the destructive medicine of his day.

"I think the administration of medicine always doubtful, and often dangerous," he wrote with great sagacity, "and would much rather teach men how to avoid the necessity of using them than how they should be used."

Not surprisingly, *Domestic Medicine* was an enormous success. "In Scotland particularly," wrote historian Barbara Griggs. "it was reckoned that almost every cottage possessed a copy of this book, with its emphasis on the importance of diet, hygiene and cleanliness, and its simple herbal remedies" (154).

Buchan leaves his discussion of cancer for last. He regards it as a "loathsome and painful" disease, which "kills by inches." This "can seldom be cured but by cutting; and even that remedy is not always certain," he writes, a sentence that, sadly, is still true for many kinds of advanced cancer. So Buchan was no mindless enthusiast for every passing cure. In fact, he warns patients that certain advanced forms of the disease "will yield to no remedy, not even the boasted specifics of quackery. These never-failing curers of disorders generally send their patients to the grave, as a complete and final remedy for every disease" (57).

He writes that cancer ought to be diagnosed early and then treated through radical surgery (in the days before anesthesia and antiseptics). He also frankly acknowledges to his lay audience that "this is one of those diseases for which no certain remedy is yet known" (57).

Buchan also had certain life-style recommendations: "The diet ought to be light, but nourishing." Strong liquors and high-seasoned or salted provisions are to be avoided. (This is straight from Galen.) He advocates moderate exercise: the patient "should use every method to divert thought and amuse his fancy," external injuries are to be avoided, all good advice, even today. But he is conventional enough to advocate bloodletting and purges with calomel (mercurous chloride).

Buchan in Maine

Buchan's influence was far-flung and long-lasting in the English-speaking world, and so too his promotion of hemlock as a cancer treatment. As a personal aside, my own "cottage" contains a well-thumbed copy of Domestic Medicine, *which I keep beside my desk. It was purchased for two dollars at a yard sale in Maine some years ago. This edition bears a copyright date of 1843, i.e., nearly 75 years after its first publication. How this 150-year-old book wound up in a small seaside village in northern New England is anyone's guess. One can imagine it brought to town by an itinerant peddler. Buchan's book was still in print in 1985, 200 years after its initial publication, a testament to the longevity of certain ideas (57).*

Buchan also mentions that "an English pint of the decoction of woods of sarsaparilla may be drunk daily" and states "I have sometimes discussed [sic] hard tumours, which had the appearance of being cancers by a course of this kind." Wild sarsaparilla (*Aralia nudicaulis*) is an American herb, a member of the Ginseng family, that was widely used as a tonic, "blood purifier" and syphilis remedy in the 19th century (153).

Buchan also mentions the treatment of cancer with "an infusion of the Solanum, or nightshade, in cancers of the breast." Solanum is another poisonous plant with anticancer potential (see Chapter 12).

However, most of Buchan's hopes center around the hemlock cure. It is the "medicine in most repute at present for this disease," he tells us. He reports that the late Baron Storck "recommended the extract of this plant as very efficacious in cancers of every kind."

Aware no doubt of its well-deserved reputation as a poison, he reports that Storck "has given some hundred weights of it without every hurting any body, and often with manifest advantage." He advises the patient, however, to begin with very small doses, as two or three grains, and to increase the dose gradually till some good effect be perceived, and there to rest without further increase. From two or three grains at first, the doctor says he has increased the dose to two, three, or four drachms a day, and finds that such doses may be continued for several weeks, without any bad consequences" (57).

How long did this supposed cure take? "The doctor [Storck] does not pretend to fix the time in which a cancer may be resolved by the use of hemlock," Buchan adds, "but says, he has given it for over two years in large doses, without any apparent benefit, nevertheless, the patient has been cured by persisting in the use of it for half a year longer."

Buchan's attitude is sensible and open-minded: "Though we are far from thinking the hemlock merits those extravagant encomiums which the doctor [i.e., Storck] has bestowed upon it; yet in a disease which has so long baffled the boasted powers of medicine, we think it ought always to be tried... This is at least encouragement for a fair trial."

Buchan's Family Physician

Instead of a "fair trial," however, the topic seems to have been simply forgotten and is entirely unmentioned in most textbooks or histories of medicine.

Conium extracts, abstracts and tinctures for a long time remained official drug preparation in the US Pharmacopoeia. They were also 'official' in the Eclectic *Materia Medica*. At the end of the 19th century, Dr. Millspaugh was still talking about its use in cancer: he himself attested to the following case of "mammary scirrhus" that he treated with it. A woman came to him with a hard tumor of the breast, about the size of a silver dollar. He prescribed "Conium in a potency, one dose per diem." Within six weeks, he says, her subjective symptoms had resolved, and four months later the tumor was much softer and the nipple less cupped. The remedy was then stopped. Four years later, he reported that he could find no vestiges of the growth whatsoever. The breast appeared entirely normal.

Conium persists as a remedy, even a cancer remedy, in homoeopathy, where the doses are so small that they presumably can cause no appreciable harm (162a). It is considered suitable for traumas of the breast and other glands. It is also used in breast swelling, for swollen lymph glands and for dizziness. In 1927, the classic homoeopathic author W. Boericke mentioned its use against tumors of the skin (46). That book is still in print in India and so I think we can assume that somewhere in the world patients are still being treated with minute doses of hemlock for their cancers.

Hemlock is also sometimes used by herbalists, as well. I found the following on the Internet: "On account of its peculiar sedative action on the motor centers, hemlock juice (succus conii) is prescribed as a remedy in cases of undue nervous motor excitability, such as teething in children, epilepsy from dentition, cramp, in the early stages of paralysis agitans, in spasms of the larynx and gullet, in acute mania, etc. As an inhalation it is said to relieve cough in bronchitis, whooping-cough, asthma, etc." (www.alternative-medicines.com/1hemlock.htm).

Please note that it is not the recommendation of this book that you give your teething child hemlock juice to drink. You may get more of a "sedative action" than you bargained for!

In addition, this chapter is not to be taken as encouragement for patients to rush out and sample the wonders of hemlock for themselves. Hemlock is undoubtedly poisonous. It contains the piperidine alkaloid coniine, first isolated in 1886. (This same compound is also present, by the way, in the pitcher plant, and appears to be its insect-paralyzing principle.)

Hemlock plants may contain as much as 2.77 percent by weight of coniine, if harvested at the proper time. (The average is 1.65 percent.) Coniine also gives the plant a disagreeable mousy odor. Ingestion of coniine causes weakness, drowsiness, nausea, vomiting, labored respiration, paralysis, and death.

Hemlock also contains some other alkaloids as well. And as if its acute poisoning effects were not enough, Conium ingestion is a well-known source of mutations and abortions in farm animals. In fact, this topic occupies almost the entirety of the scientific research on Conium at the present time. There is little scientific interest in its possible therapeutic use.

Poisonings have occurred from mistaking the leaves for parsley, the roots for parsnips and the seeds for anise seeds. Many children have been poisoned when they ate or even made whistles from the hollow stems of the Hemlock. People have died after mistaking it for parsley or wild carrots. I would strongly caution readers not to experiment with this herb.

Some foolhardy individuals have eaten hemlock leaves or roots for food or just to see what would happen. Pliny the Elder reported that "as for the stems and stalks, many there be who do eat it, both green and also boiled or stewed between two platters." A Russian botanist claimed that Slavic peasants ate it with impunity, and concluded that the colder the climate, the less poisonous the root. In 19th century England, one man ate half an ounce with no ill effects, only to be topped by another who ate four ounces "without experiencing any remarkable effect." A Mr. Alicorn countered that he ate hemlock roots in every season, without feeling any material difference. Another odd fellow boiled large roots "and found them as agreeable eating at dinner with meat as carrots, which they somewhat resembled" (277).

The hemlock craze seems to have vanished from the world of cancer research. Perhaps Conium deserves a second chance. Today, we have sophisticated *in vitro* systems which can be used to screen potential treatments, even very poisonous ones, for activity. It might be worthwhile to perform such tests and see whether Baron Storck's claims have any validity.

Chapter 4 🌹 The Rees Evans Controversy

IN GREAT BRITAIN, A MAJOR CONTROVERSY OVER HERBS AND CANCERS BROKE OUT AROUND A FOLK REMEDY IN A SMALL WELSH TOWN. LATE in the 19th century, two brothers, Daniel and John Evans, developed a serious amateur interest in herbal treatments. The Evans family lived in Penybank, a little village near Llandovery, Wales. Although Llandovery has had its moment of glory, that was 2,000 years ago, when the Romans built a fort there. In recent years, the area has been known for its dairy farms, coal mine, and rugby team (*EB* 4:101).

Out of this unlikely setting arose a cancer controversy not just for Wales, or neighboring England, but the entire English-speaking world. Daniel and John believed that "Nature had given us the means of healing all ailments, had we the wisdom to discern and apply Nature's cure for all maladies." Like many rural people, they wildcrafted and employed herbs of the field and forest for their own and their neighbors' illnesses. It was an entirely innocent, non-mercenary pursuit.

Around 1905, an older brother developed cancer. It was a natural transition for the two younger Evanses to apply their avocation to his case, especially since cancer was considered largely incurable at that time. Something happened: the Evans family believed that whatever it was they gave him cured him of an incurable disease. Word of this herbal "miracle" spread, as it tends to do, and the two brothers then began to treat and apparently to "cure" friends and neighbors in the surrounding district. The matter came to international attention and then their troubles began.

In 1906, Hugh Riddle, MD, investigated the story for the London *Daily Mail*. He reported that "for 20 years these humble practitioners have been treating all kinds of diseases with ointment and salves made entirely of herbs, but only lately has their fame spread abroad....Their method is to apply a herbal preparation to the cancer, which according to them causes the roots on all sides to withdraw into the original growth which then falls off. After this the skin heals over the wound." After this story in the metropolitan paper, patients started coming from all over Great Britain..

According to a local newspaper report, "Cardigan became the Mecca of cancer patients, during which period hundreds were cured and lived for years free from any trace of the malady..." (Llandudno *Advertiser*, 10/8/21).

There is every reason to believe that Daniel and John were simple country healers, not venal quacks. Maintaining a simple life style, they lived in the countryside outside Llandovery but every morning could be seen walking into town with their preparations in hand. They kept no books and had no fixed charges for their treatment. Under pressure, they did establish a small "hospital" where the most advanced cancer cases could stay over and by 1906, there were about 45 patients in Llandovery under their care.

All sources agreed that they "commence[d] every treatment by praying for success, and urging their patients also to put their trust in God, rather than in themselves for a cure." According to a contemporary, Rev. Morgan, they cured a "very large number of patients."

The remedy was herbal, non corrosive and had an astringent and bitter taste. After time it became acidic, probably through fermentation, according to a medical doctor of the time.

Their brown or black liquid was simply painted on the skin over a cancer of the breast. "The process of cure can be observed...." said writer Cyril Scott. "The cancer separates from the healthy tissue, and comes clean away, leaving no roots behind. The bulk of the cancer growth sloughs away in a mass and leaves a crater...which heals up by first filling with healthy tissue and then skinning over. It is not a painful process, and the patient gains in weight and improves in health" (343).

In his book on cancer (written in the 1930s) Cyril Scott reprinted several testimonial letters from grateful patients. We report these to give a flavor of the controversy. Jane Morgan of Trefach, Velindre wrote that she had a complete cessation of the pain in her throat caused by the cancer. She had survived over 30 years after her treatment. There were many other such testimonials, which were later reproduced in a privately printed book, with before-and-after photographs (343).

In 1907, the treatment was roundly condemned in the *British Medical Journal*. The reader should understand that a battle between regular doctors and herbalists had been going on in Britain for over 400 years. Two British legal scholars have commented, "Organized medicine has expended considerable energy over the centuries in an attempt to eliminate unorthodox therapies." Oftentimes, the language used on both sides was the same as during the late Middle Ages. "The language of consumer protection has invariably been invoked to mask blatant professional self-interest."

Until very recently, British doctors had to share the practice of medicine with a great many lay practitioners such as the Evans's. There was a strong demand for healers of all sorts. Well into the nineteenth century, in fact, "there was a pronounced culture of medical pluralism; it was standard practice to go outside orthodox medicine in search of relief."

England is remarkable in that it had explicitly legalized the practice of herbalism by laypersons. In the Herbalists' Charter of 1542 (also derisively called the "Quacks' Charter") King Henry VIII allowed the laity to practice herbal medicine provided that they did not charge for anything other than the herbs themselves:

"It shall be lawful for every person being the King's subject, having knowledge and experience of the nature of Herbs, Roots and Waters...to practice, use and minister...according to their cunning, experience and knowledge in any of the diseases...without suit, vexation, trouble, penalty, or loss of their goods..." (373).

Numerous battles were fought over the parameters of this Act. It wasn't until 1858 that the medical profession was strong enough to get a new Medical Act through Parliament. One of its chief justifications was to protect the public from charlatans and unskilled practitioners such as the Evans brothers. In England, however, by tradition, there was freedom for herbal practitioners, provided that they did not deceive the public by calling themselves physicians. However, this did not remove the constant state of tension that existed between the two approaches, and that erupted over the claims of the Evans brothers.

In 1919, the treatment was taken up by the son of one of the brothers, Mr. David Rees Evans, and his name has been attached to it ever since. Rees Evans had just returned from the Great War and, having seen the world, was more enterprising and ambitious than either his father or uncle. Nor did he shy away from publicity. Like Harry Hoxsey (see Chapter 5), he sought it out. In 1923 or 1924, he requested an investigation of the method by the government. The Committee for Cancer of the Ministry of Health suggested they would investigate 20 of his cases.

Since most of the literary sources are highly favorable towards Rees Evans, it is difficult to get both sides of the story. However, reporter Nat Morris says that when he was asked for 20 cases he submitted 30. The committee later reported that it was unable to even locate any of the patients for the purpose of investigating their alleged cures. Rees Evans contended in turn that the committee had failed to sincerely try, since a number of these patients told him later that no one contacted them. According to another sympathetic writer, "Mr. Evans has adequate reasons for mistrusting the activities of cancer experts" (343). The committee report was essentially negative.

In 1930, two experts from the Royal Cancer Hospital investigated the Rees Evans therapy by examining two of his patients. Rees Evans himself was not allowed to be present during the examinations. After this examination, one of the patients immediately ceased his treatment and in fact brought suit against him. This trial was long and costly. Morris reports that "a public-spirited journalist, Hannen Swaffer, assumed the cost of the trial which ended in a disagreement" (289).

Twenty years later, Swaffer summarized his experiences with Evans in a letter in the *Picture Post* (9/23/50). He cited a number of alleged "cures" that he himself had investigated. One was a woman that Swaffer himself had referred to Rees Evans and who was "cured" after all other doctors had given up hope. A doctor familiar with the case referred to this as a "miracle." However, when this doctor was urgently needed at the 1930 trial, he could not be found.

Most of the cases the Evans family treated had been given up for lost by the regular medical profession. Rees Evans would reassure the patient and tell her that they could hope for a cure in about 12 weeks. He would then apply his solution to the area above the tumor with a soft brush. This brought on sensations of penetration, burning and pulling. The treatment was given for six days a week and, except for the above sensations, was painless. An interesting note is that a lettuce leaf placed over the tumor at this point would turn black.

After twelve weeks of treatment the "roots" of the cancer came away, leaving a crater underneath that was treated by another solution. This crater then healed, leaving only a small scar (289). Although some sources say this was not an escharotic, this is very similar to descriptions of successful escharotic treatments throughout the ages (see Chapter 6).

The sociological dimensions of this struggle were particularly interesting. In the case that Swaffer referred to, the woman returned to the specialist she had first consulted. He agreed her recovery was miraculous, but then denied that she had ever had the cancer that he himself had diagnosed.

The controversy simmered for decades and in the 1950s involved the United States. Mrs. Rees Evans visited the United States around 1949 for a convention and met a woman named Mrs. Ann Lupo of Newark, New Jersey, who was very active in social work. Hearing the Evans's story, Mrs. Lupo secured an invitation from the Presbyterian Hospital of Newark for Rees Evans to demonstrate his treatment (261).

As soon as he arrived, a clinic and 16 cancer patients were assigned to him. Fifteen of the sixteen had been rigorously diagnosed and ten of them were considered "hopeless." He worked for the next eight months without compensation. The treatment of these 16 took from a minimum of nine days to the full eight months. After eight months he was finally compelled to return to England for economic reasons and resume his herbalist practice there. He arranged for publication of his results in the *Picture Post* of London (9/9/50). According to Morris, there were nine "positive indications of cure" (289).

There was naturally a flood of publicity about the treatment, yet another in the long history of "cancer cures" in tabloid newspapers. The *British Medical Journal,* which had been condemning the Evans treatment since 1907, published another severely critical editorial. On September 30, 1950, the *Picture Post* published this editorial in one column and its reply to each criticism in an adjoining column.

The *BMJ* cited a telegram from the Tumor Therapy Committee of Presbyterian Hospital: "Work entirely experimental. No definitive results obtained. Evans' statement unwarranted and unauthorized. No results to be published. Would disavow all unproven claims by Evans."

But *Picture Post* countered that as late as July 31, 1950, Presbyterian Hospital had expressed an interest in continuing the treatment. There was no doubt that the leaders of Presbyterian Hospital, including presumably its president, Royal Schaaf, MD, were irritated and embarrassed by Rees Evans's actions. But this often happens when medical professionals and lay healers try to collaborate on the evaluation of an alternative cancer treatment. Each group has its own standards, values, outlooks, and goals.

Presbyterian's leaders undoubtedly were sincere in their desire to evaluate the treatment. For them, this implied a slow building up of facts and then publication in a restrained and factual manner in a major medical journal. That process took years or even decades and in the end, when every mitigating circumstance was taken into account, the treatment in question might not appear so spectacular. In particular, at that time they had a horror of any kind of extra-scientific publicity. (Even Sloan-Kettering Institute's director, C.P. Rhoads, was censured by the New York Academy of Medicine for allowing his picture to appear on the cover of *Time* magazine.)

Lay people, on the other hand, had no ingrained habits of scientific exactitude or medical clannishness. They generally related to popular publications, not scientific journals, where they had practically zero chance of publishing their results. And they were usually driven by passions and interests that went beyond the search for scientific facts, including often an intense desire to profit from their discoveries.

Although the secrecy and cure-mongering surrounding the Rees Evans treatment were abhorrent to Presbyterian's leaders, Nat Morris is technically correct when he writes that "Mr. Evans was under no obligation to the hospital because he had in no way been compensated for his great expenditure of time and effort and certainly was within his rights in securing publication wherever he chose."

However, if Rees Evans wanted to stir up the British public with his story, he succeeded. The *Picture Post* controversy had one important fallout. Aneurin Bevan (1897-1960), the radical British Minister of Health, informed Evans that he had appointed a committee to investigate his work. The four-person committee was headed by Sir Robert Robinson, OM, FRS, president of the Royal Society and included Sir Alexander Fleming, FRS, the discoverer of penicillin.

Evans agreed but suggested what we would now call a prospective study, in which he would have a chance to demonstrate his methods and results to the committee on a group of patients chosen by them in advance. This design would have eliminated in advance the familiar charge that successfully treated patients never had cancer. The committee opted for a less convincing retrospective analysis of some British and American patients. I think most biostatisticians today would agree that Evans's proposal would have led to a more reliable outcome, but the views of the committee prevailed. It then examined the histories of 22 patients out of 34 names that were supplied. Its conclusion was as follows:

Insufficient evidence for evaluation 5
No convincing evidence of cancer at the time of treatment 3
Judged not to have suffered from cancer 7
Death from or seriously ill from recurrence after treatment 2
Rodent ulcer [i.e., basal cell carcinoma] 5
Total 22

Similarly, the committee looked at the 16 American cases and found:
Dead from cancer 8
Seriously ill from cancer 1
No convincing evidence of cancer 2
Condition doubtful 1
No recurrence, but also treated surgically or with X rays 2
Rodent ulcer 2
Total 16

The committee held a total of eight sessions, but Evans was only allowed to be present at two of these. "In his absence," says Morris, "unnamed medical practitioners testified on the Evans treatment, and their statements were accepted without the opportunity for Evans to hear or challenge them." Evans repeatedly offered to demonstrate the dramatic effectiveness of his methods to the committee, but was routinely denied that opportunity. In effect, the committee ruled that "the Evans patients who died did indeed die of cancer, while those who lived either had had no cancer or had been helped by the delayed effects of previous x-ray or surgical treatment."

One of the collateral controversies concerned the so-called "rodent ulcers." The committee threw out all such cases (which constituted over 20 percent of the British cases it evaluated). "Enquiries were not pursued" in such cases "on the grounds that it has been known for many decades that it can be successfully treated by several methods which remove the locally affected tissue; and that evidence of success in healing rodent ulcers throws no light on whether the same method will be useful in the treatment of cancer in general" (289).

Evans countered with a statement from Rupert A. Willis, a famous Australian pathologist, in which he described the progress of rodent ulcers as "slowly invasive and destructive. Untreated growths on the face may eventually destroy most of the soft tissues and bones and may penetrate to the skull or the brain" (411, 353).

But in my opinion Evans was right. "Rodent ulcer" is an old term for the most common type of basal cell carcinoma (BCC) (168). It is true that most basal cell carcinomas do not spread or metastasize and are adequately treated with conventional methods. But not all. According to *Neoplastic Diseases,* the major cancer textbook of the time (1940), rodent ulcer can maintain "a persistent ulceration which resists efforts at cure." Eventually, "it destroys the skin down to superficial fascia, where its progress is long restrained. Later it strips the tissues down to bone or muscle, where again it makes slow progress....In advanced stages, the dimensions of the rodent ulcer become very wide, involving much of the face, neck, or scalp. The destruction of tissue becomes deeper, especially with the aid of incomplete excision. The eye, ear, and nose are often completely destroyed. Cachexia results chiefly from chronic suppuration, hemorrhages, and mental depression" (125). It can be a serious form of cancer, and I can see no reason why such cases needed to be excluded. There are now over 200 cases of metastatic BCC in the literature (263).

Whether there were other methods that could cure "rodent ulcers" was entirely irrelevant to the question at hand, which was whether or not Rees Evans's treatment cured this condition. The committee refused to even consider that question.

Nor does it seem fair to say that "evidence of success in healing rodent ulcers throws no light on whether the same method will be useful in the treatment of cancer in general." Surgery, radiation and topical chemotherapy are all used conventionally to treat BCC, and their success in doing so is certainly relevant to the overall question of their effectiveness.

As to the remaining 17 British cases, the committee threw out 15 of them on the grounds that there was insufficient data or evidence that the patients had cancer. This may very well have been true, since the overwhelming majority of Evans's patients came to him with diagnoses done elsewhere. However, such elementary problems could have been avoided if the committee had taken his suggestion and done a prospective study on patients selected by them in advance.

Similarly, in the American cases, we also see the difficulty of performing retrospective analyses. Eight of the sixteen cases were found to be dead of cancer. That was no surprise, since the *Picture Post* article had only *claimed* that eight of the 16 original patients had benefitted. One of the remaining patients was found to be seriously ill from cancer. But what was his or her actual condition? Was there improvement in quality in life? Stabilization of tumor growth? We don't know, although this would have been highly relevant to the evaluation. In one case the condition was doubtful and in two cases there was "no convincing evidence of cancer." If this is true, it seems unconscionable for Presbyterian Hospital to have included such cases in the group they presented to Rees Evans to work with: this criticism rebounds on the medical profession, not on Mr. Evans.

Finally, in two cases there was no recurrence of the tumor, but the patients were also treated surgically or with X rays. Again, we would have to know when the patients had their surgery or radiation therapy and what stage they were in when they began the herbal treatment in order to make any kind of intelligent judgment.

Rees Evans was still alive in March, 1958 when Nat Morris wrote his book, *The Cancer Blackout*. Morris even interviewed one of his American patients, a woman in her mid fifties who had been operated on for cancer of the cervix. She reported that she was well, but this was presumably one of the patients thrown out by the Committee because she had had prior surgery. Essentially, the Committee report spelled the end of the Rees Evans controversy. Evans himself passed away, never having revealed the formula that his father and uncle had pioneered so many years before.

Chapter 5 ✿ Harry Hoxsey

"Of all the ghouls who feed on the bodies of the dead and dying, the cancer quacks are most vicious and most heartless." —Morris Fishbein, MD, 1965 (131)

"The distinguished author [Fishbein] had inherited from his spiritual father the technique of the big lie....Adolf Hitler was dead, but the Hitler of American medicine ranted on."—Harry Hoxsey, 1956 (194)

HARRY HOXSEY (1901-1974) WAS THE MOST COLORFUL OF ALL THE IRREGULAR PRACTITIONERS OF THE 20TH CENTURY. BY comparison, today's leaders of alternative medicine are mild-mannered milquetoasts. Hoxsey's vocal advocacy of his internal and external herbal treatments, together with his creation of a series of clinics to dispense them, set off the greatest cancer battle of the 20th century.

For nearly four decades, this ex-coal miner, who dropped out of high school and had no medical training, treated cancer patients, including the "terminally ill," with herbal-mineral formulas, which he claimed had been passed down through his family. To many Americans of the time, he was simply "the cancer doctor." To the editor of the American Medical Association's journal, Morris Fishbein, MD, he was a ghoul who feasted off the bodies of the dead and the dying.

Hoxsey's side of the story is told with surprising skill in his 1955 autobiography, *You Don't Have to Die,* which was ghostwritten by publicist Allen

69

Bernard. It has been the subject of an award-winning documentary film, *Hoxsey: How Healing Becomes a Crime* (25). Incredibly, a full-length Hollywood feature film is in the works. On the other hand, there are numerous detractors of Hoxsey, the most capable of whom was James Harvey Young in *Medical Messiahs*.

Young is a highly reputed scholar in the field of medical history and indeed his books are an excellent source of facts. However, I find his viewpoint almost as one-sided as Hoxsey's own. To me, his work is a good illustration of the dictum that "the historian is often a propagandist even when he may not be aware of it himself." I am quoting Allen G. Debus, who—ironically enough—is the Morris Fishbein Professor of History of Science and Medicine at the University of Chicago (100).

Hoxsey's Youth

The AMA has had many opponents in its day. Some of these, like Andrew Ivy, MD, held high positions in the medical establishment. But it was this ham-handed, fast-talking ex-coal miner who did more to challenge its power and credibility than any academic critic. At his peak, Hoxsey operated a chain of private cancer clinics, attracting tens of thousands of patients. In Dallas alone, he had seven licensed physicians working on his staff.

"Doctors began to tell my patients that I was a notorious quack," he once said. "My reply was—still is—that I'd rather be notorious, and save lives, than famous and bury them" (194).

To all outward appearances, Harry Hoxsey was a fast-talking supersalesman, in ten-gallon hat and cowboy boots, who courted arrest for practicing medicine without a license. He bragged that he had been arrested for this offense more times than anyone in history.

"I frequently have been accused of being a flamboyant showman and promoter, as well as a healer," he wrote. "If I am all these things, it is because the AMA forced these roles upon me" (194).

Unlike that self-described "Christian gentleman," Jethro Kloss, Hoxsey had no intention of turning the other cheek. "I ain't gonna let those sons-of-bitches kill you," was a typical Hoxsey come-on to his patients (25). In this spirit, he single-handedly took on the leader of the AMA and fought with him for 40 years.

Was Hoxsey a Quack?

The *Oxford Condensed Dictionary* defines a quack as "an unqualified practiser of medicine." Oliver Field, MD, former director of the AMA's Bureau of Investigations, called Hoxsey a classic dictionary-definition quack, i.e., "one who pretends to medical skill he does not possess" (25).

At times, Hoxsey met the definition of a quack in that he practiced medicine without a license. But was he a quack when he obtained a Doctorate of Naturopathy, valid in the state of Texas? Was he a quack when he employed seven licensed physicians, while he tended to his oil investments?

Hoxsey didn't practice surgery, radiation, or chemotherapy. What he claimed expertise in was the use of escharotics and herbal treatments. The AMA agreed that the external paste killed cancer cells. In fact, they are similar to Mohs' microsurgery, developed at the University of Wisconsin. The AMA could hardly claim that Hoxsey was a quack because he was unskilled in the use of escharotics, since he probably had more experience in their use than anyone alive.

So the question of whether he was a quack would seem to hinge on the effectiveness of his internal medication. If it was as worthless as the AMA claimed, he was a classic quack. If the formula was at all effective, however, then perhaps Hoxsey was tragically misunderstood. Or perhaps it will turn out that Hoxsey was indeed a quack, but as someone called him, "a quack who cured cancer."

In *You Don't Have to Die,* Hoxsey said that his family came to America in 1650 and settled in the Plymouth Colony. Eventually they worked their way out West. In the 1840s, his great-grandfather, John Hoxsey, established himself as a horse breeder in southern Illinois. Harry grew up in Girard, Illinois, a town of 2,000, south of Springfield.

The Hoxsey family involvement with cancer began when one of John Hoxsey's Percheron stallions developed a tumorous growth on its right hock and had to be put out to pasture. Rather than die, the horse began to graze in a deliberate fashion on various plants of the field. Subsequently, he had a remission of his disease.

Today, the study of animals' self-healing abilities is given the dignified name of Zoopharmacognosy, and it is pursued in places such as Harvard University. John Hoxsey had no advanced degrees.

But he knew enough to note down and collect the herbs that his horse had eaten. Eventually he made these into two medicines, one an external salve, the other an internal mixture. He then used these to treat horses that were similarly afflicted. People said he had the "healing tetch."

When he died he passed this formula down to his son, who eventually passed it on to his son. In fact, Hoxsey's father, John C. Hoxsey, became a veterinarian on the strength of his grandfather's original discovery, and made a living using this salve to treat animal tumors. He also started treating humans with it, although he had no formal training and did not maintain a clinic (194).

Harry Hoxsey was born on October 23, 1901. He always said that his life goal was to become a licensed medical doctor. There is a strong element of envy in his battle with Fishbein. He certainly had the intelligence and the drive for it. However, after a fall, his father became ill, and Harry was forced to quit school at the age of 15 and go to work as a "dirt monkey" in the coal mine where his older brother worked. (He obtained an equivalency high school diploma and eventually was granted an honorary doctorate of naturopathy.)

Even in the mine, Hoxsey's bent towards medicine was apparent and he was appointed to tend the mules, a skilled job for a teenager. But this quick-witted young man was far too ambitious to get stuck underground. He had a quick tongue and the winning ways of a politician. "Harry is not a man of few words," one admirer later said, "but one of many."

Hoxsey senior died in 1919. On his deathbed, his father made young Harry memorize the family's anticancer formulas by copying them out 250 times on a blank tablet. He cautioned his heir to use it only for the benefit of humanity and to disregard the opposition he would inevitably face from the "High Priests of Medicine" (420). He then passed on to his reward.

It is a lovely story, very well known in alternative medicine circles. However, there is some reason to doubt its accuracy. In a 1996 article, a naturopathic physician, Francis Brinker, ND, (who is otherwise receptive to herbal treatments) has revealed that the internal formula of Harry Hoxsey is nearly identical to what was an official National Formulary medicine known as Compound Fluidextract of Trifolium (CFT) (53. See also following discussion of formula.)

On February 22, 1921, while he was still a coal miner, Harry Hoxsey began to walk in his father's footsteps. He was approached by S.T. Larkin, a Civil War veteran "of considerable wealth and standing in the community," whose "lower lip and chin were disfigured by a hideous, running sore."

"I've been to three doctors with this," he said, "and they all told me I have cancer, they can't do anything for me, I'll be dead within the year," said Larkin. "I knew your daddy well, saw him take sores like this off other people with that medicine of his. I want you to do the same for me" (194).

Hoxsey "carefully explained" that he didn't have a license to practice medicine and that it was against the law for him to treat the elderly man. Larkin replied:

"Son, when I joined up in '61 and fought to preserve this Union for you and your children and your children's children, they didn't ask me if I had a license to kill rebs. Nobody needs a license to save lives. If I was drowning would you stand by and watch me go down because a sign on yonder tree says 'No Swimming Allowed'"?

"There's no adequate answer to that kind of logic," Hoxsey concluded, "and I didn't waste any time trying to find one." After more persuasive speeches, Hoxsey finally agreed to treat the elderly gentleman, "on condition that he would keep the treatment a secret.

"With mingled feelings of excitement and apprehension," he wrote many years later, "I applied the yellow powder to the nasty running sore on his lip and chin, plastered a clean gauze bandage over them—just as I'd seen Dad do hundreds of times in the past—and handed him a big square bottle of the internal tonic to take home with him." The treatment was a complete success, he said.

First one, then another of the town's local cancer patients came to him for treatment. Eventually, Harry Hoxsey plunged into the cancer treatment business, using the two medicines he had used on this veteran. And the old soldier frequently testified at public meetings that young Harry had cured him of cancer.

To protect himself against lawsuits, Hoxsey set up a clinic in nearby Taylorville with Bruce Miller, MD, a 57-year-old physician with a degree from the College of Physicians and Surgeons of Chicago. Miller was medical director of the clinic and Hoxsey was his mere technician. With Miller's help Hoxsey read through medical textbooks and became a kind of lay expert on the cancer problem. He could talk the talk. This first clinic did well, but Hoxsey and Miller had their eyes on Chicago, a huge medical market. To further their goal of acceptance in the big city, they met with Dr. Malcolm L. Harris, chief surgeon at a hospital in that city and a power in the AMA. (He later became its president.)

Harris was intrigued by what he heard and saw of the Hoxsey method. However, the encounter ended in disaster. Harris, said Hoxsey, offered to test the various formulas. But in exchange, Hoxsey had to shut down his irregular clinic, turn control and ownership of the formulas over to Harris and his consortium of Chicago doctors, and not expect any remuneration for a period of ten years. After that time, he would receive 10 percent of the net proceeds if the treatment panned out. It was a take-it-or-leave-it offer.

In essence, this is not all that different from the type of offer that would be made today by a pharmaceutical company interested in testing an unproven cancer treatment. But Hoxsey reacted with shock and indignation. He withdrew from the negotiations.

Still intent on penetrating Chicago, on October 1, 1924, Hoxsey, Dr. Miller and a business group headed by an insurance broker named Lucius Everhard opened a cancer clinic in Chicago, not half a mile from AMA headquarters on North Dearborn Avenue! This too ended badly. "It took me just one month to discover that Everhard and his cohorts had only one interest in my cancer treatment," said Hoxsey. "To convert it into a get-rich-quick racket" (194). The business manager had set the fees at $500 to $1,000 per case—an enormous sum in those days—and charity patients were spurned.

Hoxsey had always kept his own fees on the low end of the scale and it is probably true that he treated many people for free. As he later explained, "This policy wasn't just altruism...it was common sense business. The cases we cured for free were our best advertisement...." (194). In a stormy session with his partners, including Miller, Hoxsey accused them of "exploiting human suffering and misery for personal gain." Thoroughly disgusted and disillusioned with Chicago—"evidently just another small-town boy ripe for plucking by big-city slickers"—Hoxsey packed his formulas and went home, where he was tendered an enthusiastic reception. The Chamber of Commerce launched a campaign to make Taylorville "the cancer capital of America." Headlines in the local paper screamed that Hoxsey's clinic, the Hoxide Institute, "Will Be Mayo Clinic to Taylorville" (25).

The local Moose Lodge was converted into a handsome clinic and in early 1925, the Hoxide Institute opened its doors with another local doctor, Wilbur Washburn, MD, as medical director. Again, Hoxsey was listed as a technician. The maximum fee was set at $300 and charity cases were not turned away.

The Taylorville Chamber of Commerce then sent out testimonial brochures by the thousands to other chambers around the country. It sponsored advertisements in midwestern newspapers urging cancer victims everywhere to communicate with its Secretary "for authoritative information as to the cures that have been effected and are now being effected under strictly ethical medical supervision, painlessly, without operation and with permanent results" (194, 420).

Hoxsey put up posters, offering rewards for people who could prove that he didn't have a genuine cure for cancer. Naturally, some local AMA members were incensed and complained to the national office about these blatant promotional efforts on behalf of cancer quackery. One wrote that he had examined a patient who had been treated for a tumor on the cheek and found "necrosis not only of the soft tissue of his face, but a complete destruction of the malar [cheek] bone. This man died of hemorrhage at the hospital" (420). The death was ascribed to Hoxsey's inexpert care.

In the summer of 1925, a stranger showed up in town from the AMA Bureau of Investigations. Hoxsey invited him to visit but "a few days later I learned that he'd skulked out of town as stealthily as he had come in" (194). On January 2, 1926, a three-page attack on the Hoxide Institute appeared in the pages of *JAMA*. It was "a scurrilous, slanderous smear attack upon me, my father, the Hoxsey treatment and everyone at any time associated with us," Hoxsey later wrote. *JAMA* claimed that Hoxsey's father had himself died of cancer, a charge that was to figure prominently in the Hoxsey debate for nearly fifty years. *JAMA* also claimed that the Hoxsey treatment "ate into blood vessels," that patients had died as a result of it, and that many so-called cured patients had had "non-malignant or superficial growths."

The editor of *JAMA* at this time was Morris Fishbein, MD, and from this point on, Fishbein and Hoxsey became each other's personal nemesis.

Fishbein was the most powerful man in American medicine in his day. (His opponents called him the "Medical Mussolini.") The AMA (and Fishbein) consolidated their hold over American medicine. Subscriptions to the *Journal* had increased from 13,078 in 1900 to over 80,000 by 1924. Income from pharmaceutical advertising was already in the hundreds of thousands of dollars. Yet AMA leaders were conscious of the threat posed by irregular practitioners. Ironically, the long-time General Manager of the Association, George H. Simmons, MD, had himself been a homoeopathic practitioner in Lincoln, Nebraska, "and one of a rather partisan hue." After he "converted" to allopathy, he became a persecutor of his former colleagues (86).

Simmons was General Secretary and General Manager of the AMA from 1899 to 1911, and editor of its *Journal* from 1899 to 1924. He was considered "the greatest figure in his generation in the development of the American Medical Association...." In 1905, he established the AMA Council on Pharmacy and Chemistry. This bureau made its peace with the pharmaceutical industry. While the details of all this are very complicated, the net result, as Harris Coulter, PhD, remarks, was that "the AMA allied with, and was conquered by, the patent medicine industry."

But the "regular" doctors could not rise as a sovereign profession unless they had crippled the irregular practitioners who surrounded them. In 1901, an article in the AMA's *Journal* stated quite frankly, "Patients whose number is legion throw themselves from its [i.e., the regular profession's] arms into the embrace of quackery, and we must admit that the support is often as effective in the one case as in the other..." (86).

Although the fight against Hoxsey was initially joined at lower levels, it soon engaged the attention of Fishbein, who was Simmons' chosen successor as *JAMA* editor. It was also Fishbein who brokered the AMA's agreements and understandings with the pharmaceutical industry, and who extolled chemotherapy. He had a rather odd background: he himself never practiced medicine but went straight into medical politics. In dedicating his 1927 book to Simmons, Fishbein wrote that his "unrelenting and courageous warfare against medical quackery has been an inspiration to his successors" (132).

To put it mildly, Fishbein promoted an acerbic and self-righteous style of debate. Not content with attacking the methods of his opponents, he attacked their personalities, friends and families, as well. He was scornful of other people's belief systems. "One always finds [quacks] prating in terms of theological derivation, and usually affirming their ability to commune personally with the Deity," he wrote, in one of his milder perorations.

The fact that Fishbein was of Jewish ancestry complicated the struggle. Some of the criticism directed at Fishbein was undoubtedly tinged with antisemitism. Yet we must remember that racial prejudice was so characteristic of the times that Fishbein himself was not above making remarks that today would be considered antisemitic. For example, about a Rabbi who founded a movement called "Jewish Science," Fishbein wrote that he was "perhaps somewhat jealous of the profits of Christian Science...."

The AMA was also composed almost entirely of male doctors and there were many swipes at women in Fishbein's writing. It is interesting from a sociological point of view that nutrition and herbalism were opposed, in part, because they were associated with women. For example, Fishbein considered Eclecticism "the apotheosis of the old grandmother and witch-doctor systems of treatment." It arose out of "the medical practice of an old-woman herb doctor." Herbal remedies, built up over decades of careful observation, were mockingly derided as "veritable vegetable soups" (132).

Fishbein considered anything traditional in medicine to be abhorrent. He saw the botanical drugs of the late 19th century as "almost a replica of the herbals of the 17th and 18th century Europe." Warming to his subject, he continued:

"The woods and fields were combed for all varieties of roots and vines and grasses, and they were transformed into infusions, decoctions, syrups, tinctures, extracts and tablets. The mind of the poor medical student was bewildered by his attempts to learn the botanical names, the nature, and the alleged uses of these hundreds of drugs."

"University laboratories," he assured his lay readers, "were carefully investigating, on animals and on man, the real virtues of the remedies in use." But "most of the remedies it [i.e., Eclectic medicine] promoted have since been shown to be quite inert or utterly inadequate in the large majority of cases." Of course, the vast majority of phytochemicals now known to reside in plants and herbs (many with unique physiological effects) were undreamed of in Fishbein's day. To put it colloquially, he was simply blowing smoke. While the AMA was successful in eliminating most competition, Fishbein became concerned, and then obsessed, by "the worst cancer quack of the century," Harry Hoxsey (403).

Confrontations in Taylorville

The AMA sent copies of its blistering article on Hoxsey to every member of the Taylorville Chamber of Commerce. It send a representative to the Chamber to persuade them, individually and collectively, of their moral and financial culpability for any deaths that might result from Hoxsey's treatment. Although they were not initially frightened off, a subtle change in the administrative rules of the Chamber (which Hoxsey, of course, attributed to AMA machinations) soon put an end to their advocacy of this treatment.

In July, 1925, Hoxsey himself was visited by an investigator for the state medical board, who asked to see the clinic's medical license. Hoxsey showed him Washburn's hanging on the wall, but the man wasn't satisfied and wanted to see Harry Hoxsey's as well. Hoxsey declared, "I have none, except the license of any American citizen to work at his trade. I'm a technician. I work under the supervision of Dr. Washburn."

"That's a damned lie, Hoxsey," bellowed the investigator, "and you know it! You're the whole works here, you're practicing medicine without a license and we're going to close you down!" The next day there were headlines in the Springfield newspapers, "FAKE CANCER CLINIC RAIDED!" and "DOWNSTATE MURDER MILL RAIDED!" Oddly, no such raid had taken place—the mere fact that the AMA wished it, made it so. This was typical of the kind of problems that Hoxsey's enemies were able to generate for him over the next forty years.

In 1928, Hoxsey was sued by most of his brothers and sisters who saw his success and now wanted a share in the family formulas. (They had shown no interest in these before Hoxsey transformed them into a successful business.) This modern-day Joseph won the suit but fighting it left him virtually bankrupted. He had to close the Taylorville clinic.

Meanwhile, Hoxsey was being frequently attacked by name in the pages of the *JAMA*. Tragedy awaits "sufferers from carcinoma," the AMA's Dr. Cramp wrote, "who are beguiled by false beacons displayed by the highly respectable citizens of Taylorville." Dr. Crouch detailed alleged instances of tragedy that had already occurred. "The promoters of the scheme" were reaping "a rich harvest from gullibility and suffering" (*JAMA* 1/2/26).

The AMA had reasons to be indignant. But it had also made only a cursory investigation of Hoxsey's method. These were fighting words, and Hoxsey came out fighting. He sued the AMA for a quarter of a million dollars for libel. After some fancy legal footwork, the suit was dismissed. According to *JAMA*, Hoxsey was himself sued at this time "for the death of one his victims," and accused of practicing medicine without a license. It is said he pleaded guilty to the charge and was fined $100.

The Girard Clinic

In 1928, because of his financial difficulties, Hoxsey closed the doors of the Taylorville clinic, but, according to historian James Harvey Young, "he did not abandon the corrosive legacy inherited from his father" (420).

He soon reopened his clinic in the old Nicolet Hotel in his hometown of Girard, Illinois. Opening day, July 17, 1929 was declared "Hoxsey Day" by Girard's Chamber of Commerce. This demonstration, said Young, had "all the trappings of a Fourth of July celebration."

The Girard band played. Living testimonials from among the citizenry, including the now celebrated Civil War veteran, told of their gratitude before a large audience assembled in the town square under a broiling sun. From Indiana came one of the vanishing breed of Eclectic doctors to laud the Hoxsey method. A local minister delivered an oration imbued with religious and patriotic zeal, which compared Hoxsey to Washington, Lincoln, and Woodrow Wilson.

Hoxsey zealously addressed his former neighbors. "There is a lot of knockers," he said, "who do not know what they are talking about, and especially around a man's home town, and if those knockers are here today and have the mind of a six-year-old child and don't leave here today, a walking, talking dyed-in-the-wool Hoxsey fan and convinced beyond a reasonable doubt that this treatment is a cure for cancer they are either deaf, dumb or blind, or else they are crazy."

The regular doctors were "hard-hearted," he said, interested in "getting their hands greased with plenty of money," and unlike Hoxsey, were imbued with a desire to drive expensive Packards and Stutz Bearcats. AMA officials, he went on, had been invited to attend this rally, but had failed to show. "Why don't they fight in the open?" he demanded. "Why don't they take this platform? Why don't they prove the Hoxsey affair is a fake as they say?...But no, friends, they haven't got the guts to accept this challenge" (Gerard *Gazette*, 7/18/29).

Hoxsey claimed that his methods could cure more than 50 percent of patients (he later raised that to 80 percent), and offered a big reward for anyone who could prove otherwise. Applause was frequent and when one speaker asked those who wanted to endorse Hoxsey's efforts to stand, "those who remained sitting for any reason could be counted on the fingers."

It is true that AMA representatives did not show up for the rally, but *JAMA*'s Dr. Cramp was not slow to respond in print. "Perhaps Girard will flourish briefly—especially the local undertaker and those individuals who have rooms to rent....If that is what the citizens...want, the Hoxide fakery will doubtless give it to them. They will also get the doubtful privilege of the reputation of living in a town that fattens off the sufferings of those unfortunates who are lured there by the false hope that an ignorant faker has discovered a 'cure' for one of the most dreadful scourges afflicting the human race" (*JAMA* 8/3/29).

Enter Norman Baker

There is disagreement over the fate of the Girard clinic. Hoxsey says, "Because we saved lives our clinic prospered, and its reputation gradually spread throughout the Middle West." Dr. Young states that the clinic floundered, apparently because of the fierce AMA opposition. In any case, in February 1930, Hoxsey received a fateful telephone call from Norman G. Baker, who operated a similar hospital in Muscatine, Iowa.

Baker was an astonishing character, at one time almost as notorious as Hoxsey himself. He was (in Hoxsey's words) "a handsome, wavy-haired, middle-aged, aggressive personality with hypnotic eyes." He had previously made his living as a hypnotist on the vaudeville stage. There was even a popular biography of him called *Doctors, Dynamiters, and Gunmen*.

Baker had been experimenting with various cancer treatments but said he was unsatisfied with the results. Like Hoxsey, Baker employed an external as well as an internal remedy. The internal remedy was called a "blood purifying mixture," compounded from a secret formula of herbs, roots, and bark. Sometimes this was injected as near as possible to the tumor itself. The external remedy was an escharotic that allegedly did not burn normal tissues. Baker particularly believed in the anticancer value of onions. He was also an early crusader against aluminum, used in false teeth, which he claimed caused cancer. (Young, who does not have a good word for Hoxsey, claimed that Hoxsey learned the internal formula from Baker.)

In 1928, Baker announced in newspaper advertisements as well as over his own radio station, KTNT— "The Naked Truth"—that he had perfected a cure for cancer. Baker was given to dramatic, headline-grabbing challenges. He offered to let a committee of 12 or more from "every school of medical and health-thought" to be assembled, including laymen. This committee was then to have 30 cancer sufferers examined by independent doctors, not connected with either side, to make sure they really had cancer.

The 30 patients would be divided as follows: 20 external and 10 internal cases. Ten virgin, ten medium and ten far advanced cases. Fifteen of these patients were to be treated by the AMA-appointed doctors, with surgery, radium and X-ray, free of charge for medical services. Fifteen were to be treated by Baker using his characteristic treatments at the Baker Hospital, Muscatine, Iowa, also free of charge for medical services. The committee was then to publicly make known their findings after all treatments of the test patients had been completed.

In principle, it wasn't a bad suggestion, although (as the AMA suspected) Baker would have been unlikely to live up to his end of the bargain if he lost. It was the type of offer that Hoxsey also was to make much use of in years to come. Baker claimed that the AMA "refused to investigate, immediately condemned without investigation and continues to print discriminatory articles claiming there is no medicine that cures cancer" (343).

Two years later Baker hired Hoxsey as well as Dr. Miller to work at his Muscatine clinic. Although the association lasted only five months, it was to dog Hoxsey for the rest of his life (289). Hoxsey and Baker fell asunder when Hoxsey accused the latter man of greediness. In fact, the words Hoxsey used to describe Baker sound very much like the words Fishbein used to describe Hoxsey himself: he was a "super-salesman and past master in the art of promotion and showmanship" (194).

Another of Baker's celebrated suggestions was for a debate between a representative of the AMA and himself over either the National or Columbia radio networks. The question to be debated was "Who are the cancer quacks?" Needless to say, the AMA did not deign to answer either challenge, and rebuffed all similar challenges over the years. One doctor called Hoxsey's offers "pure showmanship and unworthy of serious consideration" (289).

Baker refused to spend money to expand the clinic or to treat those unable to pay his high fees. Eventually, Baker lost his broadcasting license but bought another station just across the Mexican border so he could reach American listeners. In 1940, he established a cancer clinic in Little Rock, Arkansas, but was convicted of unethical practices and shut down. In 1944, he was released from prison and retired to live on a yacht, and died in obscurity in Arkansas in the late 1950s.

Nat Morris, the most sympathetic of commentators on nonconventional cancer treatments, says about Baker, "He was possibly one of the most unsavory figures in the history of cancer quackery" (289). Hoxsey agreed, however his remarks on this association are revealing:

"If the Devil himself had offered me the facilities and doctors to treat cancer legitimately, and thus save the lives of thousands of victims, I would have accepted."

Hoxsey next set up a short-lived clinic in Muscatine, with Dr. Rasmussen and his own cousin, T.T. Hoxsey, ND. After that he accepted an offer from an automotive magnate and set up a free clinic in Detroit. "There's only one thing that organized medicine fears more than unorthodoxy," he wrote, "and that's free medical treatment."

Two days after this free clinic opened, Hoxsey was summoned to the office of the Prosecuting Attorney. He claims that an Assistant Prosecutor tried to shake him down for $200 a week "protection" money. Refusing to give this bribe, ten days later he was arrested. Investigators for the State Medical Board invaded the clinic posing as cancer patients and asking to be treated by "Dr. Hoxsey." Hoxsey was convicted, but the case was over-turned on appeal in December, 1932.

In the interim, the State Medical Board revoked the license of the doctor who "fronted" for Hoxsey's clinic and the free clinic closed. The same story, essentially, was repeated in Wheeling, West Virginia, where the County Medical Society had shut him down before he could see a single patient. He then moved to South Ventnor Avenue in Atlantic City. An encounter with Dr. George Dorrance, a well-known cancer expert in Philadelphia, ended in disaster, when Hoxsey refused to turn over his formulas in writing in advance of confirmatory tests. "Let me treat...25 patients," he pleaded with Dorrance. "If they get well, and you officially state that my treatment cured them, I'll release my formulas to the entire medical profession."

Hoxsey and Little

Hoxsey later had a similar encounter with Dr. Clarence Cook Little, the most famous cancer researcher of his day, and director of the Jackson Memorial Laboratory in Bar Harbor, Maine. He claims that preliminary tests at Bar Harbor showed that the Hoxsey internal and external formulas were effective. But Little called an end to the experiment, in Hoxsey's recollection, with the words, "I was not aware of your long-standing feud with the AMA....We can't afford to get involved in such a controversy. Under the circumstances, I have no choice but to terminate this experiment at once."

In almost any other sphere of human endeavor this would have been a reasonable offer. However, there is a tradition of openness in scientific medicine, which abhors secret remedies. Unfortunately, it was a distinction that Hoxsey never appreciated. And so the contact with Dr. Dorrance was broken, although Hoxsey continued to work out of an osteopathic clinic in Germantown, a Philadelphia suburb. This was during the depths of the Depression and Hoxsey says that 90 percent of the patients were charity cases. There, and later in Dallas, Hoxsey became well known for treating African-Americans. "Suffering doesn't recognize race, color or creed," he often repeated.

"Wherever he went, the AMA dogged his footsteps," wrote Prof. Young, approvingly. Finally, in March, 1936, Hoxsey headed south to

Dallas, where he took over the Spann Sanitarium. "I was heartily sick of being chased from city to city," he later wrote. "I also wanted to settle down, raise a family, become a respected citizen in the community." And for a while in Dallas he found, if not respectability, then at least relative stability and success.

As before, he left the actual treatment of patients to a succession of physicians. At one time he was convicted of practicing medicine without a license, but a higher court set aside the verdict. During this time he acquired an honorary Doctor of Naturopathy degree and was licensed in Texas as a naturopath. Hoxsey fought a string of battles with Dr. T.J. Crowe, secretary of the Texas State Board of Medical Examiners (the same body that later clashed with another nonconventional practitioner, Stanislaw R. Burzynski, MD, PhD). In 1937, Hoxsey and his wife were arrested and taken to the Dallas County Jail. There were simultaneously a flurry of warrants for his arrests from various other counties in Texas, counties in which he had apparently never set foot.

"Every time a warrant was issued it rated big headlines on the front page of local newspapers," said Hoxsey. "Dismissal of the charges invariably was buried in a few lines of fine print at the bottom of a back page of the same papers—if it appeared at all." It is a tactic not unknown to public authorities to this day.

In the summer of 1941, Hoxsey was found guilty of five counts of practicing medicine without a license, fined $2,500 and sentenced to five months in jail, which was the stiffest penalty ever handed out in any medical practice suit. This case too was thrown out in 1942, which marked a turning point for Hoxsey. When Dr. Crowe was asked why it was that Hoxsey was able to always get his convictions overturned on appeal, he said, "This fellow Hoxsey has been sued so many times and in so many States that he knows all the answers!" (194)

In all, Hoxsey was arrested over 100 times. He took to carrying $10,000 in cash in his pocket just to bail himself out. (He claimed he made the bulk of his money in oil wells, not in cancer.) Al Templeton, the assistant district attorney who issued the bulk of those arrest orders, later sent his own brother to Hoxsey for treatment. When Hoxsey seemingly "cured" him, Templeton quit his job and became Hoxsey's lawyer. He later became a County Judge. It was a celebrated conversion.

The Dallas clinic thrived and eventually moved to larger quarters. It began to take on some of the trappings of a "regular" medical center. "Documentary records of previous diagnosis or treatment, like the results of a biopsy, were solicited," even Prof. Young admits. Laboratory tests and X rays were performed by physicians in the employ of the clinic. Vitamins and other supportive treatments were also given. The cost for all of this was

$300, later $400. Hoxsey claimed that many indigent patients were treated for free.

(Present-day costs at the clinic in Tijuana are $3,500, which includes a lifetime supply of tonic, visits, medications, doctor fees; 30 percent paid on the first visit with monthly payments for the remainder. Laboratory costs, X rays, and physicals are in the range of $450 to $8,500. It is thus still at the lower end of the economic scale.)

Thousands of patients from around the country flocked to the Dallas clinic. In 1945, Hoxsey and three Congressmen visited the government's National Cancer Institute (NCI) in Bethesda, Maryland and met with its director, R.R. Spencer. He explained that for the NCI to investigate Hoxsey's methods they would need a record of at least 50 cases treated by his method, all of whom had biopsy-confirmed internal cancers that had failed to respond to conventional treatments. The patients would then have to be shown to have survived from three to five years.

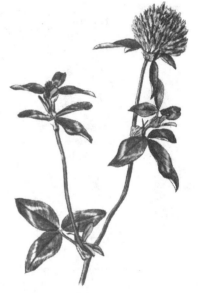

Hoxsey went back to Dallas and sent the NCI data on 60 cases. At that point NCI told him that his information did not come close to meeting its stringent criteria, being too fragmentary and incomplete to warrant any further investigation. Hoxsey apparently lacked "the type of sophisticated data from which expert scientists could draw valid conclusions." This may have been true. But Hoxsey came to believe that NCI too was under the thumb of his historic enemy, the AMA.

Trifolium pratense
(red clover)

"I was bitterly disappointed, disillusioned, and shocked," he later wrote. Hoxsey's offer to have his method scientifically evaluated is seen by Young as further proof of his deviousness. "Hoxsey's posture on having his methods tested had been used before by the cancer irregulars and would be tried again." It "impressed the layman...." but obviously not canny professionals, who could see through all the tricks of the quintessential quack (420).

(This is not my read on it at all. I believe that Hoxsey truly believed in the merits of his treatment and wanted nothing more than validation by the medical profession.)

Hoxsey managed to garner some support in Congress. Senator Elmer Thomas of Oklahoma visited the clinic and was favorably impressed. He held "a sort of formal hearing," in which he questioned some patients who had used the treatment. Hoxsey offered to put his treatment to any kind of test the Senator might arrange. Hoxsey also wrote to the Texas State Board of Medical Examiners as follows:

"If you will come out here to the clinic and we cannot prove to you that we have cured cancer after radium, X ray, and surgery had failed, we will give you $10,000 or better still, we will take 25 cases of cancer and let the entire Dallas County Medical Society or any doctor in America take 25 cases, and if we do not cure two to their one in sixteen weeks, we will donate $10,000 to any charitable organization in Dallas County" (420).

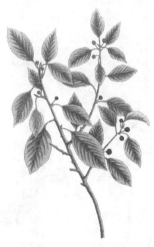

Two years later, Hoxsey also expressed his eagerness to have tests done to two scientists who visited at the behest of the American Cancer Society. In the following year he again submitted cases to NCI but again it failed to meet their basic requirements.

"Clinical tests were naturally refused," Young comments. Naturally.

Sen. William Langer of North Dakota now became interested in Hoxsey's treatment and his plight.

After visiting Dallas, Langer introduced a resolution in the Senate for a subcommittee to make "a full and complete study and investigation" to determine if Hoxsey's methods "in the treatment of cancer have proved a cure for such disease" (*JAMA* 8/7/48). Meanwhile, Hoxsey was still battling the medical establishment in the courts. A new effort to convict him of practicing medicine without a license ended in a hung jury.

Rhamnus frangula
(buckthorn)

He was also found innocent in a damage suit brought by the survivor of a woman who died after treatment at his clinic. A federal district judge refused the government's attempt to stop Hoxsey from distributing his medicines in interstate commerce.

But, most importantly, Hoxsey won two judgments in libel suits against his long-time enemy, Morris Fishbein, MD. In 1947, Fishbein had written an "excoriating editorial" in *JAMA* titled "Hoxsey—Cancer Charlatan." He also co-authored an article in the Hearst newspaper chain's weekly newsmagazine, titled "Blood Money." This was carried, among other places, in the San Antonio *Light*. Fishbein repeated his charge that Hoxsey was a charlatan, and that his father had been "a dabbler in faith cures," who himself died of cancer.

The Story of Licorice

At first sight, few herbs would appear to be less controversial than licorice (Glycyrrhiza glabra). The name "Glycyrrhiza" means "sweet root," and was given to the plant by Dioscorides. Hundreds of tons are imported every year for food and medicinal purposes, mostly from Spain and Italy. The ancient Greeks were already afficionados of various licorices, prizing especially those from the region of the Sea of Azov. Its primary medical uses are as a remedy for coughs and chest complaints, such as bronchitis. It is an ingredient in many cough remedies and lozenges, one of the few "herbal remedies" known to almost everyone.

But licorice is not without its controversies. According to the AHPA, it is not for prolonged use or in high doses except under the supervision of a qualified health practitioner. It is contraindicated for diabetics and in hypertension, liver disorders, severe kidney insufficiency and hypokalemia. It can potentiate potassium depletion of diuretics and stimulant laxatives, as well as the action of cardiac glycosides and cortisol. In some individuals, therefore, it can cause hypertension, edema, headache, and vertigo when it is eaten in therapeutic doses over a prolonged period, although it is not known if enough of this herb is contained in the Hoxsey formula to cause any of these problems.

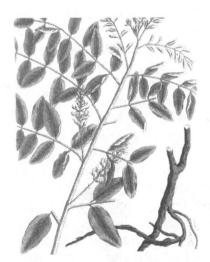

Glycyrrhiza glabra
(licorice)

The Ad Hominem Attack

It became standard operating procedure to attack the character of the opponent. Hoxsey and Fishbein's acerbic statements about each other are quoted at the beginning of this chapter. Making assumptions about Hoxsey's mental state became a regular feature and spur to action. William Grigg, FDA's spokesperson, claimed that while Hoxsey had great skill as a salesman he had "no belief that his treatment was useful." How did Mr. Grigg know? Because Hoxsey was a quack and a quack—by definition—is the purveyor of worthless treatments. This is a circularity, a fallacy exposed by Aristotle and others. But what if Hoxsey believed in a worthless treatment? Or didn't believe in a worthwhile one. In the end, to paraphrase chemotherapist David Karnofsky, MD, what mattered was not the belief system of the proponent, but whether or not his methods really worked. And that question could only be settled by scientific testing.

Astonishingly, Hoxsey won the case, although the judge, William Atwell, also ruled that Fishbein had acted from "a mistaken sense of public duty." Judge Atwell had listened to the stories of various patients, the kind of stories that had failed to impress NCI officials. He was persuaded that healing had taken place and that the circumstances brought to mind the healings performed by Jesus.

Not deterred, in 1950, FDA seized tonics being sent from Hoxsey's clinic in Dallas to a practitioner in Denver. Hoxsey fought the injunction before the same judge. "Food and Drug officials had worked prodigiously to develop a persuasive case," wrote Young. Their goal was to finally demonstrate the ineffectiveness of Hoxsey's tonics in treating internal cancer, and thereby block their distribution.

FDA's star witness was Dr. David I. Macht, professor of pharmacological and experimental therapeutics at Johns Hopkins University in Baltimore, Maryland.

"Doctor," the District Attorney asked him, "is there any recognized therapeutic use of any of these items [in the tonics]...that you are aware of?"

"Absolutely no basis for it," proclaimed the professor, "and I am speaking not only as a pharmacologist, but as a member of the American College of Physicians." Others at the trial testified that potassium iodide could actually speed the growth of tumors, and that the Hoxsey formula had no beneficial effects in animal studies.

The government also selected 16 human cases and attempted to show that either they had never had cancer, had been cured of cancer by conventional means, or had had cancer and were still afflicted with it.

Twenty-two patients took the stand in Hoxsey's defense. In fact, some of the witnesses called by the government wound up testifying for Hoxsey. (They "continued, despite the evidence," wrote Young, "to express their loyalty to him.") Despite the government's extraordinary efforts to "get" him, Hoxsey won the case, and the judge refused to grant their injunction. The government side, stung by this unexpected defeat, spread the rumor that Judge Atwell had—horror of horrors—once been a Hoxsey patient himself.

The FDA appealed the case and asked the Appeals Court to uphold the injunction. This Court acceded to their requests. A layman's opinion was "entitled to little, if any, weight." Only surgery, X ray, and other radioactive substances could possibly cure cancer, the judges declared. Such was the opinion of the "overwhelming weight of disinterested testimony." This was a matter of "general public knowledge and acceptance," they said, and Judge Atwell was remiss in not understanding this argument from authority.

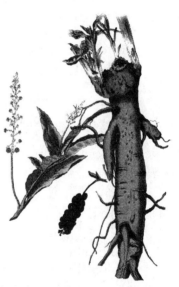

Hoxsey then appealed to the Supreme Court to reverse the circuit court's directive. But the Justices refused to hear his case, as they have refused to hear most cases touching on alternative medicine over the years. Judge Atwell yielded, but he issued an injunction that did not flatly bar Hoxsey from shipping his tonics interstate. They would have to be labeled, he said, to show that there was a conflict of medical opinion concerning their curative powers.

Phytolacca americana
(poke root)

But even this would not wash. According to Young, since the circuit court had found as fact that Hoxsey's internal remedies could not cure cancer, "no legal room existed for the assertion of differences of medical opinion." Eventually, in October, 1953, the judge was required to issue an injunction without the "conflict of medical opinion" stipulation.

Hoxsey again went to court to stop the injunction, claiming that his constitutional rights had been violated. Although the government termed the appeal "frivolous," he did raise some profound questions about the boundaries of freedom of choice in America. Hoxsey's efforts failed and in October, 1954 the injunction finally went into effect.

The publicity did not hurt business. By 1956, the Dallas facility was the largest private cancer clinic in the country. According to a story in *Life* magazine, Hoxsey treated some 8,000 patients and grossed $1.5 million.

Hoxsey remained his old militant self. "There's only one way they'll ever close the Hoxsey Clinic," he told an appreciative audience, "and that's to put a militia around it."

Hoxsey had some powerful political allies, mostly on the far right. One of these was Gerald B. Winrod, a fundamentalist evangelist from Kansas. (Winrod served as the model for Sinclair Lewis's "Buzz" Windrip, the American Nazi leader in *It Can't Happen Here*.) Winrod had a nationally syndicated radio show ("The Defender") which vociferously supported Hoxsey's claims. During the war, Winrod was indicted for sedition (but never tried). His periodical, also called the *Defender,* was infamous for its strident attacks on Blacks and Jews. The FDA later showed that Hoxsey contributed $80,000 in "donations" to Winrod (25). However, it is important to note that there is no evidence that Hoxsey himself was ever prejudiced against anyone.

Hoxsey also gained support from other non-conventional practitioners, such as the American Association for Medico-Physical Research and the American Naturopathic Association. He was involved in the formation of the National Health Federation, which continues to support alternative treatments for cancer.

Hoxsey Goes National

At his peak in the 1950s, Hoxsey had 17 clinics nationwide, the largest chain of cancer treatment centers in existence. He also won the support of, among others, Pennsylvania legislator John Haluska. Hoxsey and Haluska established a clinic in Portage, PA and such was his fame that when Hoxsey visited the floor of the Pennsylvania Senate he was greeted with resounding applause from the legislators.

In 1955, the FDA sent agents to Portage, deceptively posing as patients. They then used a fallacious "diagnosis" of cancer as a pretext to seize half a million pills from the clinic. But when they emerged, the agents found themselves surrounded by "a hostile throng of townspeople" (420). After a prolonged trial, the Portage clinic was unable to get the pills back and was eventually shut down.

But the FDA would not wait for a repeat of Dallas. While the Pennsylvania case was in progress, they exercised their right under Sec. 705 of the 1938 Federal Food, Drug and Cosmetic Act relating to the gross deception of the consumer. Employing this never-before utilized provision, in April 1956 they issued a press release declaring Hoxsey a public menace. Then in January, 1957 they printed up inflammatory "Public Beware!" posters, in red and black, and displayed them in 46,000 post offices and substations, as well as in innumerable other public institutions throughout the country. These included churches, lodges, and, ironically, Chambers of Commerce. (Twenty years later, FDA did much the same to destroy the credibility of laetrile.)

Ausubel has told me that in preparing his documentary on Hoxsey, he interviewed "the fellow whose idea it was—a nasty little man with a tight mustache and bow tie. With trembling hands, he told me Hoxsey was a 'murderer.'"

FDA officials were gratified by the result. This action, they concluded, cut down on at least 3,000 Hoxsey customers. By October, 1957, the government could claim that it had "now been successful in all pending Federal court actions involving the 'cancer remedies' known as the Hoxsey treatment."

The FDA had limitless financial and publicity resources. When Hoxsey employed physicians to give his treatment, Texas courts revoked their licenses and forbade him from operating a clinic. When he turned the clinic over to someone else, FDA secured a court order requiring the Hoxsey clinic to write individually to all patients and inform them that the treatment was no longer available. The final blow came on October 29, 1958 when the FDA simultaneously padlocked his clinics in a single day. "In no way did Harry have the money to fight that state by state," said his longtime nurse, Mildred Nelson (25).

By the early 1960s, when James Harvey Young's book was written, the Hoxsey treatment appeared dead. In fact, Young's book was its literary tombstone. This was a victory over one "quack" treatment, said Young. However, "among the fearful and the desperate, these false prophets continued to find victims for their worthless wares."

Yet in 1963, Mildred Nelson reopened a Hoxsey clinic in Tijuana, Mexico where there was a freer regulatory atmosphere and a generally more receptive atmosphere for herbal treatments. Ms. Nelson in fact started the migration of irregular practitioners to the Mexican border towns. Hoxsey decided to stay behind and tend his oil business. He gave Ms. Nelson the formulas, but requested that she not use the Hoxsey name, which in his view was a red flag for the medical authorities. However, even though she called her institution the "Bio-Medical Clinic," the patients to this day still call it the "Hoxsey Clinic."

Hoxsey died in 1974, allegedly of prostate cancer which his treatment failed to cure (202). However, his treatment lives on. Mildred Nelson's clinic continues to draw many patients and, as in days of old, many followers who believe that it has been an effective treatment for their malignancy. Like Hoxsey she has at times claimed an 80 percent "cure" rate, although there are some indications she has modulated those claims in recent years.

At the Bio-Medical Center, the internal and external remedies are combined with a rather stringent diet that forbids patients pork, vinegar, alcohol and most salt. It also emphasizes psychological factors since, as Nelson said, "the greatest success comes with the patient's attitude" (25).

The Hoxsey treatment has appealed to some intellectuals as well. At one time, famed "attorney for the damned" Clarence Darrow was numbered among its defenders. Among those who have written favorably about it in recent years are filmmaker Ausubel, researcher Catherine Salveson, RN, investigative journalist Peter Barry Chowka, historian Patricia Spain Ward, and naturopathic physicians Francis Brinker, ND, and Steven Austin, ND.

I have deliberately omitted the anecdotal material which has been the mainstay of Hoxsey's promotional literature. I should note, however, that I myself have been told by a number of individuals that they or a loved one were cured by this treatment. One of these was an acquaintance who happens to be among the wealthiest people in America. He told me in great detail about his own child's recovery from cancer on the Hoxsey treatment, after conventional medicine had given up all hope. And there are others. While much work must go into turning an anecdote into a genuine case history, I find it difficult to dismiss all such stories as error, self-deception, or wishful thinking.

The Hoxsey Formulas

In Young's view, Hoxsey only used escharotic pastes for external cancers in his Illinois days but had added internal cancers to his repertoire by the time he reached Dallas. "Exactly when he began using his 'tonics' for hidden cancers within the body is not clear," says Young. "Perhaps he acquired his formulas from Norman Baker during the tempestuous joint operation in Muscatine. To a public increasingly fearful of cancer and increasingly hopeful of chemotherapy," said Young, "such an appeal offered a gleam of hope" (292). Filmmaker Kenny Ausubel strongly disputes this claim, and believes that Hoxsey's story of a family remedy is fundamentally true.

Hoxsey the empiricist admitted that he did not know why the internal medicine worked; simply that it did. According to his detractors, his tentative explanations were "a complicated fantasy of irrelevant scientific and pseudo-scientific jargon that sounded very impressive to the layman but caused genuine cancer experts to grieve" (420).

A "Syrup Trifolium Compound" was produced by Parke-Davis & Co. starting in 1890. A similar Compound Fluidextract of Trifolium (CFT) was first described in 1898 in a standard Eclectic text, *King's American Dispensatory,* where it was recommended as an "alterative" (an old-fashioned medical term that means something that cleans the blood or changes the metabolism) and widely prescribed for scrofula and skin eruptions in secondary and tertiary syphilis. CFT was produced by William S. Merrell Chemical Co. (now part of Marion Merrell Dow, Inc.). As the name implies, it contained red clover blossoms (*Trifolium pratense* being the scientific name of red clover).

Although exact dosages are not known, a comparison by James Duke revealed that Hoxsey's dosages were rather low compared to those of the CFT that was listed in the 1898 *Dispensatory* (113a). CFT continued to be listed in the *US National Formulary,* 5th edition (1926) and 6th edition (1936) as an official pharmaceutical remedy.

How did this confluence come about? It is impossible that Merrell copied the Hoxsey internal formula, since this was kept in a safe deposit box at the People's Bank of Girard. So either both the Hoxsey family and the pharmaceutical company were drawing on a common folk tradition or else Hoxsey (or his ancestors) lifted a popular botanical formula, converted it into a proprietary "secret cancer remedy," and then made up a cock-and-bull (or rather cock-and-horse) story as an attractive cover. A third possibility is that the story was essentially true, but that Hoxsey later improved the original formula by adding ingredients learned from studying Merrell's CFT. This is the explanation that I favor.

There is independent confirmation of the fact that there was indeed a traditional Hoxsey family formula, which John C. Hoxsey used. In the spring of 1927, after Hoxsey had had some success in the cancer business, all of Harry's many brothers and sisters (except one) sued him for $500,000 for their share in their father's estate which he, according to the complaint, had "illegally appropriated." Hoxsey senior had had no property except the formulas, and the other children ganged up to get their share. Judge Thomas Jett threw out the case. However, I think it proves that there was some sort of formula in the family. Since it was, by its very nature, a secret formula, it is impossible for us to compare it to CFT.

In 1949, in the course of the Fishbein law suit, Hoxsey agreed to the court's demand that he make public the formula. Here is what he claimed it consisted of:

Hoxsey formula #1 (1949):

Scientific name	Common name	Part Used	AHPA
Cascara amarga	Cascara	Bark	—
Zanthoxylum americanum	Prickly ash	Bark	2b
Rhamnus frangula	Buckthorn	Bark	2b,2d
Trifolium pratense	Red clover	Blossoms	2b
Medicago sativa	Alfalfa	Leaves	1

Note: This formula should only be used under a physician's direction. Please see the warning in the front of the book.

These herbs were in a base of potassium iodide and honey drip cane syrup for flavoring. He obviously did not tell the court everything, however, for in 1954 he added several more herbs to the content list:

Hoxsey formula #2 (1954):

Scientific name	Common name	Part Used	AHPA
Glycyrrhiza glabra	Licorice	Root	2b,2d
Arctium lappa	Burdock	Root	1
Stillingia sylvatica	Stillingia	Fresh root	2c
Berberis spp.	Barberry	Root	2b
Phytolacca americana	Poke	Fresh Root	3

It also contained Aromatic USP 14, an artificial flavor.

To further confuse matters, literature from the contemporary Hoxsey clinic in Tijuana lists the ingredients as:

Current Hoxsey Formula (394):

Scientific name	Common name	Part Used	AHPA
Glycyrrhiza glabra	Licorice	Root	2b,2d
Trifolium pratense	Red clover	Blossoms	2b
Cascara amarga	Cascara	Bark	—
Arctium lappa	Burdock	Root	1
Berberis spp.	Barberry	Root	2b
Phytolacca americana	Poke	Fresh Root	3
Stillingia sylvatica	Stillingia	Fresh root	2c

Note: These formulas should only be used under a physician's direction. Please see the warning in the front of the book.

There are yet other versions of the Hoxsey formula available in the world of herbalism. Every herbalist seems to have his or her own "take" on the actual composition of the mysterious internal formula.

But does the murky liquid of Hoxsey's internal formula really contain these herbs? The answer is yes. The presence of most of them was independently confirmed by an analysis by the Hipple Institute at the request of Dr. Richard Early of the American Cancer Society, not an individual favorable towards alternative methods.

Potassium Iodide

In the companion volume to this book we shall analyze in detail most of the above herbal ingredients for possible antitumor effects. Our conclusions are essentially the same as those reached by Patricia Spain Ward, PhD, historian of the University of Illinois at Chicago. Ward investigated this question as a contract researcher for the Office of Technology Assessment's

report on unconventional cancer treatments. Dr. Ward (who had previously reported in a derogatory fashion about an alternative cancer treatment,
Krebiozen) surprised the OTA staff when she concluded that there was both
historical and laboratory evidence to support a possible antitumor role for
Hoxsey's ingredients.

The only ingredient we shall not analyze at length is potassium iodide, a
mineral product which actually constitutes three-fifths of the formula.
Potassium iodide has many historical associations with cancer. However,
according to an outdated American Cancer Society diatribe against Hoxsey,
consuming it may result in toxic reactions such as "pimples, excessive secre-
tion of the eyes or nose, impotence, and a mumps-like condition of the
salivary glands" (10).

By contrast, many of the herbs in the formula (seven out of nine, by
Ward's calculation) have folk histories as cancer treatments. This is particularly so for red clover, barberry, burdock, and poke. There are scientific
rationales for the possible activities of some of these, including the presence
of genestein in clover, of the "B factor" and other compounds in burdock,
and of powerful (but toxic) mitogens in poke. These do look like the kinds
of plants that might be expected to exert an antitumor or anticancer effect.

External Formulas

In addition, Hoxsey had several external formulas for cancer. We shall
deal with this subject more fully in our chapter on escharotic salves (see
Chapter 6). However, we should record that Hoxsey's external medications
included the following:

External yellow powder #1: Talc, flowers of sulfur, arsenic trisulfide,
sweet elder, magnolia flower, bloodroot, and antimony trisulfide. This list
was submitted to the courts by Hoxsey. (Hoxsey's nurse Mildred Nelson
reports that sweet elder and magnolia flower are no longer part of the
formula.)

External yellow powder #2: Vaseline, lump rosin, refined camphor,
refined beeswax, tincture of myrrh, and oil of spike. (This is an additional
Hoxsey formula cited by Dr. Brinker.)

External yellow powder #3: Arsenic sulfide, yellow precipitate (USP
sulfur per Mildred Nelson), sulfur, talc. Said to be selective for cancerous
tissue.

External red paste: Antimony trisulfide, zinc chloride, bloodroot (not
selective for cancer, but reputedly works more rapidly). Used on melanomas
and cancers under the skin.

The question every reader would undoubtedly like answered is: "Does
the Hoxsey treatment really work?" The brief answer is, We don't know.

The escharotic salves almost certainly are capable of burning away tissue. As to the internal formula, I think the scanty evidence points in a positive direction.

Folk Usage

Seven of the main ingredients have folk usage as cancer treatments as well as some scientific support. The long historical use of red clover, burdock, barberry root and other herbs as historical cancer treatments certainly lends some credibility to the treatment. There is also a strong association between some of the phytochemicals in these herbs and cytotoxic or anti-tumor activity in the laboratory.

There have been one or two studies on a limited number of patients that have shown promising results (24). One of these was a prospective cohort with no controls. It was carried out by Steve Austin, ND, with survival as the endpoint.

During 1983-1984, he conducted a site visit to three alternative clinics in Tijuana—that of Gerson, of Contreras, and the Biomedical Center of Mildred Nelson, which utilizes the Hoxsey formulas. Patients were questioned about the location of their primary tumor, whether it was biopsy confirmed or not, whether it was diagnosed in the US or Mexico, and whether the cancer was known to have spread to lymph nodes or distant organs.

Patients who were diagnosed by a Mexican clinic or by any means other than biopsy were excluded. Patients were then queried by letter once a year and the relatives or friends (reached through previously obtained addresses) were queried if the patient stopped responding. Patients were followed for four to five years or until death.

The outcomes at the Gerson and Contreras clinic, in this study, were not good. But there was a suggestion of benefit at the Hoxsey clinic. Of the 39 cancer patients Dr. Austin met there, 23 (59 percent) were lost to follow-up. Most of these never returned their questionnaires and were excluded from any evaluation of the group. Many of them probably died, but they cannot be statistically included in any tabulation of effectiveness.

Ten of the remaining 16 patients died after an average of 15.4 months. Given the diversity of their diagnoses, it is impossible to say if this is better or worse than average.

The six remaining survivors claimed to remain disease-free, with an average follow-up of 58 months. I heard Dr. Austin state in 1998 that five of the six remain cancer-free. These six long-term survivors included two lung cancer patients (one with advanced disease), two melanoma patients (one with level 5 disease), one with recurrent bladder cancer, and one with labial (lip) cancer. Given these types of cancer, the extent of disease, and the likely outcome without treatment, this is impressive. Dr. Austin was impressed enough to use a form of the Hoxsey internal formula in his own medical practice.

Similar results were reported by Mary Ann Richardson, DrPH, of the Center for Alternative Medicine Research at the University of Texas, at a medical meeting in 1998. This is unpublished data, which is still undergoing review. Nevertheless, I think it provides a rough estimate of what is going on at the Hoxsey clinic.

Richardson's center studied patient outcomes dating from the first quarter of 1992. First of all, as one might suspect, few records contained patient histories or copies of results from their biopsies, X rays, scans, or other diagnostic tests. Patient followup was also poor: only 57 percent were either known dead or had been contacted in the last year, compared to 90 percent in US tumor registries.

During the quarter in question, 149 patients had been treated for cancer at the Hoxsey clinic in Tijuana. Of these, 52 were known via patient records or the Social Security Death Index (SSDI) to have died, which left 97 last known to be alive. Of these 97, 64 were lost to follow-up (usually because of an invalid phone number), while 33 had active phone numbers. Of these, 16 were dead while 17 were still alive (more than five years later) and were interviewed.

It is likely that many of those lost to follow-up had died. But there were 17 long-term survivors out of 149 people, yielding a long-term survival rate of 11.4 percent following this treatment.

Depending on the analysis, this 11.4 percent figure could be significant. Obviously, a much deeper analysis of those 17 survivors is both necessary and warranted. The Texas center is currently analyzing the nature of their diagnoses, the extent of their disease when they were seen at the Hoxsey clinic, and what other treatments they have taken. The result could be illuminating (327).

Other questions are:
● Is the treatment safe? There has been no reported toxicity from the formula itself, although questions have been raised about potassium iodide and of course a few of the constituent parts, like berberine, can be toxic if taken in great enough concentration.
● Do patients have an intrinsic right to utilize treatments like the Hoxsey formula, against the wishes or advice of their regular physicians?

• Do uncredentialed persons ever have the right to treat cancer patients? In Hoxsey's terms, does one need permission to throw a rope to a "drowning" person?

In the course of this struggle, the AMA raised a number of objections to the Hoxsey treatment. These are in fact applicable to most non-conventional cancer treatments.

First of all, at one time it was claimed that the treatment was intrinsically dangerous. The AMA used to instigate or publish obituaries on virtually every clinic patient who died after their treatment. There is no doubt that the escharotics used in the Hoxsey treatment could be dangerous, since they indiscriminately burn away tissue, cancerous or normal (see chapter 6). I am against any self-administration of these agents by cancer patients. However, whether they were particularly dangerous depends on one's assessment of the skill of physicians at the Hoxsey clinic. My suspicion is that at times the Hoxsey doctors were very experienced and therefore probably skilled in the use of these agents.

A second objection is that the treatment raised "false hope" in patients. This argument begs the question of whether or not the treatment had any effectiveness at all. We might compare the use of chemotherapy in many forms of advanced cancer. There is no data that such treatment actually leads to an increase in overall survival for many kinds of disseminated cancer. Yet chemotherapy is given—oftentimes to give the patient the feeling that something, at least, is being done. Is this "false hope," or a legitimate attempt to assuage a patient's distress at the end of life? If one is for using a toxic drug in this context, then one cannot logically be against the use of a relatively non-toxic herbal combination.

A third argument is that recourse to a "quack" treatment such as Hoxsey will cause patients to delay getting proper and proven treatment. I agree with this argument in principle, although the danger here is often exaggerated. I have known several people who opted for unproven treatments for small tumors that could have been surgically removed. They then had to deal with disseminated cancers which killed them. I think these were tragic cases. However, in the vast majority of cases, people use such treatments as adjuvants to conventional care, or after they have completed standard treatment, or in situations in which the efficacy of conventional treatment (e.g., chemo- or radiotherapy) is a matter of scientific dispute. In such cases, the proper treatment becomes a matter of debate and there is a wider scope for exercising personal choice.

To summarize, the argument between Hoxsey and the medical authorities brought out the worst in both sides. Neither could see any justice in their opponent's position. Yet there was plenty of blame to go around. I think much of Hoxsey's behavior was reprehensible, such as his secretiveness, public posturing, and exaggerated claims. On the other hand, Fishbein was equally guilty—of making *a priori* judgments about the treatment, of refusing to conduct serious trials, and of making gross personal attacks on an opponent.

Officials of the University of Texas School of Public Health in Houston have examined this entire controversy in a dispassionate way. Like Dr. Austin, they have identified some individuals who appear to be surviving far past the statistical norms for their disease. They have concluded that animal studies of both the internal and external formulas are needed. In addition, they have recommended a formal retrospective review of patients attending the Bio-Medical Center. They also want to help develop a prospective monitoring and follow-up system. Catherine Salveson, RN, PhD, who coproduced the Hoxsey film, has obtained a list of all registrants at the Clinic from 1990 to 1995. If this project gets funded, completed and published, then the Hoxsey treatment may finally get the evaluation it most emphatically deserves.

Chapter 6 🌲 Escharotics

N UNUSUAL FEATURE OF THE HARRY HOXSEY STORY IS THE
PRESENCE OF A CLASS OF COMPOUNDS KNOWN AS "ESCHAROTICS."
To readers familiar with medical history, escharotics are treatments
that went out with the use of leeches. In fact, not only are escharotics still
part of the Hoxsey treatment given in Mexico, but they continue to be one
of the more popular "underground" treatments. This includes various
pastes, salves, and poultices applied either to an external tumor or to the
normal skin that overlies a superficial tumor.

It is generally assumed that such pastes are merely burning agents—like
putting a strong acid on the skin. However, according to a lively folk tradition, these salves have a mysterious ability to "draw out" cancerous
tumors from their interior location, selectively destroy malignant tissue
(while sparing the normal skin), and then restore the body to health once
more, leaving a healthy patch of new skin.

A 'salve' is defined as an ointment made up of herbs and/or other substances as well as some fat or oil. A paste is a preparation of herbs and other
substances made with water, but no oil or fat. It is thick and malleable. A
plaster is also an oil or water-based medication, which is thick, soft and easy
to handle. Finally, a poultice resembles a plaster except that the herbs are in
a water or tincture base.

Any one of these can be an "escharotic" (es-ka-rótik). This is defined as
any caustic or corrosive substance that causes an eschar (es'kar). This eschar
is a thick, coagulated crust or slough which develops following any thermal

burn or the chemical or physical cauterization of the skin. In conventional medicine, an "eschar" is also the overlying dead skin on a full-thickness burn.

Today, escharotics have gone almost completely out of use in orthodox medicine. A cancer dictionary does not list any of these terms, nor is it mentioned in the indices of five of the leading cancer textbooks.

Yet the use of escharotics is very old and interest in them has never entirely died out in folk medicine. Part of this interest was undoubtedly due to their use in the Hoxsey treatment. More recently, medical anthropologist Ingrid Naiman, PhD, has been researching these unusual treatments and has written a book on them titled *Cancer Salves: A Botanical Approach to Treatment* (296). There are also Websites on the Internet both discussing, promoting and/or selling various escharotic products, including Dr. Naiman's own.

For centuries, the use of such escharotics was quite common in cancer treatment. Some ancient Egyptian source mentioned the use of an external application of garlic (*Allium sativum*) for indurations (256). But the widespread use of cancer salves (including escharotics) dates from the 18th century. Members of the Allium species figure prominently in these remedies, including roasted red onions. I am told that the use of chopped onions on external cancers continues as an American folk remedy to this day.

It may seem senseless, in this day and age, to turn to such primitive treatments for a disease as serious as cancer. But the reasons patients have turned to such salves are many. These include an "aversion to the knife, fear of surgery and mutilation, and a sincere desire for less drastic ways to treat cancer..." (296). While cancer surgery has improved vastly in the last 150 years, such motivations are certainly still understandable in many cases.

There are some famous historical escharotics. Mr. Richard Guy, an 18th century English cancer surgeon, purchased the secret remedy for an external poultice from the Plunkett family and began treating cancer patients with it in the 1750s. In 1762, he published a paper on his alleged successes with this treatment, including 100 cases, especially of breast cancer (159). "His powers of observations were remarkable," says Naiman. "It is difficult to read such a work and continue to believe that all medical practices of previous eras were based on mere superstition" (296).

But a major controversy erupted over Guy's extraordinary claims. A major sticking point was Guy's refusal to reveal the composition of the Plunkett formula which he had purchased for a considerable amount of money. He was particularly faulted by his chief rival, Mr. Thomas Gataker, surgeon to the British royalty, for purchasing a treatment from laypeople. Guy refused to give up for nothing what he had paid good money for, and to this day we know nothing about the nature of Guy's plaster. Obviously, it is impossible for us to evaluate whether there was any basis to his treatment.

The question of secrecy crops up again and again in the history of herbal medicine, and in particular, of salves. "Here is one of the marks of the charlatan in medicine," wrote Morris Fishbein, MD, the *JAMA* editor, in a diatribe against Eclecticism. "The true medical scientist has no secrets that he guards from other physicians; his knowledge is broadcast through the medical periodicals so that physicians everywhere may use it in alleviating the ills of mankind" (132). In an ideal world, all useful knowledge would be freely available. In reality, people seek to profit from what they know, especially if they have invested money or time in its acquisition.

Pharmaceutical companies and research institutes are extremely secretive until they secure patents on their work. Then they may speak freely about it. But herbal remedies cannot be as securely patented as isolated pharmaceuticals. Hence there is an understandable tendency to keep its nature secret, or to complicate it artificially in order to make duplication more difficult. As a general rule, I do not bother investigating treatments whose ingredients are secret. A possible exception are those formulas whose patents are pending.

Elsewhere, we have alluded to the use of arsenic in cancer. This also figures in the history of cancer salves and involves one of the most famous figures in American medicine, Benjamin Rush, MD. On February 3, 1786, Rush, signer of the Declaration of Independence and first Surgeon General of the US Army, read a paper to the American Philosophical Society in Philadelphia. It was called "An account of the external use of arsenic in the cure of cancers." In this paper, Rush explained to the assembled savants that a Dr. Martin of Philadelphia had advertised a cure for skin cancer which he claimed to have learned from North American Indians. After Martin's death, Rush managed to get some of his powder and found that its active ingredient was arsenic. Rush dissolved the powder in water and then painted it on tumors with a feather.

As Patrick Logan has remarked, "In the days before anesthesia was available, the use of arsenic in treating skin growths was a significant advance and until surgery became safer, at the end of the 19th century, cancer plasters were as satisfactory as anything else available" (264).

Most external salves have as their main component arsenic and one of two North American herbs: bloodroot or goldenseal.

Bloodroot and Cancer

Bloodroot (*Sanguinaria canadensis*) was unknown to Europeans before the colonization of North America, but soon came to the settlers' attention.

Capt. John Smith reported the colorful tale that attractive Indian women were offered for his pleasure; what made them particularly attractive was that their bodies had been decorated with this dye.

It is also said that the Indian women used this herb internally to bring on the menses or even trigger abortions. In the eighteenth and early nineteenth centuries bloodroot also became a popular treatment for cancer in the United States and then in Europe as well.

Its fame as an escharotic was due mainly due to the activities of J. Weldon Fell, a New York doctor who emigrated to England and set up a very successful practice there. Fell reported the use of a paste made of the red sap of the bloodroot, zinc chloride, flour, and water. Fell had been on the faculty of New York University and was one of the founders of the New York Academy of Medicine. In the 1850s, he moved to London to work at Middlesex Hospital. It was there that he first carried out these cancer experiments.

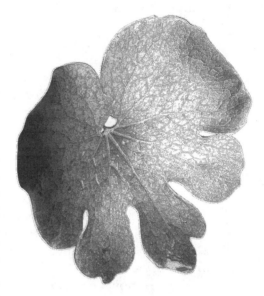

Sanguinaria canadensis
(bloodroot leaf)

As with Richard Guy, many of his patients had advanced breast cancer. But, unlike Guy, Fell never kept his formula secret.

According to an account he later published of the many patients he treated with bloodroot paste, all showed evidence of remission of their original growths. There was even a primitive attempt to set up a control group in the study. Eight out of ten patients treated by surgery had to return for treatment within two years, whereas only three out of Fell's ten bloodroot patients had a recurrence during this same time.

Fell received a generally favorable reception from his peers. Many felt that the new method was relatively safe and could be used in inoperable cancer (the majority in that pre-Listerian era). They observed that, after the treatment, tumors hardened and could be removed in one piece in a process called "enucleation." Following this, there was healthy granulation of new tissues (296).

As late as 1916, Fell's approach was still being given some positive evaluations, and it continues in a very modified form to be used today (Mohs' chemosurgery) (374). However, there were obviously naysayers as well, including very skeptical accounts in the 1880s. The general consensus turned out to be that "if it produces any effect in such cases, it must be very small indeed, and that it is, therefore, practically useless for such a purpose" (36).

Like most of these treatments, Fell's approach was ultimately traceable to Native American practices. He said he was taught it by traders, who in turn learned it from North American Indians living along the shores of Lake Superior.

"On hearing of this plant [i.e., bloodroot], Fell developed a treatment far superior to any other," wrote the authors of a standard textbook on medical botany. In applying this treatment, the paste was smeared onto a cloth or cotton and then placed on the tumor daily. If there was healthy tissue over the tumor it was first eroded with nitric acid. When the tumor became encrusted, incisions were made into it about one-half inch apart. The paste was then inserted into the cuts. Generally, Dr. Fell said, the disease was destroyed within two to four weeks. The mass fell out in an additional 10 to 14 days, "leaving a flat, healthy sore that usually healed rapidly" (256).

Although this treatment may seem to belong to the magical trend in cancer therapy, there may be a scientific rationale. There are several alkaloids present in bloodroot, sanguinarine and chelerythrine in particular, that have a necrotizing (destructive) effect on carcinomas and sarcomas in mice. Sanguinarine is present in from 6,000 to 60,000 parts per million.

A lesser-known contemporary was John Pattison, MD. Like Fell, Pattison was a New York physician who emigrated to England. But unlike Fell, he was not as successful a transplant. His relative failure may have been due to the fact that he was more Eclectic and holistic than his more celebrated contemporary. In 1866, Pattison also reported on his treatment of over 4,000 patients with cancer using escharotics.

He claimed to be the first person to employ another herb, goldenseal, in the treatment of cancer. He said this possessed "to a certain extent, a specific effect on the disease itself, but has the important advantage of preventing, in great measure, the pain that would otherwise arise, while the destructive power of the zinc is increased." Pattison also called his process enucleation, and considered this a kind of bloodless 'operation' for the removal of diseased tissue. To get at internal cancers, Pattison also first applied a dilute solution of nitric acid. He claimed this was no more painful than a blister or a mustard plaster. Ingrid Naiman, PhD, is currently attempting to resurrect Pattison's approach to cancer, which she finds most promising.

Dr. Eli Jones, the Eclectic, also used escharotics quite liberally in his practice. It is important to note, however, that the outspoken Jones called doctors who relied exclusively on escharotics, quacks. He was convinced that cancer, in essence, was a constitutional disease, a disease of blood, and had to be treated internally as well as externally.

"There is no plaster, caustic or salve that can be applied to a cancer," he wrote, "that will cure it without internal treatment for the blood" (296). In this he anticipated not just laymen like Harry Hoxsey, but also most medical oncologists who increasingly emphasize the need to eliminate micrometastases after surgery, with chemotherapy or immunotherapy.

In the period before World War One, escharotics were not entirely ignored by the regular medical profession, either. William Stuart Halsted, MD, developer of the "Halsted radical" operation for breast cancer, once wrote:

"I have several times had occasion to operate upon cancer which had been vigorously and repeatedly treated with caustics [escharotics] and to note the comparatively admirable conditions, the freedom from cancer permeation of the surrounding tissues and of the axilla; whereas, after incomplete operation with the knife, the local manifestations of recurrence were almost invariably deplorable, and the prognosis, of course, invariably hopeless" (*Annals of Surgery* 7/07).

Johanna Brandt, popularizer of *The Grape Cure* (see Chapter 8), was another non-credentialed healer who extolled the use of escharotics. These apparently were quite popular in South Africa in her day.

Perry Nichols, MD, operated a popular cancer sanitarium in the 1920s and 1930s. Like Norman Baker and Harry Hoxsey, he was part of that breed that refused to divulge the nature of his formula. Each year, however, he published a handsome annual of testimonials from satisfied customers.

"One has the sense," wrote Naiman, "that discharged patients felt themselves to be members of a club of persons fortunate enough to have heard of the Nichols Sanitarium and to have had treatment there..." (296). Nichols relied exclusively on escharotics and then transplanted skin grafts to cover the scars resulting from the treatment. He said it took four years to learn the proper use of escharotics. Those who jumped into this practice overnight were, in his opinion, quacks. Of course, to his foes in conventional medicine he was a quack. (There was a lot of quacking going on in those days.)

Mohs's Microsurgery

One of the strongest indications of the value of cancer salves was the concurrent development within conventional medicine of an escharotic-like treatment for skin cancer. This was, and is, the celebrated Mohs's chemosurgery, a treatment that involved the carefully controlled microscopic monitoring in the excision of skin cancer (281, 168).

Frederic E. Mohs (b. 1910) was a dermatologist affiliated with the University of Wisconsin. When he was still a medical student, he observed that an injection of 20 percent zinc chloride into tissues resulted in a fixation and preservation of the histologic structures (104). Mohs performed extensive research on this "fixative paste," which was an external preparation containing not just zinc chloride, but bloodroot and stibnite (an ore consisting mainly of antimony trisulfide).

By using different-sized granules of zinc chloride he could control its tissue penetration. He first used this mixture in animals bearing transplanted tumors. When he sectioned these tissues, he found that the killed tissues were well preserved or "fixed."

A problem with conventional surgery for skin cancer is that doctors may remove too little or too much of the tissue. If they fail to remove all the cancerous tissue, the cancer will grow back. If, conversely, they are too aggressive, they remove too much healthy tissue, delaying recovery and possibly mutilating the patient. Mohs applied his fixative paste and then removed very thin slices of the affected tissue. He would then examine the removed tissues under the microscope, until he reached a specimen that was no longer involved with cancer.

Mohs found he could remove malignancies with complete microscopic control if the borders between the cancer and the normal tissue were clearly demarcated. Chemosurgery thus bridged the gap between traditional escharotics and modern surgery. After removing all the visible tumor, another layer of paste was then applied to the open wound.

Dr. Stephen Snow, a disciple of Dr. Mohs, also described the paste as a kind of "regional hyperthermia," since it heats up the local tumor site. He felt it also might have an immunological effect, although this aspect of the treatment has never been adequately explored (296).

Mohs's microsurgery is considered the most definitive surgical procedure for all types of skin cancer. The problem is that it requires a skilled practitioner, more time and equipment, and more cost for the patient and/or insurance companies.

In recent years, Mohs's original "fixed-tissue technique" which involved the use of bloodroot and zinc chloride, has given way to the less labor intensive "fresh-tissue technique," in which tissues are not chemically treated *in situ* but are rather examined in a special manner as frozen sections. The vast majority of cases are now done through fresh-section technique. However, one standard cancer textbook states, "the fixed-tissue technique may be better" for very large basal cell and squamous cell carcinomas (BCCs and SCCs).

This text also points out that "the cure rate of recurrent lesions treated by chemosurgery is markedly superior to that of other modalities." In various series, it was found that while the cure rate for conventionally treated recurrent BCC was as low as 41 percent, with Mohs's microsurgery it ranged from 95 to 97 percent (168). Mohs was himself an outstanding clinician, who personally treated 8,000 primary basal cell carcinomas from around the world—most of them cases referred to him because of their extreme difficulty. Using the fixed-tissue technique, his personal cure rate was 99.8 percent, with a follow-up of over five years (282). Yet, according to an ACS-sponsored textbook, "the fixed-tissue technique (using zinc chloride) is rarely used today and is mainly of historic interest" (335).

The relation of Mohs's technique to the escharotics is puzzling, to say the least. To my knowledge, Mohs himself never discussed the unconventional history of escharotic use in his extensive bibliography. His explanation of how he arrived at bloodroot is bizarre.

He claimed that he experimented with a great many agents, but finally settled on bloodroot to prevent the zinc chloride from settling to the bottom of the container. If so, this is one of the most extraordinary coincidences in the history of medicine, since bloodroot and zinc chloride was precisely the combination that most of the nonconventional practitioners (like Hoxsey and Baker) were using for that very purpose at that very time. That out of thousands of agents, Mohs just stumbled upon bloodroot by complete happenstance strains credulity.

Equally odd is the fact that bloodroot has entirely disappeared from all standard discussions of this technique, and in fact from the technique itself. The DeVita cancer textbook states that "zinc chloride paste is used to fix the tumor *in situ*" [in place]. No mention of bloodroot.

Haskell's textbook, which describes and praises Mohs's technique in unstinting fashion, never reveals the nature of the compound used in the superior fixed-tissue technique. Nor does Holland's *Cancer Medicine*, which complains however that the procedure is "time consuming and probably has no place in the treatment of early, clear-cut [BCC or SCC] lesions" (189).

Present Day Practices

One of the big surprises for me has been learning about the extent to which escharotic pastes, salves, creams, etc. are still in use. There are numerous such formulas available on the market or simply handed down as family recipes, especially in the American South, Southwest, and Western states. If you surf the Internet, you find many solicitations to buy "black" or "yellow salves."

Some of these are expensive while others sell for under $10 a bottle. Often, as in the days of Dr. Guy, the ingredients are kept secret or partially revealed. One such "Black Ointment" formula claimed to contain the following:

A Typical Modern "Black Salve" Formula

Scientific Name	Common Name	Part Used	AHPA Class
Larrea tridentata	Chaparral	whole plant	2d
Lobelia inflata	Indian tobacco	whole plant	2b
Symphytum officinale	Comfrey	leaf	2a
Hydrastis canadensis	Goldenseal	root	2b
Plantago major	Plantain	root	1
Trifolium pratense	Red clover	whole plant	2b
Verbascum thapsus	Mullein	whole plant	1
Althaea officinalis	Marshmallow	root	1
Stellaria media	Chickweed	whole plant	1
Commiphora myrrha	Myrrh	gum	2b, 2d

Note: This formula should only be used under a physician's direction. Please see the warning in the front of the book.

These are contained in a base of olive oil, beeswax, pine tar, and vitamin E oil. Although none of these herbs is poisonous enough to rate an AHPA class 3 rating, some are rated as 2a, 2b or 2d. 2a indicates that the plant is for external use only (which would be the case here), 2b that it is not to be used during pregnancy, and 2d that there are other specific use indications, such as in the case of myrrh, a contraindication in the case of excessive uterine bleeding. All in all, if these are the true ingredients, this formula would seem reasonably safe for external use.

Whether such treatments do more than just destroy tissue, cancerous and normal both, remains to be seen. It would require a simple experiment to find out, but to my knowledge no one has performed it.

Ingrid Naiman says that in her opinion, "salves, elixirs and suppositories are not cures for cancer, but they are reasonable alternatives to the procedures and protocols offered by modern science. If used properly, and this is a most important point, they do not have harmful side effects" (296).

At the same time, she is well aware of the many abuses that exist. She has published on her Website the case of a young woman named Janis who seriously harmed herself with the use of a black salve she purchased over the Internet. She had apparently gotten rid of a previous melanoma tumor with this salve, but when the tumor seemed about to recur, she smeared the salve all over a three-inch square area on her cheek.

Consulting the salve company's Website she felt reassured. "The info said nothing would happen if there was no cancer and I wanted to make sure I got it all," Janis reported. "Nothing cautioned me as to the aggressiveness of the product."

Immediately, she had a horrendous reaction. "Aside from severe pain," she wrote, "my face swelled up, my eye swelled shut and my cheek area drained around the edges of the eschar (bloody) for several weeks. Then the huge tortoise shell-like scab fell off and then rescabbed for two months, I am left with extensive scarring on my face. Needless to say, I am devastated." In effect, Janis burned off part of her lovely face.

"I am being followed by a local burn center," she reported, "who are treating it as chemical burn. I wear a pressure bandage at home and a...bandage that I cover with flesh makeup when I go out. I have become a recluse...." The presence of the scar tissue now makes it impossible to do a standard biopsy to find out if the melanoma is actually gone.

And Janis is not alone. "I know at least three other people who have also experienced scars on their face from using this product," she wrote, "and they are also distraught and feel the instructions were not clear." She informed the Bahamas-based company of what happened, but they never changed the instructions at the Website or warned other patients of the potential for harm. "There are days that I wish I had my little bump back," she concluded, pathetically.

The manufacturer of this salve operates outside the boundaries of the United States, in a regulatory climate that is, to put it mildly, lax. Since Lawrence Burton, PhD, ran away to the Bahamas in the 1970s to start his Immunoaugmentative Therapy clinic there, Freeport has become a haven for savvy entrepreneurs who know how to negotiate the moral shoals of the offshore islands.

The manufacturer's attitude towards scientific evaluation is provided at their Website. "What studies have been done to prove that [their product] is a proven skin cancer treatment system?..." they ask. "How many have we done? Not a damn one," they defiantly proclaim. "And we proudly never intend to, just like the US FDA never intended to fulfill the court's order to investigate the effectiveness of Hoxsey's topical formula in the Fifties, after hundreds of proven cancer cures managed to stop the government's case against him dead in its tracks."

Thus, the government's failure to seriously, carefully, and fairly evaluate Hoxsey and the other non-conventional herbal treatments serves as a cover for medical adventurers to evade the evaluatory process entirely, and make their fortunes in the name of "freedom of choice." So what if a few unlucky individuals have their faces burned off in the process? That apparently is all part of the glorious tradition of freedom.

Who cannot see that this is a sorry situation? But where does the blame lie? With the entrepreneurs who will do anything to make a buck? Or with the bureaucrats in the "cancer establishment" who scoff at the scientific method? There is plenty of blame to go around.

Chapter 7 ❧ Essiac Tea

URING THE SAME PERIOD THAT HARRY HOXSEY WAS ROILING THE WATERS OF AMERICAN MEDICINE, A PARALLEL CONTROVERSY erupted in Canada. This was the struggle over Essiac tea, the brainchild of an Ontario nurse named Rene M. Caisse (1888-1978).

Today, Essiac is still the most popular herbal mixture used for treating cancer in North America. Caisse's original proprietary formula is trademarked and manufactured by the Resperin Corporation of Canada. There is also a competing formula called Flor·Essence, and innumerable variations and "knockoffs." Resperin's formula contains four simple herbs: burdock root, sheep sorrel, slippery elm, and Turkey rhubarb. Flor·Essence has these, plus four more: watercress, blessed thistle, red clover and kelp.

Essiac has exercised the imagination of Canadians for almost 75 years. It has been the subject of five books, innumerable articles, radio and television shows, audio and videotapes, and Websites. It is generally one of the first things cancer patients learn about herbal treatments, especially in Canada, where it is legally available under their Emergency Drug Release Program. In America, it is widely sold in health food stores.

The reader has possibly heard the extravagant claims made for this product. In my opinion, some of this is not just incorrect, but exploitative of cancer patients. Essiac is not a "cure" for cancer in the sense that most people conceive of that term. By all indications, the numbers of people who experience a total disappearance of their tumors after taking it are very small (if they exist at all). The woman who produced it was not a saint, but a very fallible human being. Unfortunately, none of the books on Essiac give an adequate introduction to the subject. Three have no references or bibliographies at all, even for key documents, and some statements in these books sound like puffery.

For example, on the cover of one of them there is a bold quote from a doctor who used Essiac: "The results we obtained with thousands of patients....definitely proves Essiac to be a cure for cancer" (385). Another ascribes to Essiac "an incredible recovery rate of 80 percent!" (306) A third describes Essiac as "nature's cure for cancer" (146).

Most such claims are unverified, and may, upon closer examination, turn out to be illusory.

On the other hand, there are many anecdotal accounts of pain relief, improvement in general well-being, and occasionally tumor shrinkages. In rare cases, I have heard of complete and lasting remissions, although usually there are many confounding factors that make valid interpretation extremely difficult.

The facts have to be pieced together from a variety of sources. Rene Caisse was a secretive woman who, unlike Hoxsey, never left an authoritative account of her ideas. The job of reconstructing her history fell to journalists, to her friend Mary McPherson, and then to Dr. Gary I. Glum, a Los Angeles chiropractor, whose previous experience had been mainly in treating professional athletes for muscle injuries. Glum did a creditable job in his out-of-print book, *The Calling of an Angel*. But the title and subtitle (*Nature's Cure for Cancer*) reveals that this book is more hagiography than biography.

One problem is that Caisse was always very tight-lipped about her formula. Both Resperin and Flora, makers of the two main competing formulas, present credible cases that they have the real thing. If there was one single authentic formula, she took it to the grave with her at the age of ninety. The story of Essiac tea is as slippery as any brew of slippery elm.

Rene Caisse (pronounced 'Reen Case') was born in Bracebridge, Canada in 1888 into a Catholic family of 12 children. Bracebridge is a solid little town of 9,300 surrounded by wooded hills and built near the banks of the Muskoka River. It is 175 kilometers north of Toronto. Rene's father was the local barber, her mother active in Catholic Church affairs. Rene became a surgical nurse and got a job at the Sisters of Providence Hospital in Haileybury, Ontario, a small

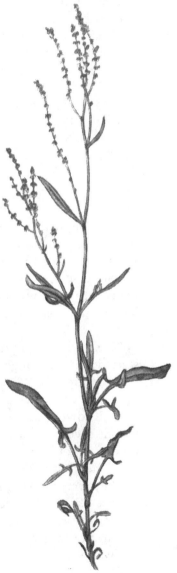

Rumex acetosella
(sheep sorrel)

town further north. Although she was trim and strikingly beautiful as a girl, in her twenties she let herself go "and became terribly overweight, well over 200 pounds, and she stayed that way for the rest of her life" (146).

In 1922, she had a life-shaping experience. While she was going about her duties in the hospital she noticed an elderly patient with a strangely scarred breast. She asked the woman how this had happened and was told that thirty years before, the woman had come from England to join her husband prospecting in northern Ontario. Shortly after her arrival, she detected a hardened mass in her breast. An Ojibwa Indian living in the area "diagnosed" her as having breast cancer and then, in the spirit of charity, offered to cure her with a "holy drink that would purify her body and place it back in balance with the great spirit" (385).

The woman and her husband rejected the Indian's advice as "superstition" and went instead to the nearest big city, Toronto, where she was also diagnosed as having a malignancy. A mastectomy (surgical removal of the breast) was advised. Frightened, and also unable to afford the expensive operation, the woman returned to northern Ontario and took up the Native American's offer. What he gave her was a pleasant-tasting herbal tea, which she was instructed to drink twice a day. He also gave her the formula and instructed her on its preparation.

Supposedly the breast tumors gradually diminished, she never had a recurrence, and was 80 years old at the time Rene Caisse met her (306). The woman had been effectively healed of her cancer. At least that is the story.

Needless to say, nurse Caisse was intrigued. The breast of the woman was scarred but no longer cancerous. Caisse asked for the formula and the woman complied. Caisse was later quoted as saying:

"I was very interested and wrote down the names of the herbs she had used. Knowing that at that time doctors threw up their hands when cancer was discovered in a patient, my thought was that if I should ever develop cancer, I would use it" (385).

Shortly thereafter, Caisse was visiting a retired doctor of her acquaintance. As they were walking in his garden, he took his cane and lifted up a weed. "Nurse Caisse," he said, "if people would use this weed there would be little or no cancer in the world" (146). It happened to be one of the weeds that had been given to her in the formula.

Two years later Rene's aunt Mireza, her mother's only sister, who lived in Brockville, was diagnosed as having cancer of the stomach with liver involvement. Since this form of cancer was incurable by conventional means, Rene asked her aunt's physician, Dr. R.O. Fisher of Toronto, if she could try the old Indian remedy. Although Dr. Fisher was understandably skeptical, he admitted that he had nothing better to offer and consented.

Rene Caisse gathered the herbs and brewed the tea according to the instructions.

After two months of daily oral doses, Mireza appeared cured. She lived for twenty-one more years after being given up by the medical profession. There was no recurrence of cancer (306). Caisse and Fisher had reason to be astonished.

Rene Caisse was living with her mother in Toronto at this time. "Dr. Fisher was so impressed that he asked me to use my treatment on some of his other hopeless cancer cases," she later said (146). When these patients were treated with the herbal tea, they too supposedly showed dramatic improvement. We have no details on these cases, but word spread. It should be emphasized that then and later on, Rene Caisse never charged for the treatment, although she occasionally took small gifts of gratitude.

Dr. Fisher reasoned that if oral administration was so good, then an injectable form would be even better. And so they injected it directly into the tongue of a man from Lyons, New York, who was suffering from oral cancer. The immediate reaction was unsettling. According to Caisse:

"I was scared to death. There was a violent reaction. The patient developed a severe chill; his tongue swelled so badly the doctor had to press it down with a spatula to let him breathe. This lasted about twenty minutes. Then the swelling went down, the chill subsided, and the patient was all right. The cancer stopped growing, and the patient went home, and lived quite comfortably for almost four years" (306, 385, 16).

To inject unpurified herbs into a patient was foolhardy, to put it mildly, and the patient understandably refused all further treatment. Herbs like this contain many proteins and impurities which can easily cause fatal allergic-type reactions if injected. Institutional Review Boards didn't exist back then. However, Caisse and Fisher were encouraged enough by their results that they attempted further research along these lines. And so, in 1925, she converted the basement of her mother's house on Parkside Avenue, Toronto, into an impromptu laboratory in which she and Fisher tested various versions of the formula in tumorous mice:

"It took Dr. Fisher and I [sic] about two years to find out just what ingredients could be given hypodermically without a reaction, and by elimination we found the ingredients that directly reduced the growth of the cancer. However, I found that the other ingredients, which could not be injected, were necessary to the treatment in order to carry off the destroyed tissue and infections thrown off by the malignancy. So by giving the injection to destroy the mass of malignant cells and giving the medicine orally to purify the blood, I was able to get the best results."

These experiments were not intended for any scientific journal. It was during this period, also, that Caisse named the tea "Essiac." Although the name has a vaguely Indian sound, it is actually her own family name, Caisse, spelled backwards. During this time she kept a day job as hospital nurse, working on her formula during the nights and weekends. (She was not to get married until the 1930s and never had children of her own.)

Other doctors began sending her their hopeless cases. It is said, for instance, that an 80-year-old man named J. Smith showed up with a "hideous, hemorrhaging malignant growth on his face." Within 24 hours of starting on the tea, the bleeding stopped. Eventually the growth began to reduce in size and the large holes in the man's chin started to heal (385).

I assume this is the same old man, mentioned by author Cynthia Olsen, who was expected to live about ten days but then actually lived six months. The reader should understand that such prognoses, although they go on all the time, are actually quite meaningless. Doctors, then and now, cannot accurately predict how long an individual cancer patient will live. Patients who are expected to live only days sometimes survive for lengthy periods without treatment—and vice versa. Cancer is an idiosyncratic and unpredictable disease.

Yet clearly there was an impression of benefit for many people. In 1926, eight doctors felt strongly enough that something important was happening to petition the Department of National Health and Welfare in Ottawa (the equivalent of the United States Food and Drug Administration) to allow Rene Caisse to do independent research on her discovery.

Their petition read as follows:

"We, the undersigned, believe that the treatment for cancer given by Nurse R.M. Caisse can do no harm and that it relieves pain, will reduce the enlargement of tumors, and will prolong life in hopeless cases.

"To the best of our knowledge, she has not been given a case to treat until everything in medical and surgical science has been tried without effect and even then she was able to show remarkable beneficial results on those cases at that late stage.

"We would be interested to see her given an opportunity to prove her work in a large way. To the best of our knowledge she has treated all cases free of any charge and has been carrying on this work over the period of the past two years (146).

The Department of Health and Welfare was not impressed. In fact, having detected a "quack," it quickly sent two investigating doctors empowered with the documents they needed to have Caisse arrested:

"When they arrived and found that I was working with nine of the most eminent doctors in Toronto and heard their opinions, they did not arrest me. In fact, one of them [Dr. W.C. Arnold] became so interested that he arranged to have me work on mice at the Christie Street Hospital Laboratories with Dr. Norich and Dr. Locheed. These mice were inoculated with Rous sarcoma. I kept the mice alive for 52 days, which was longer than anyone else had been able to do so" (385, 306).

Arnold later became a supporter of Caisse, and a steady correspondent, always trying to persuade her to release her formula.

A typical case from the 1920s is presented in a letter from Dr. J.A. McInnis, one of the petition signatories. It concerned a Mrs. DeCarle, who in 1928 was found to have a tumor in her upper abdomen. "The tumor was hard and nodular to the touch," wrote Dr. McInnis, "There was also another mass which could be distinctly palpated in the region of the uterus....From the history of her case, symptoms and physical examination, I had no hesitation in arriving at a diagnosis of carcinoma." Her specialist physicians "believed [she]...had only several months to live."

Since she was considered inoperable, the doctor decided to ask Rene Caisse to administer her treatment. The medicine was given orally, twice daily. After ten days, the woman's abdomen was less rigid, her appetite was improved, and her discomfort and pain upon eating were considerably lessened. Over the next few weeks, the tumors became smaller and she felt much better. Within a few months not only had her general health improved but the growth in the upper abdomen was reduced in size by more than two thirds, her swollen lymph nodes entirely disappeared, and the tumor in the pelvis was scarcely palpable at all.

This is impressive. However, we must temper our enthusiasm by observing that this diagnosis of cancer was not made by biopsy or X rays. The best that Dr. McInnis could offer were his subjective impressions, bolstered by a "gastric series" taken before the treatment, which indicated the presence of two masses. Dr. McInnis considered these "strongly indicative of carcinoma." Today, such diagnoses would be considered inadequate, although they were fairly typical for the time and place.

Dr. McInnis concluded that the Essiac treatment was "decidedly remarkable" and "apparently restored the patient to normal health." Many other similar cases could (and are often) cited. Thus, we hear of a Mr. F. Maxwell who "appeared" to have "malignant disease in his pancreas" but was still alive five years after taking Essiac. But what does "appeared to" have pancreatic cancer mean? Without a biopsy, no one can reliably diagnose pancreatic cancer or distinguish it from non-malignant diseases. Yet in the 1920s doctors routinely did so and drew conclusions about Essiac's value in cancer based on such cases.

By the early 1930s, word had spread throughout eastern Canada about the herbal cancer "cure." Caisse was able to give up her nursing job, move out of her Toronto apartment (the neighbors were complaining about the steady stream of patients, as many as 30 per day), and move to Petersborough, just east of the city. After she was again threatened with being arrested for practicing medicine without a license, Caisse boldly took five physicians and twelve patients and visited the Minister of Health, R.J. Robb. Dr. Robb saw them and agreed that Caisse would not be arrested if she limited herself to patients who had written diagnoses of cancer from their doctors and if she made no charge. She agreed to both terms and was generally good to her word.

In 1932, the Toronto *Star,* an internationally respected newspaper, caught wind of her activities and published the first major article on the controversy. It was titled, "Bracebridge Girl Makes Notable Discovery Against Cancer." The "girl" in question was then a 44-year-old woman, "under heavy stress carrying her patient load, and on her feet all day and half the night in the kitchen of her apartment cooking up Essiac."

Needless to say, she was quickly besieged by patients and various entrepreneurs. A Toronto businessman offered her $2,000 per year if she would "assign and set over all her right, title and interest in the said formula above referred to" (146). Apparently, she never answered his letter, for the pristine contract was found in her files after her death. From then until the end of her life, people tried to coax, cajole, purchase, or scare the formula out of her. She steadfastly refused almost all offers, and certainly was not cowed by any threats.

In the mid-1930s, a doctor in her hometown of Bracebridge, Dr. A.F. Bastedo, persuaded the Town Council to turn over the British Lion Hotel to Rene for $1.00 per month rent. (The town had seized the hotel for back taxes.) In 1935, the Prodigal Daughter returned home and opened the doors of a large, municipally sponsored outpatient facility. (Shades of Harry Hoxsey.) She was given an office, dispensary, reception room, and five treatment rooms. There was a large "Cancer Clinic" sign on the door and thousands of patients began flocking to Bracebridge, some from the United States.

Whatever the townspeople's humanitarian motives may have been, as with Hoxsey's supporters, it was also a shrewd business decision. Everyone knew how a thriving clinic could help the economy of a Depression-era town. Years later, a few older people in Bracebridge recalled the days of Nurse Caisse and her clinic. According to a 1977 article in *Homemaker's* magazine:

"Dominion Street took on an atmosphere reminiscent of the famous Shrine of Lourdes, as hopeful pilgrims sought a new lease on life. Cars were parked solidly along its shoulders. People from all walks of life waited patiently to enter the red brick building. Some were carried. Others were pushed gently up the steps, while the rest managed on their own. Occasionally, an ambulance would shriek its arrival as it double-parked. Rene would be seen coming quickly down to it to treat a stretcher case.

Always with a doctor standing by, she injected scores of patients every day" (358).

At about the same time, Rene Caisse's own 72-year-old mother was diagnosed with inoperable liver cancer. Four doctors attested that she was too weak for surgery. According to Caisse, a specialist, Dr. Roscoe Graham, said that her mother's liver was a "nodular mass," and she had only a few days to live. Rene did not tell her mother she had been diagnosed with cancer but gave her daily injections of Essiac. Her mother subsequently recovered and died after her ninetieth birthday. This was enormously satisfying to Caisse, who said it "made up for a great deal of the persecution I have endured at the hands of the medical people" (146).

Once again, the diagnosis was apparently made on the basis of clinical signs and symptoms, which can be unreliable. Today, such a diagnosis would require a biopsy by a qualified pathologist. Because of that lack, no firm conclusions can be drawn about Essiac from this anecdote either.

On September 14, 1935, the Ontario Minister of Health, Dr. J.A. Faulkner, wrote to Caisse that if she expected the government to take measures to legalize her treatment, "It is necessary that a full statement be submitted indicating the exact nature of the materials suggested for use, the manner in which they are to be used including dosage and the experience which has attended their use, with such detailed reports on pathological diagnosis, treatment, and present condition of patients as exist."

Eleven days later, he again wrote to Caisse that he had "chosen an outstanding scientist to investigate your treatment. If you will submit the information desired it will be referred to him for investigation and report." This seemed like a reasonable offer. What could any honest person have to fear in revealing useful formulas?

Yet Rene Caisse wouldn't do it. She called demands to release the formula "putting every obstacle in my way." Dr. Glum states that although she was "wide open about her work" she "wasn't about to turn over the formula." But what then does "wide open" mean in this context? Like Hoxsey, she demanded that doctors conduct a retrospective analysis of her cases and then admit publicly that she had cured people of terminal cancer. After that, she would make the formula known. It was a "Catch-22." From Caisse's point of view, once she revealed the formula, its very simplicity would be used to discredit her. One can imagine the howls of disbelief at the claim that sheep sorrel or the other weeds could "cure" a dreaded disease like cancer.

On the other hand, the doctors were opposed to secret remedies in general, and secret cancer nostrums in particular. What would happen, for instance, if they confirmed that she had indeed cured some cases of cancer...and then she still refused to release the formula! An erratic,

unpredictable "girl" would then have a world monopoly on an acknowledged cancer cure. It was unthinkable.

And so the medical profession grew increasingly hostile. Caisse's supporters responded in turn with a mass petition of local residents as well as
of nine physicians (only two of whom had signed the original 1926 petition). By 1936, there were numerous articles and letters to the editor about
Essiac in the Ontario newspapers. An increasing number were from people
who claimed to have been brought back from the brink of death by Caisse's
treatment. The word "cure" was heard often in reference to her remedy.
According to Glum:

"This was really the beginning of the notion that Rene Caisse was
preaching that she could cure all cancer. She wasn't. She was saying that
Essiac caused regression in tumors, prolonged life, relieved pain and—in the
right circumstances with patients whose organs weren't already destroyed—
could cure cancer" (146).

But the patients, and her cadre of referring doctors, were not splitting
hairs. They thought cures were taking place. It is necessary to repeat, however, that, on one point at least, the medical establishment was right: many
of these patients did not have biopsy-confirmed malignancies and so, despite
what their doctors may have told them about their cases, we can draw few
factual conclusions.

The mayor of Bracebridge, Wilburt Richards, next visited the Minister
of Health, Dr. Faulkner, with a petition containing 2,700 signatures requesting the government legalize the treatment. This would have removed the
fear of arrest from Caisse's head and allowed her to be compensated for the
treatment.

On July 10, 1936, Caisse and her patients met face to face with the health
minister. Faulkner's brilliant idea was to have Sir Frederick Banting (1891-
1941) investigate the treatment. Banting was at that time Canada's greatest
scientist. He was a Nobel Laureate, a humanitarian who was internationally known as the co-discoverer of insulin. In late July, 1936, Rene Caisse
actually met with Banting, one of the oddest encounters in the history of
cancer. He appeared to be intrigued, and generously offered her facilities to
test her compound doing animal research there under his supervision.

What was particularly magnanimous was his offer: "You will not be asked
to divulge any secret concerning your treatment." However he also stipulated: "All experimental results must be submitted to me for my approval
before being announced to anyone, including the newspapers, or published
in medical journals." One can sympathize with his nervousness: Caisse was
a woman who either sought or attracted publicity, and this was an era in
which doctors could be censured for simply allowing their pictures in the
paper.

There was one "catch" to his offer, however. Caisse would have to devote herself full-time to working in the Toronto laboratory, 170 kilometers from Bracebridge. She would have to give up the rigorous schedule at her clinic. This she refused to do. In a letter to Banting she explained an additional reason for refusing his offer, "My relatives and friends do not approve of my going back to animal research, when I have already proved the merit of my Cancer Treatment on human beings." She explained that she was entirely dependent on these same friends for her financial support, since she was unable to charge patients for the treatment. Without them she would have no financial resources whatsoever as "I have never had a hundred dollars I could call my own.

"I appreciate the fact that you are doing what you think is best for me," she wrote, "and to please you I wish I were in a position to accept this offer, but there is a saying, that you can't get blood out of a stone, and that is my position at the present time."

In fact, we know that some of her staunchest friends disapproved of this rejection. Dr. Arnold wrote her about the offer: "I think it is fair enough. It is the same proposition I made to you many years ago when we put the mice into the Christie Street lab." Banting's letter is "as much as you could have expected." But Caisse was convinced of the efficacy of her treatment and was also convinced that many people would die for lack of it. "It was an agonizing decision," she later said, "but I refused his offer."

The world thus lost a chance to see what could have come from the collaboration of two remarkable individuals, one the distinguished leader of Canada's biomedical community, the other her country's major proponent of herbal cancer remedies.

Caisse's argument that Toronto was too far away was undercut by what followed. In October, 1936 she accepted an offer from doctors in Chicago to demonstrate her treatment there. She shuttled between Bracebridge and Chicago every week, treating patients in both locales. In Chicago, she worked under the supervision of Dr. John Wolfer, director of the Tumor Clinic of Northwestern University Medical School. How she could commute to Chicago but not to Toronto is never explained by her admiring fans.

These roundtrips to and from Chicago were, however, wearing on her health, and expensive. Some cancer patients reported dramatic decreases in their level of pain. But before Dr. Wolfer could reach any conclusions about the treatment, Caisse terminated the relationship. The trip was undermining her health and finances, she said. Another physician then offered her facilities at Chicago's Passavant Hospital if she wished to move there. However, she decided to stay in comfortable Bracebridge.

Caisse's flirtation with American medicine inflamed nationalistic passions north of the border. The tempo of comments in the newspaper was build-ing to crescendo, as were the letters pouring in to the Ministry of Health. The Toronto *Evening Telegram* reported on March 8, 1937 that "matters soon will reach a final stage in the effort of Miss Rene Caisse, Bracebridge nurse, to obtain Canadian medical recognition for her cancer treatment methods."

A new petition drive, this one with 17,000 signatures, had now been launched, and had been signed by a number of new doctors, including B.L. Guyatt of the University of Toronto. A Bracebridge delegation to Toronto was given a tumultuous send-off in the high school auditorium, chaired by the town's mayor. Doctors and patients fired up the crowd with the amaz-ing results they had experienced. The delegation that finally converged on Toronto consisted of local officials, 18 patients and 40 doctors. Both Dr. Faulkner, the Minister of Health, and Dr. Banting met with member of the delegation, and this made front-page headlines across Ontario. After the meeting Dr. Faulkner told the press that the government was considering legislation to allow such putative cancer "cures" to be tested.

In July, 1937, with an election pending, Premier Mitchell Hepburn agreed to meet with Caisse, who had become a populist force in the province. The Premier later told the press, "These people are sincere, clear-thinking people, and it seems to me that something must be done to make this treatment available....The onus is now on the medical profession...." He suggested extraordinary legislation allowing this single non-physician, Rene Caisse, to practice medicine without a license.

As the number of Caisse's patients increased so, too, did public reports of reputed "cures." This further agitated the newspapers, which led to fur-ther public outcries. It is one of the most extraordinary facets of this herbal treatment that because of it an obscure, small-town registered nurse became a power in the land, and was courted by top politicians and scientists. By 1938, it looked as if Essiac might actually gain official acceptance and legalization.

The political struggle, as it often does, came down to a question of two competing bills. In February, 1938, the Premier himself introduced a bill, that "Rene Caisse be authorized to practice medicine in the Province of Ontario in the treatment of cancer in all its forms and of human ailments and conditions resulting therefrom." (For a parallel, one would have to imagine President Franklin D. Roosevelt meeting with and proposing leg-islation on behalf of Harry Hoxsey.)

The Caisse bill was adamantly opposed by the organization of doctors in the province, the Ontario Medical Association. Obviously, such a bill would have punched a hole in the Association's legal monopoly on the practice of medicine in the province. Many others, including naturopaths, chiropractors and an assortment of uncredentialed laypeople, could be imagined gleefully rushing through that loophole. The Medical Association, and its allies in the Department of Health, therefore offered a counter-proposal. This was called the "Kirby Bill," after the new Health Minister, Harold Kirby. It called for the establishment of a Royal Cancer Commission, composed of members of the thoroughly orthodox Canadian College of Physicians and Surgeons. If Rene Caisse's evidence was persuasive, they said, the Commission would then have the power to legalize Essiac. The same applied to several other non-conventional treatments then in use.

But, as Gary Glum states, "there was a catch." The nature and composition of all such formulas had to be turned over to the Commission. Anyone refusing to do so could be fined $100 to $500 the first time they were caught treating a patient, and from $500 to $2,500 the second or subsequent times. Failure to pay such fines could result in 30 days to 6 months in jail.

And although members of the Commission were required to maintain the confidentiality of the formulas put in their trust, there was no penalty if they failed to do so. Caisse's comments were acerbic:

"I have developed and proven a cure right here in Bracebridge, and I am running a clinic where hundreds of cancer sufferers are being treated and helped. Why then should I be asked to give my formula over to a group of doctors who never did anything to earn it?"

Rene Caisse declared that if the Kirby Bill were passed, she would move to the United States, which did not yet have such laws on the books.

In late March, 1938, the bill to allow Caisse to practice medicine came before the Private Bills committee of the Ontario legislature. It was accompanied by a growing petition that now numbered 55,000. Fifty of her patients observed the proceedings from the visitors' gallery, and the debate was fierce, with J. Frank Kelly, MP, from Bracebridge, arguing vigorously in Caisse's defense. Some MPs vigorously defended the medical association's position and shouting matches erupted between MPs and the patients in the gallery. The chairman threatened to clear the chamber.

When the time came for a vote there was virtual pandemonium on the floor. Although no accurate head count could be taken, newspapers the next day reported that it had been defeated by three votes. Soon after this historic defeat, the opposing Kirby Bill was passed into law by the full legislature. Despite verbal support by the Premier himself, Caisse and her supporters had been bested by the medical establishment.

There followed a kind of "phony war." Rene Caisse would announce that she was closing her clinic because of the Kirby law; the media would then flock to the door of the eponymous Kirby himself, only to be reassured that he had no intention of closing the Bracebridge clinic.

Some time later rumors would circulate that Kirby was about to crack down on her. Caisse would then shut the doors of the clinic, leading to panic among existing patients and consternation among her tens of thousands of supporters. The same scenario would be acted out again between the media and the health minister. This harlequinade lasted for two years, during which time the clinic was opened and shut at least half a dozen times. For a provincial nurse, Rene Caisse turned out to be a very adept practitioner of hard-ball politics.

The focus of struggle next shifted to the Royal Cancer Commission, whose creation had been mandated by the Kirby bill. This body consisted of six highly credentialed doctors, chaired by a non-physician, Mr. J.G. Gillanders, judge of the Ontario Supreme Court.

Two members of the Commission visited Rene Caisse's clinic in Bracebridge and then in March, 1939, the full Commission held public hearings at the Royal York Hotel in Toronto. An extraordinary 387 Essiac patients showed up to present, as one might expect, overwhelmingly positive testimony. There were so many potential witnesses that Caisse had to rent one of the ornate hotel's massive ballrooms as a waiting room. Ultimately, however, the Commission allowed only 49 such patients to testify, presumably because of time constraints. Gary Glum has summarized this testimony as follows:

"The hundreds of pages of transcript of those 49 sworn witnesses is filled with heart-rending testimony. To a person they were convinced that Essiac had helped them to regain their health. Some of them told of partial and continuing recoveries when all else had failed; others described complete, almost miraculous, recoveries after they had been near death."

Whatever one might think of the accuracy of these patients' assessments of their own conditions, there is no doubt that they were passionately convinced that they had been helped. The sheer numbers of people willing to make difficult and expensive trips during history's worst Depression, is itself eloquent testimony to the depth of their convictions.

If any of the members of the Commission were moved, however, they didn't show it. A few weeks later, representatives of the College of Physicians and Surgeons got to present their testimony. This consisted of cases that, they said, had *not* benefited from the treatment. Logically speaking, such cases were even more absurd than unsubstantiated claims of cure, for no treatment on earth is foolproof. They could just as easily have "proven" the inefficacy of Banting's insulin by citing instances in which it did not work.

One has to sympathize with Rene Caisse's plight. The agreement she had made with the prior Minister of Health, R.J. Robb stipulated that she limit her treatment to patients who had written diagnoses of cancer from their doctors. By definition, most of these patients had been given up for lost by their physicians. But now, if they died, she was held accountable.

In newspaper coverage, Rene Caisse responded:

"The Commission would not consider any recovery due to Essiac unless there had been no other treatment previously taken....[But] I have been obliged to treat so many cases sent to my by doctors after everything in medical science had been used ineffectively. I have not been allowed to take a cancer case without a doctor's diagnosis, and in the majority of cases, a doctor will not give me a diagnosis unless he considers the patient beyond the help of medical science."

There was also the familiar charge that any benefit seen had to be due to the residual effects of radiation therapy. Again, it was the same old story: the orthodox physician irradiated until he could irradiate no more. He then dismissed the patient to the care of the "quack." If the patient recovered, the orthodox physician claimed the cure.

"In other words," Caisse defiantly told the assembled doctors, "if the patient lives, you take the credit for radium, but if the patient dies, radium has nothing to do with it." It was a sharp retort, indeed.

But one thing emerged from these hearings. Even in those cases in which it was claimed that Essiac had no objective benefit, many patients reported pain relief. This point was usually glossed over by the Commission. "Subjective" responses did not count at all.

The Commission once again was demanding the formula. (Supporters asked why they would want it, if Essiac was worthless?) Caisse again stubbornly refused: she told the assembled doctors that she did not want the formula taken from her and then immediately shelved as worthless. "I want to know that suffering humanity will benefit by it. When I can be given assurance, I am willing to disclose my formula, but I have got to know that it is going to get to suffering humanity."

The Chairman replied that he wouldn't admit any merit before receiving the formula—so there was a deadlock. "If you had heard Dr. Noble and Dr. Richards [two of the Commissioners, ed.] pull my work to pieces you would believe me to be a criminal," she later wrote to her ally, Premier Hepburn. Then Caisse and her supporters waited.

It wasn't until nine months later, in December, 1939, that the Royal Cancer Commission finally delivered an Interim Report to parliament. Not surprisingly, they denigrated the treatment. They dismissed several of the diagnoses as incorrect. (But of course Caisse did not make any of these diagnoses—this was an indirect indictment of their own colleagues.) Other cases were ruled out because they had received prior x-ray or radium treatment. "In the 49 cases presented, there were only four in which the diagnosis was accepted and in which recovery occurred apparently from Miss Caisse's treatment," the report stated.

This might look like a success rate of 8.2 percent in so-called terminal cases. But, unable to accept the implications of this, the Commissioners found reasons to doubt the validity of their own judgment. In one case, they reported, "The Commission now has a signed statement from the surgeon to the effect that the growth he removed was not cancer." The most likely scenario was this: the patient was told she had cancer, was operated upon and possibly irradiated as well. She was then told she was terminally ill and sent for an herbal treatment. When she got well, her surgeon re-examined her records and had a change of heart. She never had cancer!

An almost identical scenario was played out in the evaluation of the Rees Evans and Hoxsey's cases, down to the recantation of a surgeon under pressure. No safeguards were taken in any of these cases against the obvious possibility of bias on the part of the evaluators.

There was no "blinding" of the judges (i.e., so that they would not know the nature of the treatment patients had undertaken), the deliberate inclusion of 'ringers" among the cases (i.e., adding patients cured by conventional means), or the inclusion on the Commission of members sympathetic to non-conventional medicine.

The Report also unfairly implied that these 49 cases represented the sum total of positive cases that Caisse was able to muster, while 338 other patients in the Royal York ballroom waited to testify. The Report concluded, "...the evidence adduced does not justify any favorable conclusion as to the merits of 'Essiac' as a remedy for cancer..." (146).

Once again, however, in their written report the Commissioners demanded the "worthless" formula. Caisse called this report "one of the greatest farces ever perpetrated in the history of man."

With this defeat by the Commission, however, the first phase of the Essiac movement ended. The Depression was over and World War II had come. Rene Caisse disappeared from public view for the next 20 years. Propelled by the same Depression-era energies that had lifted Harry Hoxsey to prominence, Caisse almost gained legalization for her herbal treatment. But there were critical flaws in her argument (especially her insistence on secrecy), and the medical establishment proved more powerful. As Richard Thomas wrote, "she had taken her fight as far as any one person could against the awesome power and limitless resources of the Medical Establishment."

The struggle left her both physically and emotionally exhausted. Although she kept the Bracebridge clinic open for a while, she could no longer procure written diagnoses from doctors and finally "in a state bordering on collapse" she permanently closed the clinic and left Bracebridge. She retreated to the town of North Bay, with the husband that she had married in the 1930s. At some point it is said that she had a nervous breakdown, but the facts concerning her activities during this period are sketchy. We know that her husband died in 1948, and she returned to Bracebridge. It appears that Caisse was quietly treating patients throughout the Fifties and that she was once again under surveillance by agents of the Ministry of Health (385).

Yet, surprisingly, near the end of her life, the Essiac drama flared up once again. In February, 1959, she was approached by editors at the sensationalist *True* magazine, who, in turn, introduced her to a doctor named Charles Brusch, MD. Dr. Brusch was one of Senator John F. Kennedy's physicians and was director of the Brusch Medical Center in Cambridge, Massachusetts. At the age of 70, Rene Caisse signed an agreement with him to develop and market Essiac. She presumably gave him the formula at that time, the first person she had ever shared it with.

Rene Caisse then started to treat patients at Dr. Brusch's clinic. In addition, he arranged to have her treat some mice that had been sent from Sloan-Kettering Institute in New York. At first, Sloan-Kettering scientists seemed enthusiastic about the result. But then they backpedaled, saying they would need to have the formula in order to continue.

Dr. Brusch seriously considered their proposal but Caisse held firm to her inveterate stance. The National Cancer Institute was next approached but made the same precondition—Give us the formula! And so Brusch's animal experiments continued without the imprimatur of any major cancer center. He concluded that when injected into animals, Essiac caused "a decided recession of mass, and a definite change in cell formation." This data was never published or subjected to peer review, however.

On human patients with confirmed tumors, Brusch believed that Essiac "reduces pain and causes a regression in the growth; patients have gained weight and shown an improvement in their general health." These initial conclusions were modest and probably accurate. Years later, however, in the midst of a commercial promotion, Brusch claimed that Essiac was in fact a "cure for cancer."

In the 1960s, Caisse continued to supply Brusch with Essiac and also to secretly treat some patients out of her home in Bracebridge.

In 1973, at the age of 85, she made one last stab at scientific validation. She wrote to Sloan-Kettering Institute, reminding them of the encouraging results they had previously achieved with this product. She heard back from Dr. C. Chester Stock, the vice president and associate director for administrative and academic affairs. He said they would be willing to test Essiac on mice. What she sent, however, was not Essiac, but one ingredient, sheep sorrel. She knew from prior experience that they were primarily interested in tumor regression. Sheep sorrel was the active cytotoxic ingredient, while the other herbs were primarily ancillary "blood purifiers."

On June 10, 1975, Dr. Stock wrote to Rene Caisse: "Enclosed are test data in two experiments indicating some regressions in sarcoma 180 of mice treated with Essiac. With these results we will wish to test enough more that I should ask if you can send more material. If you have questions about the data, please don't hesitate to ask them" (146).

The reader should understand that this was the era of openness towards non-conventional treatments at Sloan-Kettering, including the examination of amygdalin, or laetrile (an era I detail in my book, *The Cancer Industry*). It is intriguing that SKI achieved "some regressions" with sheep sorrel. However, as with laetrile, some follow-up tests were said to be negative. Caisse complained about the manner in which the sheep sorrel was being handled. Instead of boiling the herb, Sloan-Kettering, she said, was freezing and then thawing it. Stock apologized for the error but she scrawled on his explanation, "All wrong. Rene M. Caisse," and sent it back to him. "They might as well have been injecting distilled water," she complained.

She then withdrew from the Sloan-Kettering testing. In 1978, after Sloan-Kettering's involvement with non-conventional treatments had ended in a fiasco, some patients went to court in Detroit to win the right to legally import Essiac for their own use. At that time Dr. Stock filed a sworn affidavit in which he said, "We have tested Essiac in a very limited way against sarcoma 180. We have not seen any consistent activity." This was technically correct but managed to convey a negative impression.

In 1977, the editors of *Homemaker's*, a national Canadian magazine, learned about Essiac and investigated the issue intensively. They had concluded that "Essentially, Rene's story was true." But they were very nervous about publishing anything positive about a non-conventional cancer treatment. (I can attest to that: I was Sloan-Kettering's spokesperson at the time and was called on an almost daily basis by the increasingly nervous author, Sheila Snow.)

Yet the magazine's editors became convinced, as many others have, that there was some merit to this treatment, and they generously offered to set up a Trust to represent the elderly nurse in her dealings with the medical profession, government, and industry. To their dismay, Caisse turned them down flat. She appeared to have her own agenda, although no one could ever figure out what it was. (She also failed to tell *Homemaker's* about her arrangement with Dr. Brusch.)

The editors concluded: "There's a tragic and shameful irony in the Essiac tale. In the beginning, a simple herbal recipe was freely shared by an Indian....In the hands of more sophisticated...healers, it was made the focus of an ugly struggle for ownership and power." It was an eloquent indictment of both sides in this struggle, both of whom frequently lost sight of the best interests of the patients.

Nonetheless, the magazine's story produced a sensation which, in a sense, has not died down yet. As was anticipated, patients besieged Rene Caisse's home in Bracebridge, demanding treatment. Television and newspaper teams arrived at her doorstep. Some individuals actually threatened the 90-year-old nurse if she wouldn't turn the formula over to them and at one point she actually had to seek police protection!

In the fall of 1977, Rene Caisse was approached by David Fingard, a "distinguished-looking 70 year old gentleman" who was vice president of something called Resperin Corporation. This was described as a Canadian company with interests in the pharmaceutical field. "Fingard couldn't believe that in over 50 years, no one had been able to capitalize on Essiac," wrote Thomas. "He set out single handedly to obtain the formula."

Of course, Rene Caisse turned him down but he was persistent and nearly ever day arrived at her house with a new proposal. He promised to bring Essiac to "suffering humanity," and so forth. He then apparently told her that if she gave him the formula he would open five fully staffed clinics across Canada and give Essiac free to terminally ill patients who couldn't afford it. Swayed by such arguments, on October 26, 1977, Rene Caisse turned the formula over to Fingard. She received a token payment of $1.00 and $250 per week for six months. Out of this money she was supposed to buy herbs and furnish them to Resperin. Resperin in turn would undertake the human, clinical testing of Essiac.

The Department of Health and Welfare Canada, under great public pressure after the *Homemaker's* article, agreed to register Essiac as an experimental drug available for the treatment of terminal cancer patients with approval of the Health Protection Branch of the Department of Health and Welfare. But within several months it was apparent there were problems. The two hospitals that had agreed to give Essiac a try, Princess Margaret and Toronto General, now insisted on using the tea in conjunction with other treatments—chemotherapy or radiotherapy—that their clinicians deemed appropriate. This of course would have made evaluation of the final results nearly impossible.

It was a classic dilemma. As Thomas remarks, "if the treatment worked they could claim it worked because of the other therapies employed and not Essiac...If the treatment did not work they could simply blame it on Essiac, and not on the damage done by conventional therapies...." And so the plan was changed: Essiac would be evaluated by private doctors. However, many of these doctors were reluctant to comply with the stringent guidelines that had been set forth by the government agencies. Rene Caisse, not fully understanding the circumstances, was bitterly disappointed and blamed Resperin.

Then, after breaking her hip in a fall, Rene Caisse had surgery but died on December 26, 1978, at the age of 90. At her funeral, her priest concluded, "History may have further to say about her work someday."

Dr. Brusch also became disillusioned with Resperin. He belatedly hired private investigators who told him that Resperin was a shadowy corporation with few assets other than David Fingard's charm. One of Resperin's two employees was in fact brewing Essiac in his kitchen.

Rene Caisse's Original Proprietary Herbal Formula From Resperin Corporation ®

ESSIAC

HERBAL TEA/TISANE

La recette de marque déposée originale de Rene Caisse des Sociétés Resperin

AUTHORIZED BY

Rene M. Caisse

1888-1978

Net Weight 1.5oz/42.5g Poids Net

To make the story more bizarre, that employee was Dr. Matthew Dymond, who had been the Minister of Health responsible for the surveillance of Rene Caisse!

In April, 1981, an internal memo of the Health Protection Branch spelled out its extreme disappointment with Resperin's testing program. Essiac was being distributed to 160 physicians across Canada. However, it wrote, "to date, the Health Protection Branch has received a small number of incomplete clinical case reports, but no data which would establish that the product distributed is uniform in composition batch to batch...The results of the clinical studies are *impossible to evaluate*" (italics in original).

On August 30, 1982, the Minister of Health and Welfare moved to shut down this "shoddy test." There were howls of protest from patients on the treatment, but Resperin had thoroughly discredited Essiac in the eyes of much of the public as well. The government then made Essiac available, but only through the Emergency Drug Release Act. This meant it was only allowed on a compassionate basis for terminally ill patients. This obligated doctors to fill out a considerable amount of bureaucratic paperwork, something many were unwilling to do.

In November, 1984, Dr. Brusch was interviewed by a radio talk show host and producer in Vancouver, British Columbia—Elaine Alexander. Ms. Alexander had had some prior interest in holistic health. Over the next two years she produced seven two-hour shows on Essiac. She interviewed people who claimed to have been cured of cancer on the tea. With Rene Caisse's death, a vacuum had been created. "The public began to treat Elaine as if she were Rene herself," wrote Thomas. (I saw this phenomenon several times at Canadian health expos.) Elaine Alexander conceived the idea of selling a form of Essiac as a harmless "detoxifying" tea in health food stores, with no cancer claims whatsoever. Brusch agreed. Their thinking is ably summarized by Richard Thomas:

"Drugs are designed to block or change some function of the body. Essiac is, in fact, a natural substance that was always meant to simply purify and detoxify the body, not block or change its function in some unnatural way.

Drugs are, by their very nature, toxic. Essiac is, by its very nature, non-toxic. And therein lies its real power. Essiac is the ultimate body purifier. Thus, the body, once it is cleansed of toxic disease-producing impurities, has the power to heal itself" (385).

In November, 1988, Brusch and Alexander officially became partners. Brusch than signed over to Alexander the herbal formulas he had been given by Rene Caisse. In 1992, they settled on the Flora Corporation, a German company, as their manufacturer. The company owns a huge manufacturing facility in Bavaria and a chain of health food stores in Germany called "Salus Haus." They also own large farms in Bavaria, Chile, and Florida. There followed a period of intense promotion and competition for the Essiac market. In a familiar pattern, instead of the companies themselves making claims for its product, they allow or encourage journalists to do so.

Thus, a company called the Alternative Treatment Information Network published the book, *The Essiac Report* by Richard Thomas. In a biographical note, Mr. Thomas describes himself as "a highly sought after copy writer in the burgeoning field of health and fitness." While his book is a valuable source of documents on Essiac's history, at times it reads like copywriting for Flor·Essence, with pages of color pictures of Flora's manufacturing facilities. A 1997 tape called *Keeping Hope Alive,* also produced by the above organization, is being distributed by Flor·Essence. I have seen no mention in any of the promotional literature for Flor·Essence that Elaine Alexander herself died of ovarian cancer in the mid-1990s, unable to save herself with her own product.

Meanwhile, the Resperin formula continues to be sold under the registered Essiac name. It comes in a package of four dried herbs: burdock root, sheep sorrel, Turkey rhubarb and slippery elm, which the consumer must then make into a tea. Burdock seems to be the chief ingredient by weight while sheep sorrel is allegedly the most active against cancer.

In 1991, Resperin assigned its rights in the product to Mankind Research Foundation, with David Dobbie of New Brunswick as their distributor. The Canadian Trademark "Essiac" is held by Mankind of Maryland (7). It has been no less aggressive in its marketing. Its advertisements warn consumers, "Beware of Counterfeits." One also finds endless variants, such as Easy-ac, Essi-ease, etc. from a variety of companies, some of them mom-and-pop herbal suppliers. Resperin has gone to court to stop infringements on their brand name.

Today's patients are regaled with tales of success with Essiac in the pre-war era. But it is important to note that in Rene Caisse's hands, Essiac was always given as both an oral tea and also as an injection. We don't know what this injection consisted of or how it was prepared. All of today's products are only meant to be taken as oral preparations, a fact which changes the biochemical effect considerably.

Knowing this, and no doubt being perplexed by the difference between today's rate of response and the historical claims, some individuals have drawn the wrong conclusion: that they should start injecting Essiac tea into their veins. Nothing could be further from the truth!

Injecting an unpurified vegetable substance into the body is courting disaster. We have already alluded to one such instance. In that case, Sandor Olah, DO, of Hamilton, Michigan was treating a 54-year-old woman named Petra Hall for chronic leukemia.

According to newspaper accounts, on January 1, 1996, Dr. Olah administered Essiac intravenously to Ms. Hall. She began to experience shortness of breath as well as other symptoms following this treatment. Nevertheless, he sent her home. Later that day, however, she checked into Hackley Hospital in Muskegon, Michigan, where she experienced multiple organ failure. She died eleven days later and the cause of death was listed as "respiratory distress syndrome due to vitamin [sic] therapy" (The Holland [Mich.] *Sentinel,* 4/18/97). Dr. Olah's medical license was suspended.

In addition to being tragic for the individuals involved, this case was a fillip for the quackbusters. "This story is typical of a persistent type of cancer quackery involving a willingness to try anything," crowed Dr. Stephen Barrett. It thus damaged the very cause it was trying to promote.

Essiac's Indian Connection

One thing that bothers me is that Essiac is universally described as a traditional Ojibwa cancer remedy. "To begin to understand the essence of Flor·Essence," Richard Thomas says, "it is important to remember and appreciate its true originators, the proud Ojibwa" (385). The books of both Dr. Gary Glum and Cynthia Olsen feature pictures of Native Americans on their front covers.

But is Essiac (or Flor·Essence) really an old Ojibwa formula, as claimed? This is far from proven.

The Ojibwas (also known as the Chippewas) are an Algonquin-speaking tribe who were formerly concentrated along the northern shores of Lake Huron and on both sides of Lake Superior, from Minnesota to North Dakota. There are also about 50,000 Ojibwa Indians in Canada on reservations in Manitoba, Saskatchewan, and Ontario (with one just outside Bracebridge).

There is no disputing that the Ojibwas were celebrated for their healing practices and the annual meeting of the Midewiwin, or Grand Medicine Society, was the major Ojibwa ceremony of the year (102, also *EB* 8:895).

Thus, an Ojibwa herbal treatment for cancer seems quite possible in theory. However, there are several obstacles to accepting such an attribution for Essiac. First, it is uncharacteristic of Indians to combine multiple herbs into a single formula. Genuine Indian remedies were usually single herbs. It was the pseudo-Indian patent medicine men of the 19th century who popularized the practice of combining many herbs together, and ascribing to them an Indian ancestry. They may have done this to preserve the secrecy of their formulas (see Chapter 2).

In this book's companion volume, I shall deal with each of the herbs in the Essiac formula in greater depth. They are fine herbs, both individually and collectively. But are they an authentic Ojibwa remedy, as Rene Caisse said? There are reasons to doubt it.

Ulmus fulva, or slippery elm, was definitely known and used by Ojibwa, who called it "gawakomic." It was a medicine for sore throats (a usage that is continued today in Thayer's throat lozenges). There is no mention of any connection to cancer in any of the standard sources, including Hartwell.

Arctium lappa (burdock): There have been several studies showing antitumor activity of burdock in animal systems (134, 110). (Other studies showed no such effects.) An antimutation factor has also been isolated, which is resistant to both heat and protein-digesting enzymes. Scientists at Kawasaki Medical School, Okayama, Japan, called this "the burdock factor" (287). Burdock has also been found to be active in the test tube against the human immuno-deficiency virus (HIV) (416). Benzaldehyde, also present in burdock, has been shown to have significant anticancer effects in humans. (Intriguingly, burdock independently was included in the Hoxsey treatment.)

A related species, *Arctium minus,* was used among the Ojibwa as a medicine for coughs, as a tonic, and for stomach pains. However, burdock root is unmentioned as a cancer treatment in many standard works on traditional Ojibwa medicine (279).

Acetosella vulgaris, or sheep sorrel, is probably the key ingredient in Essiac. It is in fact a historical anticancer remedy with many citations in Hartwell. There was a particular upsurge in such citations in the 1920s. NCI is said to have tested one sample of Taiwanese sorrel and found no activity against mouse leukemia. But again, aloe emodin, isolated from sorrel, does show "significant antileukemic activity" (242, 287).

Yet sheep sorrel was not included in a 1915 Canadian government study of medicinal plants (2). It was not mentioned in a classic 1928 work on Ojibwa medicine. Nor is it mentioned as an Ojibwa plant in the *Field Guide to American Indian Medicinal Plants* (279). Two related plants, *Rumex obtusifolius* and *Rumex crispus* (bitter dock and yellow dock) were used as medicines for cuts, ulcers and eruptions, but again there is no mention of any use against cancer by the Ojibwas.

Rheum palmatum (Turkey rhubarb): This to me is the most suspicious inclusion. This plant has indeed been demonstrated to have antitumor activity in the sarcoma 37 test system (35). (Again, conflicting tests did not show such activity.) Certain chemicals in rhubarb, such as emodin, catechin, and rhein, "have shown antitumor activity in some animal test systems," according to the Office of Technology Assessment report on unconventional cancer treatments (394).

But how could Turkey rhubarb possibly be part of some traditional Ojibwa formula when it is not even an indigenous American plant? Its history is well known. Traditionally, it was grown in China and then laboriously (and expensively) imported via Turkey, hence its popular name. According to all classic sources, Turkey rhubarb was unknown to the Ojibwas. I conclude that whatever their power, the four-herb Essiac tea formula could not have been a genuine Ojibwa Indian "cure for cancer." How it actually originated is anyone's guess.

A Foreign Medicinal Plant

At one point, Rene Caisse claimed that enough of Essiac's component herbs grew in Ontario to supply the whole world. This is probably true of the first three ingredients, but could not have been true of Turkey rhubarb. As late as 1915, this was listed as a "foreign medicinal plant" in an official compendium. There were some speculations on possibly cultivating it in parts of southern Ontario where the winter is not too severe. However, in northern Ontario, where this formula allegedly originated, it probably would not grow. So, on all accounts, it is absurd to think that Turkey rhubarb was part of any truly indigenous Ojibwa cancer treatment.

Toxicity

It is nearly universally agreed that Essiac is relatively harmless. Even the Canadian Department of Health and Welfare, in shutting down Resperin's research project in 1982, commented, "It is acknowledged that Essiac is not harmful to a person's health provided it is not substituted for proven forms of cancer therapy" (385).

I personally have never heard of anyone being harmed by taking Essiac tea as a drink. It has a mild and pleasant taste. (Injecting it in any form can be fatal.) However, from a purely theoretical basis, there are some concerns that should be addressed.

First of all, there is oxalic acid present in several ingredients: Turkey rhubarb, sheep sorrel, and (in the Flor·Essence formulation) watercress. Sorrel has about 0.3 percent oxalic acid in the leaf (6). Therefore, individuals with a history of kidney stone formation should use these herbs cautiously. That said, they should also eat spinach, garden sorrel, rhubarb pie, etc. with similar caution.

Both Turkey rhubarb and sheep sorrel also contain between 7.0 and 15.0 percent tannins. The biological effects of tannins are complex and contradictory. Thus, both carcinogenic and anticancer activity has been reported for tannin. Tannic acid, a derivative of nutgalls (*Quercus spp.*), can be quite dangerous; however the adverse effects of other plant tannins is generally limited to digestive irritating properties (6). It can be assumed that if one does not get stomach upset by drinking a tea of such ingredients, then no damage is being done.

Rhubarb (*Rheum spp.*) is contraindicated in cases of intestinal obstruction, abdominal pain of unknown origin, or any inflammatory condition of the intestines. It is not indicated for children less than twelve years of age, not for long-term use in excess of eight to ten days, nor for individuals with a history of kidney stones (see above). Chinese physicians sometimes prescribe up to 12.0 grams per day of the rhizome or root. It is not clear whether or not there is enough rhubarb present in Essiac to rank as an area of concern or danger. Probably not.

Slippery elm is a class 1 herb, which can be safely consumed when used appropriately. So, too, is burdock. However, the reader should be aware that there was a single poisoning reported with burdock. This turned out to be almost certainly a false alarm, caused by the adulteration of burdock with another (and dangerous) plant, *Atropa belladonna,* or the deadly nightshade. However, it is occasionally still cited in the negative literature on herbal remedies.

Essiac is relatively non–toxic, inexpensive, and accessible through almost every health food outlet. One can brew Essiac tea at home for about five cents per day, and so it appeals to the budget-conscious who may have been financially drained by other cancer treatments.

Clinical Results

We have seen the essentially negative conclusions reached by the Royal Cancer Commission. The Resperin "clinical trial" ended in fiasco in 1982. In 1987, the Health Protection Branch of Canada contacted 150 physicians who were known to have received supplies of Essiac from Resperin. Replies from 74 of the physicians concerning 86 patients showed that "47 patients reported no benefits; eight of the reports were not evaluable; 17 patients had died; one patient was reported to have had a subjective improvement; five patients were reported as requiring less analgesia; four patients were said to have an objective response; and four patients were in a stable condition." This would seem to indicate that 10 out of 80 evaluable patients (12.5 percent) received some benefit from the treatment. Of these, four had tumor shrinkages of greater than 50 percent, which is the standard oncological definition of "objective response" (five percent).

Five years later, in 1982, the eight patients who had either an objective response or who had remained stable were re-examined by their physicians. The following results were reported: in three of the eight cases, the disease had progressed, but the patients were still alive; two patients had died; and three remained stable.

As with the Royal Cancer Commission, the Health Protection Branch re-examined the three stable patients' histories. It was their "impression" that in these cases the stability was due to other forms of treatment. Their overall conclusion from these 86 patients "must therefore be that Essiac had not altered the progression of cancer in these patients, and did not show any specific benefit with the exception of a possible placebo effect in some cases."

There was no description on the part of the Health Protection Branch (itself an interested party in this dispute) of what steps it took to eliminate the possibility of bias on the part of its own evaluators.

In May, 1993, official Essiac was tested twice in very small animal studies. The NCI confirmed a "moderate" effect on the HIV virus. A 1993 report from Vetrepharm Research also showed a moderate ability to enhance immune response.

The Bottom Line

Does Essiac exert any objective effects beyond that of placebo? Like the Canadian authorities, I have been disappointed by the paucity of research on Essiac. This is in the face of an almost irresistible tide of good publicity. In the 1980s and '90s, there were no less than five books on the topic of Essiac tea. These were *The Calling of an Angel* by Gary Glum (1988); *The Essiac Handbook* by James Percival (1994); *The Essiac Report: Canada's Remarkable Unknown Cancer Remedy* by Richard Thomas (1994); *The Essence of Essiac* by Sheila Snow (1994); and *Essiac: A Native Herbal Cancer Remedy* by Cynthia B. Olsen (1996). With Elaine Alexander's death, the Essiac craze seems to have abated somewhat.

I once received from the manufacturer an unpublished report on 162 patients treated with Essiac in Israel. Approximately 50 percent reported relief from the side effects of chemotherapy; 20 percent were said to have had some regression of their tumors (including cancers of the liver, lungs, lymphoma, leukemia, etc.); while five percent were allegedly "healed completely." But half of this last group were also on chemotherapy. Thus, only 2.5 percent (4 patients) were "healed completely" on Essiac alone. When I tried to get more data from the Israeli clinician, I got no response to repeated faxes and phone calls. I do not set great store by this report, but present it as typical of the "data" that is occasionally provided in support of the mixture. It would not surprise me at all if the remission rate with Essiac alone was in fact around 2.5 percent.

In other words, I believe there is an effect, but a small one. The most telling quote comes from the afterword to the book, *Essiac: A Native Herbal Cancer Remedy.* It is by Jim Chan, ND, a well-known Canadian naturopath. Obviously, he is considered pro-Essiac if his statement is sought out by advocates of the tea. Yet he states, "Based on the observation of thousands of cancer cases, I have not found Essiac to be effective across the board. However, there were cases that showed promising results. The majority of other cases needed other forms of support and intervention" (306). This is reasonable.

I also agree with the statement of Keith Block, MD, a well-regarded Evanston, IL oncologist who also uses complementary treatments in his medical practice. He has characterized Essiac as a "weak combination of anticancer herbs." Robert Atkins, MD, of New York calls Essiac a "mild...therapeutic" tea that can "contribute to feelings of well-being which in turn influence the patients' quality of life and potential for recovery" (401). Each of these clinicians has seen innumerable cases of cancer and a wide variety of treatments and situations. The fact that they are still using Essiac is telling; but claims for the product are deliberately kept low key.

But what about all those cures? Well, the historical record is very difficult to interpret. There are many changes in medical procedures and terminology that make reading and interpreting old medical records difficult. Not all of this is the fault of Essiac's proponents.

For example, in the late 1980s, Gar Hildenbrand and colleagues at the Gerson Research Institute, San Diego, California, undertook a retrospective analysis of the melanoma cases treated according to the methods of the late Max Gerson, MD. This analysis was finally published in 1995 (180). It took more than six years to produce. Obviously, then, accurate epidemiological evaluations of patient outcomes in a non-conventional setting require painstaking and time-consuming work. Glib demands for "proof" based on such records underestimates the difficulty.

In some instances, too, sources of historical data disappeared, as doctors who initially were enthusiastic about Essiac "recanted" or went silent when Caisse lost her battle with the Medical Society.

We must also recognize that the general situation of today's cancer patient is quite different than what it was in Caisse's heyday. In those times, many of Caisse's cancer patients were treated with just surgery. But before they get around to taking Essiac, today's patients have probably received high dose chemotherapy, and hormonal, or radiation treatments. These can have disastrous and unpredictable effects on the immune system and other organs. Thus, any host-mediated effects of the herbs would probably be dissipated in trying to overcome the immune-suppressing effects of conventional approaches.

The physical, sociological, and psychological climate are strikingly different today, as well. Caisse's patients were part of a mass movement, and this could have influenced their will to survive and thrive. As another example: there are the deleterious effects of food additives, food colorings, herbicide, and pesticide residues and other chemicals in the food, air, water, and workplace. These have an undetermined effect on immunity.

Furthermore, today's patient is likely to utilize not just conventional anti-cancer drugs, but other pharmaceuticals, over-the-counter medications, food supplements, and a variety of non-conventional approaches, herbal and otherwise. In the pre-war period, most patients just took Essiac—or nothing. The prevalence of polypharmacy makes any outcome almost impossible to interpret.

Another important factor, usually glossed over by promoters and enthusiasts, is that traditionally Essiac was simultaneously injected and taken orally. Today, it is only taken as a brew of some sort. One would expect that the injected formula would have stronger and more rapid effects than any oral preparation, although as we have seen, it carries real dangers of its own.

I have vowed not to buttress arguments with unconfirmed anecdotes: there are certainly more than enough of these to go around in the promotional literature.

However, I would like to share some stories about Essiac I have heard over the years. To be truly scientific, the details of these stories would have to be carefully tracked down, something I do not have the resources to do. Nevertheless, I think they at least give some of the flavor of the claims that underlie the surprising persistence of Essiac.

There was a well-documented case in the *Townsend Letter for Doctors & Patients* of a man who seems to have thrown off prostate cancer with Essiac (401). The manufacturer once put me in touch with a man who seemed to have had a very similar remission of a stage III bladder cancer in the same manner. He came to my lecture in Toronto with photographs of necrotic material he had expelled with his urine. It was very dramatic. Another person of my acquaintance had a partial remission of a widely disseminated non-Hodgkin's lymphoma after taking Essiac. In 1995, he finished eight rounds of CHOP chemotherapy, when the tumors started to grow back. He then started to take Flor·Essence, two ounces three times per day on an empty stomach. Three weeks later all tumors had stabilized and a few had begun to shrink.

In mid-March, 1996, he added another non-conventional treatment, hydrazine sulfate. After several months on this dual regimen, the lymph nodes in his groin and armpit were markedly smaller. He had regained the muscle mass that he had lost in the previous year. He was still in partial remission about six months later, when I lost touch.

I once met a woman who had had stage IV breast cancer. As she was getting out of her car one day, her husband impatiently told her that he wished she would die, since she was slowing him down. The next day she filed for divorce and determined to get well to spite him. To do this, she mainly relied on Essiac. When I met her in Toronto it had been many years and she was in good health. I did not see her medical records, but she seemed like a credible witness.

A friend of mine who is a professor at an Ivy League medical school took me aside once and asked, "What is this Essiac tea?" He told me of a woman, also with stage IV breast cancer, who had a complete remission of her cancer on Essiac. The two professors who had sent her home to die were quite astounded when she walked back into their office some months later, free of cancer.

Mistaken diagnoses? Residual effects of conventional treatment? Spontaneous remission? Outright fraud? Who knows? The fact is, such questions cannot be answered outside the context of carefully designed clinical studies. But historically, neither side in this dispute has evinced much interest in designing studies that could fairly evaluate the treatment. Both sides potentially have had much to lose from such studies.

Proponents who claim that Essiac yields an "incredible recovery rate of 80 percent" will be deflated if that rate turns out to be a modest five to six percent (306). On the other hand, the "cancer establishment" has gone out on such a limb that even a modest five or six percent success rate will be devastating to the pretense of infallibility. It is only intelligent cancer patients and their loved ones who have sufficient motivation to demand factual evaluations of this and similar treatments.

Chapter 8 ❧ The Grape Cure

AS FAR BACK AS ONE GOES IN HISTORY, THERE HAS BEEN AN ASSOCIATION BETWEEN GRAPES AND HEALTH. WHOLE GRAPES, GRAPE seeds, leaves, raisins, juice, wine, brandy—and recently grapeseed extract—have been touted as special healing substances.

While we don't normally think of grapes as "herbs," they are included in most herbals and botanical gardens. They are among those special foods that occasionally come to the fore as nearly miraculous healing agents, and therefore play an important role in our history.

Grapes are so familiar that they hardly would seem to need any introduction. They are a woody vine, which climbs by means of tendrils (i.e., modified branches), and can reach a length of 50 feet or more. In arid climes, grapes may take the form of a semi-erect shrub. Grapes have small, greenish flowers, in clusters, that precede the fruit. The fruit varies in color from nearly black to green, red or amber. This fruit is technically a globular berry, within whose juicy pulp lie the seeds. In many varieties, the fruit develops a white powdery coating, called the blush.

Fossilized grape leaves, stem pieces, and seeds have been unearthed from Miocene and Tertiary deposits in the Northern Hemisphere, indicating the prehistoric existence and wide distribution of the vine. The species that are native to North America include *Vitis labrusca* and *Vitis aestivalis,* the American wild bunch grape; and *Vitis rotundifolia,* the popular muscadine of the American Southeast. *Vitis vinifera* is the species most widely used to make wine. It was successfully cultivated in the Old World for thousands of years and eventually brought to California (*EB* 5:428).

At the present time, grape and wine production are notable in France, Italy, and Spain, as well as Turkey, Algeria, Argentina, Chile, Greece, Hungary, Portugal, Romania, and the United States.

Grapes are incredibly complex, or perhaps because of their economic importance they have just been better studied than other plants. In either case, science knows of about 350 separate constituents, including many which are unique to this plant. We are only at the beginning of our knowledge of grapes' physiological effects.

The grape is mentioned in most of the major herbals, but it is mainly considered in its role as a food and beverage. However, there is another less known aspect to grapes, and that is, its use as a medicinal herb.

Dr. Solomon Solis Cohen's 1901 *System of Physiological Therapeutics* tells the reader about a dozen Central European sanitaria that practiced what he called "the grape cure." The grape cure consisted of visiting a resort near a region of vineyards, and then gorging on grapes. Autumn was the natural time to pursue such a pleasant course.

One of the centers of the cure was in Baden-Baden, in the Black Forest region of Germany. This lovely town was chosen not just for its charming location, mild climate, and Celtic-Roman baths, but because of its close proximity to the vineyards of the nearby Rhine river valley.

Although in Germany the grape cure is now mainly history, Baden-Baden retains its reputation as a shrine of complementary medicine. It is quite fitting that the nutritionally-oriented German Society of Oncology holds its annual convention there every fall.

Johanna Brandt

The grape cure would probably have gone the way of the horse-drawn coach if it hadn't been for an enterprising South African lady named Johanna Brandt. She was born in South Africa in 1876, and as an adult experienced a "gnawing pain at the left side of her stomach." At that time the American socialist writer, Upton Sinclair, had written a popular book titled *The Fasting Cure*. So Brandt started fasting, but the pain only got worse. She had no diagnosis, but she believed that a "growth was now pushing its way through the diaphragm, toward the heart and left lung." She had a vivid imagination. "I seemed to see it like a red octopus feeding on the impure blood at the base of the lung," she wrote. "Breathing became difficult. I spat blood occasionally."

In November, 1921, she finally admitted herself to Johannesburg's General Hospital for an x-ray examination. Many images were taken and finally a noted surgeon pronounced his verdict. "The stomach was being divided in two by a vicious, fibrous growth. An immediate operation was recommended as the only means of prolonging my life." However, the adamant Mrs. Brandt refused this advice. Instead, she fasted some more, drinking only pure water and lying in the morning sun. When she returned to the hospital six months later, in mid-1922, followup X rays revealed that "no trace of the growth could be found!" (51)

Assuming the facts are as she reports them, we are still left with many questions. The x-ray photographs showed a "vicious, fibrous growth." But what was the nature of this growth? X-ray plates alone generally cannot distinguish a malignant from a benign tumor. Mrs. Brandt reported that she was often subsequently asked, "How do you know that you had cancer?"

"This could not be proven in my own case," she admits, "because I had not been surgically examined." Bear in mind, also, that Mrs. Brandt's "remission"—if that's what it was—was truly spontaneous in nature. It may have been the result of fasting, sunlight, and prayer, but at this point she still had not discovered any special healing herb or food.

Nevertheless, she was still in pain, although, from her doctor's point of view, there didn't seem to have been anything physically wrong with her. Three years later, in 1925, she "accidentally discovered a food that had the miraculous effect of healing me completely within six weeks." That food, of course, was the grape. She began lecturing in South Africa about grapes and about her miraculous recovery.

In 1927, she left her family and set off for the United States to publicize her big idea. She had a letter of introduction to Benedict Lust, MD, ND, DO, who was considered the father of Naturopathy in America. He suggested that she speak to Bernarr Macfadden (1868-1955), a famous physical culturist who made a fortune in the publishing business. Among his enterprises was a sensationalist New York newspaper called the *Evening Graphic*.

Ms. Brandt's story was published in the magazine section of that paper (1/21/28). This created a sensation and a book-length version of the article was published shortly thereafter. It was endorsed by Lust and his backing certainly helped establish Brandt's story as an iconical part of the Naturopathic movement. (Seventy years later, *The Grape Cure* is still readily available, with Lust's endorsement, in most health food stores.)

For virtually every condition, Johanna Brandt recommended the following: First the patient should fast for two or three days, drinking plenty of pure, cold water and should take an enema of a quart of lukewarm water daily. (She recommended a little pure white soap in the enema, but few doctors would make that recommendation today.)

After the fast, the patient drinks one or two glasses of pure, cold water the first thing in the morning. Half an hour later the patient has his or her first meal of well-washed grapes. "Chew the skins and seeds thoroughly and swallow a few of them as food and roughage." Starting at eight AM and having a grape meal every two hours until eight PM, this would give seven grape meals daily. This is kept up for a week or two, even a month or two, in chronic cases of long standing, but not longer.

Mrs. Brandt said that any good variety of grape could be used. Hothouse grapes were better than none, and the seedless varieties were excellent. "The monotony of the diet may be varied by using many varieties," she writes. The quantity varies according to the condition, digestion, and occupation of the patient. Most patients begin with one, two or three ounces per meal, gradually increasing this until they double the quantity. In time, she says, about half a pound may be safely taken at a meal. A minimum quantity of one pound per day should be used, while the maximum should not exceed four pounds. Invariably, she writes, the best results have been effected when grapes have been taken in small quantities. A "loathing of grapes" may indicate the need for a fast, she writes. Indeed.

To verify her claims, Mrs. Brandt called upon "the medical council [sic] to have an exploratory operation performed" on herself. This was "the only way the efficacy of the cure can be established." It was a dramatic offer, to be sure. Although she dreaded being "hurried to the house of slaughter," as she called the hospitals of her day, she needn't have feared. No hostile physicians were about to respond to her challenge.

I must repeat, the efficacy of grapes to cure cancer never was an issue in Brandt's own case, since the tumor disappeared three years before she started eating grapes. If anything, grapes helped her deal with the residual pain, yet oddly, Mrs. Brandt concluded that all her fasting had been unnecessary. "The mistakes I made need not be made by other patients," she concluded. Yet it seems to have been the fasting, not the grapes, that cured her (if she ever really had cancer at all, which is not certain).

Ms. Brandt was convinced that she had found in grapes a panacea for all human ills. "A method that will cure cancer may cure almost any other disease," she wrote. "What is more, it may prevent cancer and almost every other disease." She exulted, "I have watched our old people getting young and our young people becoming superbly beautiful." All by virtue of eating pound after pound of grapes.

The inevitable next step was that in 1927 Mrs. Brandt set herself up in the cancer business in New York City, not just advocating but treating people with the grape cure. This was the time that Hoxsey was hitting his stride in Taylorville, Illinois, and Rene Caisse was developing her Essiac treatment in Toronto. That same year, Morris Fishbein, MD, editor of the AMA *Journal,* published a book titled *The New Medical Follies.* "Cult follows cult," he complained, "and quackery succeeds quackery, frequently with amazing rapidity" (132).

Since Mrs. Brandt had no medical credentials, she took the time honored course of allying herself with a medical doctor. "Our test cases will go down in history," she wrote, with no false modesty. Although she says "the details of all our test cases have been carefully tabulated for publication," these are nowhere to be found in her book, or anywhere else, to my knowledge.

Mrs. Brandt also states that all the cases she saw in New York recovered under her treatment. "After beginning the grape diet," she wrote about one woman, "the pus poured from her. When she began to pass worms, I knew that the terrible ordeal was nearly over....Sanctified by suffering, this woman has emerged from the abyss of premature death to be a witness to the divine healing properties of the grape." The grape seemed to regain the religious significance it had at the time of Dionysus.

In another case, she visited a patient in the Bronx who was clearly dying of advanced colorectal cancer. Brandt therefore wrapped her swollen limbs in grape compresses, in order to open the pores. This worked and "wonderfully to relate, the hard mass in the ascending colon had been disappearing gradually. Nothing was left of that...."

Brandt used grape poultices as an escharotic for the treatment of external cancer. "The grape apparently eats its way deeper and deeper into the diseased flesh and the wounds do not heal until all the poisons have been eliminated. Then the healing seems to proceed from within."

Brandt did admit that, as in her own case, "some of our test cases may likewise be disputed...." In fact, she seemed aware that her anecdotal accounts of cured left much to be desired.

Here is her idea of a sure-fire case: a woman had one breast removed because it was cancerous. The other, she says, was "heavy with suppuration, ready to be removed." There was "pus forming again in the scarred remains of the tissues on which the operation had been performed—these ominous signs striking a chill to the heart." Once again, grapes to the rescue. But did the woman have cancer in the second breast? Pus alone is not a sufficient diagnostic sign.

In fact, all of the cases in *The Grape Cure* are like that—unconvincing from a scientific point of view. Grapes may cure cancer. But there is certainly no convincing proof of that in Johanna Brandt's book.

Toxicity

Grapes are an excellent food and are non-toxic. One can safely take fairly large amounts. However, grapes and grape products (e.g., wine) are often heavily sprayed with pesticides, which is a limiting factor.

There has been little research until recently into the potential anticancer effects of grapes. However, recent research has taken two directions. The first has been into certain antioxidants called procyanidolic oligomers (PCOs) found in grape seeds.

The second has been the discovery of a substance named resveratrol, a natural phytoalexin found in grapes, which may play a role in preventing heart attacks. Resveratrol appears also to inhibit cellular processes that are associated with tumor initiation, promotion, and progression (276).

Most of the known vitamins and trace minerals are present in grapes.

Resveratrol (which is related to another compound found in health food stores, quercetin) is found in wine at twice the level of grape juce. It is almost entirely absent from white wine (except champagne) but is found in abundance in most of the reds, especially Pinot Noir, Merlot and a German wine called Zweigeltrebe. (It is also present in peanuts.)

Scientists have concluded that "resveratrol has a direct antiproliferative effect on human breast epithelial cells that is independent of the estrogen receptor status of the cells. Thus, this dietary compound is a potential chemopreventive agent for both hormone responsive and non-responsive breast cancers" (338). So maybe Brandt was onto something.

In addition, there has been a considerable amount of epidemiological support for the notion that people in areas of high wine consumption have lower rates of cancer than other areas.

For what it's worth, a few years ago I was contacted by two individuals in California who claimed to have totally cured themselves of advanced cancers by following the advice in Brandt's book. They weren't trying to sell me anything, but asked that I use their cases to educate my readers. I found them both credible people, with good stories to tell, but unfortunately I was unable to obtain solid documentation of their cases.

Chapter 9 ❧ Mistletoes and Medicine

T HE CANCER HERBAL CONTROVERSY IN GERMANY HAS FOCUSED ON PREPARATIONS MADE FROM A SINGLE PLANT, MISTLETOE *(VISCUM album,* or 'Mistel' in German). To its advocates, mistletoe preparations are useful adjuvant cancer treatments that occasionally result in remarkable "cures." To detractors, they are quack remedies propounded by a mystical sect for commercial and ideological reasons. For a long time, the mistletoe therapy was on the American Cancer Society's "unproven" or "questionable" methods list, although it is not discussed in the current version on complementary and alternative treatments.

At the moment, mistletoe is out of the doghouse, but not yet fully accepted in the United States as a legitimate treatment. However, mistletoe treatment is legal in Germany, on the official *Rote Liste* of drugs, and is also registered with the Swiss Inter-Cantonal Office for drug control. It is available in Germany, Switzerland, the Netherlands, the United Kingdom, Austria and Sweden. Commercial preparations of mistletoe can be legally prescribed by licensed physicians in these countries, according to the US Office of Technology Assessment report (394).

However, because of FDA regulations, no injectable mistletoe preparations are available in the United States. In my discussions with officials of the European manufacturers, it became clear that seeking FDA approval would be too onerous and expensive. And so American patients must either go abroad to receive such treatment at a foreign clinic or else import three-months' worth for their personal use from a European company.

Mistletoe is quite unique in that it is a green parasitic plant that does not normally grow in the ground but on the branches of trees, where it forms pendant bushes, two to five feet in diameter. As Nicholas Culpeper (1616-1654) said, its seed "was never yet known to spring being put into the ground, or anywhere else to grow" (90).

Viscum album is a European plant that survives and thrives in a broad swath from western France up to Scandinavia and all the way into Asiatic Russia. Unlike other parasites, it is a green plant, which engages in photosynthesis. Mistletoes can grow on a variety of hosts. In the 1850s, scholars cataloged their occurrences. Apple was the most common, followed closely by black poplar. But mistletoes were also found on horse chestnut, maple, poplar, acacia, laburnum, pear, large-leaved sallow, locust, larch, Scottish fir, spruce, service, olive, vine, walnut, plum, common laurel, medlar, and gray poplar (58, 85). The most significant historically was also the rarest, oak (see below).

The mistletoe is a kind of "infection" of the tree. But a host can live for many years with such unwanted fellow travelers. After about 50 years, the burden of mistletoes may become so great that they simply overwhelm the host tree, which then dies. As afflictions go, it is relatively benign, and many trees die of other causes before they die of their mistletoe.

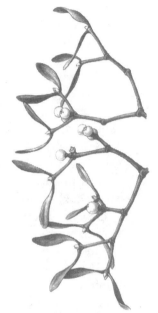

Viscum album
(mistletoe)

Mistletoe has an unusual means of propagation, which was already recognized in antiquity: its shiny white berry is swallowed by birds, particularly the mistle thrush. The bird digests just the outer skin and part of the pulp and within five or six minutes deposits it on a branch, commingled with its dung (221). In 1532, the early English herbalist, William Turner (1520-1568), wrote with the candor typical of his day, "The thrush shiteth out the miscel berries." In fact, the Old English mistel (mistletoe) is a diminutive of *Mist*, which in German means dung.

It is impossible to discuss mistletoe without noting its extraordinary role in mythology, ritual, and folklore. All around the world, but especially in central Europe, there have been ancient traditions about the mystical and magical uses of this plant. In fact, some consider it the single "most sacred and magical of plants" (154).

"From time immemorial," wrote the great anthropologist Sir James Frazer (1854-1941), "the mistletoe has been the object of superstitious veneration in Europe" (138, 389). It has been used in magic, religious ritual, and medicine—ancient societies did not always clearly distinguish between the three.

"In winter," says Frazer, "the sight of its fresh foliage among the bare branches must have been hailed by the [pre-Christian] worshippers of the tree as a sign that the divine life which had ceased to animate the branches yet survived in the mistletoe, as the heart of a sleeper still beats when his body is motionless" (138).

Frazer's life work, *The Golden Bough*, is named for the mistletoe, since he was convinced that the branch with which Aeneas sought the underworld was made of this plant. The mistletoe sometimes has golden berries and the whole branch turns golden when it is cut and left to dry.

Mistletoe also plays an important role in Norse mythology, where it had unexpected powers. The myth recognized its uniqueness from all the other plants in the vegetable kingdom. In giving the benificent god Balder protection from harm, the gods overlooked the insignificant mistletoe. The dart with which the evil god Hoder killed Balder was made of "Mstelteinn."

In mythology, mistletoe was frequently identified with the sun (and with the oak). There was a cult of Apollo Ixius, at Ixiae in Rhodes, that was allegedly named for the mistletoe (90). Even Culpeper knew of this association in the 17th century, for he wrote "This is under the dominion of the Sun, I do not question."

Mistletoe berries ripened in October, and were present throughout the winter, which itself generated awe. It was called the "winter flower" that killed the sun. The berries were also worshipped as the fertilizing dew of the supreme spirit. They were thought to be drops of the gods' semen.

In an oft-quoted passage, the ancient encyclopedist Pliny the Elder (23–79 AD) wrote that mistletoes, especially those growing on the oak tree, were worshipped by the Celtic priesthood, the Druids, who "went forth clad in white robes to search for the sacred plant, and when it was discovered, one of the Druids ascended the tree and gathered it with great ceremony, separating it from the Oak with a golden knife" (319).

They apparently thought that the fact that the mistletoe grew in a tree's branches, rather than on the ground, gave it a more "ethereal" nature. The Gallas of Africa said the mistletoe is grafted onto the tree the way the soul is grafted onto the body (71).

The Druids called it "all-healer." Nearly 2,000 years later, their modern Celtic descendants in Brittany, Wales, Scotland, and Ireland still call mistletoe "an t'uil," which means "all healer." This tradition continued into the 20th century (155).

All mistletoe were believed to have their uses, but the variety that stimulated the greatest interest, to the Druids and others, were those that grew on the oak. Culpeper also states "that which grows upon oaks, participates something of the nature of Jupiter, because an oak is one of his trees." This fascination with oak mistletoe had something to do with its rarity: mistletoes grow on oaks in only one in one hundred thousand cases.

Pliny also tells us that the efficacy of mistletoe was dependent on the manner in which it was harvested. It was to be gathered on the first day of the new moon. In harvesting, it was not allowed to touch the ground and no iron was to be used in separating it from the tree. To accomplish this, the Druids used the famous golden scythe to separate it from the host. It is thought that Pliny was referring not just to northern priests but to the practices of his contemporaries in Italy as well (138).

To my knowledge, Druids no longer file into the countryside by the light of the moon. Today, the company that manufactures Iscador advertises in French rural newspapers, offering generous rewards for the discovery of oak mistletoes. The location of these trees is a carefully guarded secret.

In more modern times, in many parts of the Continent, mistletoe could not be cut in the ordinary way, but had to be knocked off the tree with stones. A noteworthy center of belief in mistletoe was in the Aargau region of Switzerland. There, the peasants "shrink from cutting it off in the usual manner. Instead of that they procure it in the following manner: when the sun is in Sagittarius and the moon is on the wane, on the first, third, or fourth day before the new moon, one ought to shoot down with an arrow the mistletoe of an oak and to catch it with the left hand as it falls. Such mistletoe is a remedy for every ailment of children" (274).

How extraordinary that present-day mistletoe medicines are manufactured just a few miles west of the Swiss district in which the above practices were recorded in the mid-19th century.

Skeptics make fun of the manner in which mistletoe is gathered. A quack-baiting Website sneers at claims that "the time of picking the plants [is] important because they react to the influences of the sun, moon, and planets." However, there is a core of rationality to many traditional practices. Certain chemicals in mistletoe can combine with metals to form organometallic compounds, which have different biological or medicinal properties than the ones naturally found in the plant. This is probably why the Druids and others empirically forbade the harvesting of mistletoes with iron knives, but insisted on using the (chemically inert) golden scythes. Similarly, by not letting the mistletoe touch the ground, they avoided contact with other substances that might lessen its power.

The time and manner in which a plant is gathered can affect its chemical composition. For example, the yield of podophyllin from mayapple (*Podophyllum peltatum*) has been known for over a century to be affected by the time of year in which it is gathered (42). (It is high in April, but scanty in July.) Similarly, there are different chemical properties to the summer and winter saps of mistletoe. In current practice they are mixed together in an elaborate and costly way.

Wherever it occurs, mistletoe is the object of awe. The 19th century Ainu of Japan held the mistletoe in "peculiar veneration" (Frazer) and regarded it as a virtual panacea. They esteemed the variety that grew on the willow, their sacred tree (28). Africans in Senegal and Gambia venerated a kind of mistletoe called "tob." A 19th century traveler remarked that there is "...something supernatural in a plant which grows and flourishes without having roots in the earth. May they not have believed, in fact, that it was a plant fallen from the sky, a gift of the divinity?" (31)

Mistletoe and Cancer

In his chapter on "Misselto," Nicholas Culpeper states that "the birdlime [associated with mistletoe] doth mollify hard knots, tumours, and imposthumes; ripens and discusses them, and draws forth thick as well as thin humours from the remote parts of the body, digesting and separating them..." (90). (An impostume is a purulent swelling, cyst, or abscess.) This may be the first literary reference to the use of mistletoe against a kind of neoplastic growth.

Throughout history, there have been scattered references to the use of mistletoe against cancer, although epilepsy has always been its main indication. In the late 19th and early 20th century, an herbalist named E.F.W. Powell used half an ounce each of red clover blossoms, yellow dock root, dandelion root, violet leaves, and mistletoe as a cancer treatment. He added to this one-quarter ounce of goldenseal root and licorice. These herbs were gently simmered in three pints of boiling water for 20 minutes, and then strained. Patients took a wine glassful every two hours.

However this plant's introduction into modern cancer therapeutics was the work of a man who had no training in medicine. Rudolf Steiner, PhD (1861-1925) was one of the most extraordinary intellectual figures of the early 20th century. His friends and disciples (and there are still about 50,000 of them around the world) called him the "scientific seer."

His original area of study was the scientific work of the poet Johann Goethe (1749-1832), the greatest figure of German Romanticism. This choice of work shows that Steiner straddled the usually separate worlds of literature and science. He was also a mystic, clairvoyant, and a system-builder in esoteric philosophy.

Steiner considered the myth of Balder true on a symbolic level. "Deep truths lie hidden in the Mysteries," wrote one of his disciples. "In the distant past during the time of the creation of the myths, people were still able to describe, in picture form, what took place in the Cosmos and on Earth" (265).

Kissing under the Mistletoe

Most readers will be familiar with the custom of kissing under the mistletoe, or kissing bunch, at Christmas time. Legend has it that if two people kiss under a mistletoe branch they will fall in love. Millions of people lightheartedly perform this ceremony without stopping to consider its ancient roots. In ancient times, kissing under mistletoe was a sign not just of love but of atonement, good will, and reconciliation. The reasons for this are obscure. Mistletoe, as a plant that thrives in winter, has long been associated with Christmas. In the so-called tree calendar, it is associated with December 23. Its connection to kissing is a carry-over of various pagan beliefs in the plant's generative powers. Frazer said it was connected to Saturnalia, a festival which took place during what is now Christmas.

Balder, the Nordic god of Peace, was slain by an arrow made of mistletoe. He was then restored to life at the intercession of the other gods and goddesses and the mistletoe plant was put under the protection of the goddess of Love. It was then ordained that everyone who passes under this plant should receive a kiss to show that the branch had become an emblem of love, not hate (153).

Needless to say, the fact that mistletoe therapy has its roots in "occult-based practices" has not endeared it to the quackbusters. In fact, they deride him and his ideas as a prime example of "New Age" medicine.

Steiner's insights into cancer medicine were based more on tradition than modern science. Yet, as we shall see, he had good intuition. In 1900, he began working with the physicians among his followers, suggesting ideas about the treatment of illness. In 1907, he referred to mistletoe as "ein bestimmtes Heilmittel" (a definite remedy or cure). He discussed mistletoe as treatments for uterine and breast cancer before World War I. In 1917, he proposed to a Zurich medical doctor Dr. Ita Wegman (1876-1943), that she investigate the use of mistletoe in the treatment for cancer.

She began to treat patients with it in that year (172). In Anthroposophical terms, this event was regarded as a kind of "world-compensation....A human being, familiar with the light realms of the gods and consciously united with the world of the spirit, suggested mistletoe as a cancer remedy to a physician..." (265).

In 1920, Steiner gave a course of lectures for both allopathic and homoeopathic physicians, called "Spiritual Science and Medicine." As a result, an increasing number of doctors began to work with him. At that time Steiner put forward the revolutionary suggestion that cancer was not just a cellular disease, but a disease of the whole organism:

"In our organism we fight in a permanent way against the life of the cells. The worst misconception is brought about by cellular pathology which considers the human organism as an edifice made out of cells, whereas the human being is an entity connected with the cosmos and has really a constant fight with the obstinacy of the cells" (251).

After Steiner's death in 1925, Dr. Ita Wegman published a book on their mutual work, called *Fundamentals of Therapy*. During those years, she worked with a Zurich pharmacist, A. Hauser, to produce a mistletoe cancer remedy The use of this was expanded by N. Kaelin and then by Drs. Alexandre Leroi and his wife, Dr. Rita Leroi von May (217). The end result was a product that came to be known as "Iscador," as well as other companies' products, Helixor, Iscucin, Vysorel, and ABNOVAviscum (92).

Iscador was the first commercial preparation of Mistletoe, and remains the best-known of the five modern-day remedies derived from the plant. There also are several different Iscadors, depending on the method of preparation and intended use. Thus, Iscador M refers to a preparation made from mistletoe growing on apple trees; Iscador Qu, oak tree mistletoe, is used mainly for men. Iscador P, from pine trees, is used for men and women, as is Iscador U, made from elms.

There are also homoeopathic doses of metals added to some of these preparations, which are thought to enhance the activity of the botanical. Copper is used for primary tumors of the liver, gallbladder, stomach and kidneys. Iscador with tiny amounts of mercury is used to treat tumors of the intestines and lymphatic systems. Iscador with silver is used to treat cancers of the urogenital system and the breast. And Iscador without any additives is used to treat tumors of the tongue, oral cavity, esophagus, nasopharynx, thyroid, larynx, and extremities (394).

The Anthroposophy movement already owned a pharmaceutical and cosmetic company named Weleda, which was founded in 1921. While Iscador was made in Switzerland, Weleda became the distributor of Iscador and other such medicines around the world. Presently, it operates a five-story factory in Swäbisch Gmünd (Bavaria). It produces many cosmetics, toothpastes, and herbal mixtures, which are famous around the world for their high quality.

There are many subtle differences between the Iscadors as well as different indications for their use. It is a life work to master all the intricacies of this science, a field of study that is unknown to the vast majority of oncologists. In 1978, it was estimated that almost 2,000,000 ampules were sold in countries where Iscador is legal and that about 30,000 patients are treated with it each year. I think this number is much higher today.

Dr. Wegman also founded a small hospital in Arlesheim, Switzerland, just a few miles from the world center of Anthroposophy in Dornach. It was there that Iscador was first used in the treatment of cancer. This was a time of great hope in cancer. Anthroposophists hoped that in Iscador they had found a true cure for cancer. However, "when the first great hopes that many of his friends had placed upon mistletoe therapy were dashed in the 1940s, [Dr. Alexandre Leroi] steadfastly continued his investigations and treatments with the mistletoe preparation, Iscador" (172).

Steiner the Visionary

Steiner was involved with esoteric trends, such as Rosicrucianism. (His grave in Dornach, Switzerland is adorned with a rosy cross cut in stone.) Under the sponsorship of a wealthy Russian princess, he founded a movement called Anthroposophy (the wisdom of man), which emphasized Central European traditions of Christian mysticism, such as those of Meister Eckhart (c. 1260-1327) and Novalis (1772-1801).

Steiner was clearly a brilliant man and a polymath, whose interests included virtually every sphere of human activity. He founded the Waldorf Schools, which spread from their original base in Stuttgart all over the world. He was a pioneer of organic farming (Biodynamic Agriculture), at a time when most of the world was yielding to artificial farming practices. He was also a sculptor and architect, who designed the astonishing cathedral of Anthroposophy, the Goetheanum in Dornach.

The Wegman Clinic still exists as a general hospital run along Anthroposophical lines. However, in 1963, Leroi established another small hospital across the street. This they called the Lukas Klinik, after the gospel writer who was also the first Christian physician. Administration of this clinic was in the hands of Dr. Leroi's physician-wife, Rita, who cared for cancer patients for the next 25 years. The Lukas Klinik expanded to in-patient status in the late 1960s. They also added a facility to train physicians in the use of mistletoe therapy.

Although most conventional treatment is administered before patients arrive at Arlesheim, clinic doctors sometimes do administer less-toxic forms of chemotherapy at the clinic itself. They claim that patients suffer far fewer side effects when their treatment is combined with Iscador and other forms of holistic treatment.

Nor is Iscador the sole treatment given there. The overall approach is mainly spiritual, not biochemical. Some of the "treatments" patients are encouraged to participate in include a kind of dance-exercise called Eurhythmy, also invented by Steiner. Eurhythmy is designed to raise patients' spirits and simultaneously stimulate circulation. The Lukas Klinik has facilities for light therapy (which mostly involves staring at screens of different colors in a darkened room), art therapy, and music therapy using a variety of instruments, some of them quite strange.

Like all Steinerian institutions, all Anthroposophical hospitals eschew straight lines and artificial building materials. Common day items are crafted out of expensive woods. Unlike American hospitals, all electronic instruments are hidden out of sight. There are no televisions in the rooms but there is a well-stocked library. Thomas Mann's *Magic Mountain* would be a particularly good choice of reading material.

Gathering Mistletoe

Production of Iscador requires an international effort. Various kinds of mistletoe are gathered by teams of Anthroposophical workers in both summer and winter from southwestern France. Special procedures and precautions are used in gathering the plant, similar to those mentioned by Pliny 2,000 years ago.

I was told that French farmers are happy to get rid of their mistletoes, since they regard them as worthless parasites. The plants are carefully cut and then trucked to Switzerland, where they are processed at the Helixor laboratory in Arlesheim, across the street from the Lukas Klinik. This sterile facility is built around an enormous centrifuge, which mixes the summer and winter mistletoe saps in carefully defined proportions. There is also research into the medical and scientific properties of the product. In some ways, this looks like a typical scientific laboratory that could be found anywhere in the world. In other ways, however, it is quite different, since its activity is almost entirely centered on a single herb.

The mistletoe sap is tested for purity and strength and freed of any bacteria or other contaminants that could cause untoward side effects or interfere with its action. From the Arlesheim laboratory, the processed liquid is shipped to the Weleda factory in Swäbisch Gmünd, Germany, a small city outside Stuttgart. Here it is put into glass ampules in a special clean room on the top floor. When I visited in 1997, several technicians were hard at work in what looked like Mylar space suits. The entire factory seemed remarkably well organized.

The machines were not run at high speed, in order to allow ample time for checking and rechecking the products. The workers I met were clearly intelligent and highly motivated. The physical surroundings were clean and attractive. (There was even a huge mural in the stairwell depicting the evolution of life from the mineral world on the first floor to the spiritual world on the top.)

Everything connected with Iscador's production struck me as sanitary, well-organized, and infused with a sense of purpose and responsibility. I was informed that the price of Iscador is kept low so that it will be available to all cancer patients and in effect is subsidized by the popular Weleda line of sanitary and cosmetic products. Weleda maintains among the highest quality standards of any "alternative medicine" in the world.

In a book on Rudolf Steiner's Anthroposophical medicine, *Spiritual Science and the Art of Healing,* Victor Bott, MD, gives various explanations of the process of biological growth: "It is the result of two activities, one of multiplication arising from the etheric forces, and the other of form-building, the sculpturing activity of the forces of the astral body and the ego which transforms the etheric forces into formative forces" (50).

In his first course of lectures on medicine, Steiner put forward a philosophy of cancer that was similar to the 19th century theory of "embryonal rests" that is associated with the name of Julius Cohnheim (1839-1884) (367, 83).

Cohnheim was a scientific materialist, whose theory presupposed the existence of physical residues of embryonic material, which could be triggered to grow into cancer.

Steiner, being a philosophical idealist, thought that etheric forces constituted the "islets of organization."

Steiner had other very strange and provocative ideas about cancer. He regarded cancer as an "ectopic sense organ." That is because in sense organs, and in a more general way in nerve-sense systems, "form production is pushed to an extreme at the expense of the powers of regeneration." The organizing forces of the ego and the "astral body" withdraw to a greater or a lesser extent, and the organ is exposed to external influences and "becomes the plaything of chaotic forces." Steiner suggested mistletoe as a means of strengthening the defenses of the organism "in the direction of structuration" (50).

Steiner's disciples have taken issue with some of the basic assumptions of Western biology. Friedrich Lorenz, MD has written "Cellular pathology and cellular physiology are under the crassest misconception when they designate the cell as the basis of all life and regard the human organism merely as a conglomeration of cells. The truth is that the human being is to be seen as an entirety, in relation to the cosmos...In reality, it is the cell which constantly disturbs our organism instead of building it up" (265).

Needless to say, these ideas are not typical of modern oncology. I quote them here to show how profound is the gulf between the conventional and the Anthroposophical views of this disease, indeed of life. Yet Iscador has been adopted by hundreds, possibly thousands, of physicians in Europe as an adjunct treatment for cancer. For example, in Switzerland, among 160 consecutive patients in a conventional oncology clinic, 35 were taking herbal teas and 13 were found to be taking Iscador (286). Even at the top of Norway, investigators also found considerable Iscador use. We might therefore ask why this approach has been so popular in the northern countries, but so little known or accepted anywhere else (330, 329).

Germany has traditions and a legal structure that favor the use and acceptance of complementary and alternative medicine. In her outstanding work of popular anthropology, *Medicine & Culture,* Lynn Payer ascribes this to the "lingering influences of Romanticism" in German medicine. While Germans have a reputation for efficiency, they also tend to see health and the body as going hand in hand with Geist (spirituality) and nature. Payer writes that the German health care system "accommodates both the efficient and romantic aspects of the German character...."

One can see both trends in Iscador: a medicine chosen by the most intuitive of means, which is produced in a sterile and precisely calibrated manner.

Postwar Germany has been pluralistic in its approach to medicine. There is a reluctance to impose a one-party dictatorship of allopathic medicine. In Germany, drugs are approved only for safety, not effectiveness. Hence there are 120,000 different drugs on the market in Germany, compared to about 1,000 in some other countries. Furthermore, drugs are frequently put together in complex combinations. Germans see their doctors on average once a month, or three times more frequently than the average American.

Germans are also familiar with the concept of preventative tonics. As one professor told Payer, German medical practice stems from their central European cultural perspective on physiology. "There is a basic assumption," he told her, "of equilibrium or balance—that antagonistic forces should be kept in balance." It is also not uncommon for conventional doctors in Germany to send their patients to spas like Baden-Baden. Hydrotherapy, or water therapy, is still a going concern, since it "fits in perfectly with German romantic ideas of polarity and balance."

Even Rudolf Virchow, the "God" of German science, considered a lowered resistance to be a necessary precondition for illness. And herbal medicine has never died out in Germany. Of the 8,250 preparations listed in a recent edition of the German pharmacopoeia, the *Rote Liste,* 1,400 were of herbal origin (313).

Anthroposophical medicine was suppressed under the Third Reich. However, the attitude of the Nazis towards medicine was contradictory. On the one hand, they fostered the German chemical complex, I.G. Farben, and the beginnings of chemotherapy. On the other hand, the Nazis demagogically mimicked popular trends. As Barbara Griggs remarked, "Adolf Hitler's enthusiasm for all things Aryan raised folk traditions to near-religious status. Folk medicine became respectable." The plant-drug industry, already well established, was encouraged "as a patriotic duty." New chairs in Pharmacognosy were created in universities. Learned papers explored the significance of this "sunken culture."

In 1933, the Nazis passed a law giving naturopaths and herbalists nearly equal status with doctors and surgeons. Nazi leader Rudolf Hess remarked, "I have had experience of the value of natural healing on my own body. Science admits that it is faced with failure. The natural remedy, it seems to me, is to return to Mother Nature."

The country was flooded with natural remedies and books on plant therapy. Similar trends were seen of course in other countries: "Fitness classes were crowded; yoga became popular; and homoeopaths, osteopaths, naturopaths, and herbalists were all busier than before" (154). But the back-to-nature trend was strongest in Germany.

Today, about one-fifth of all German MDs practice either homoeopathy, Anthroposophical medicine, or phytotherapy (the German name for herbalism). Government commissions smoothly regulate homoeopathic, herbal and Anthroposophical medicine (313).

Rudolf Steiner's world view may seem hopelessly esoteric to an American, yet it is shared by a significant proportion of the German population, according to Johns Hopkins University professor Paul Unschuld. Many Germans apparently believe that the spiritual realm can be grasped as one grasps geometrical propositions.

There is an endowed chair at a German university devoted to the subject. There are half a dozen hospitals in Germany operating along Anthroposophical lines. When I visited one of these, the Filderklinik, south of Stuttgart, it had just opened a new wing financed by a government grant of about $30 million. It was strange to see a hospital that so seamlessly merged conventional and "alternative" approaches.

Is there anything to Iscador? Historically this has been denied by various orthodox cancer agencies in both the United States and Europe. According to statements from the Swiss Society of Oncology and and the Swiss Cancer

League, there was no evidence that mistletoe products such as Iscador "has an activity against cancer in human beings." They sternly warned patients against using it as a treatment for cancer.

For many years, the US medical establishment agreed. In 1979, the American Cancer Society was presented with 17 papers on the topic, which they submitted for evaluation to two unnamed expert consultants. They concluded that all apparent cures ascribed to mistletoe could be explained by other factors. "No evidence had been provided that Iscador has anti-cancer activity against human cancer," they declared. In the following year, they were given more clinical data and a bibliography of 25 publications and 14 unpublished manuscripts. A *Summary Review* of this data was resubmitted to the same consultants, who once again concluded that "there was little change from the material previously reviewed" (15).

In 1998, ACS replaced all its old negative statements on "quackery" or "unproven" methods with more tolerant statements on complementary and alternative medicine (CAM). At this writing there is no new statement on Iscador or other mistletoe products.

In fact, Iscador has been as well studied as any "alternative" cancer treatment. There are 140 references to "mistletoe and cancer" in the standard Medline database and 74 references to Iscador alone. There is a lengthy book in English published in India. Many studies never make Medline because they are published in obscure German publications. For example, I have on my desk a two volume compendium of articles from the years 1986-1988, collected and translated by Paul Scharff, MD of the Fellowship Community in Spring Valley, NY.

Dr. Scharff is one of America's leading practitioners of Anthroposophically Extended Medicine (AEM). There are a total of 24 articles in these compendia. Thirteen originally appeared in English, but the others were published in German or occasionally in French. They deal with such topics as the biochemical and immunological effects of mistletoe, clinical results, and properties of the various components.

I would like to briefly summarize some of the scientific literature.

In the 1970s and 80s, it was demonstrated beyond a reasonable doubt that there are cytostatic and immune-modulating chemicals in mistletoe extracts. Crude mistletoe contains a cytotoxic lectin called viscumin or mistletoe lectin I. There are other similar lectins as well and a few cytotoxic non-lectin proteins called viscotoxins. There are also potentially anticancer compounds among the component polysaccharides and alkaloids.

One of the mysteries of mistletoe is that some of these lectins are lost in the course of fermentation. Yet it appears that other antitumor compounds take their place, although this is not as well studied. Iscador seems to contain a compound related (but not identical) to viscumin, along with some other additional cytotoxic materials similar to the viscotoxins found in unfermented mistletoe (243).

Mistletoe, and particularly Iscador, were found to kill cancer in cell cultures. In particular, significant anticancer activity was found in mice with lung, colon, and breast cancer. However, no such activity was found in mouse leukemias, Ehrlich ascites, melanoma and a few others. I don't think anyone would suggest that human clinical results would be exactly the same as in the mouse models.

Many studies have also shown that mistletoe extracts increase the activity of natural killer cells and increase the size of the thymus. Rather than enumerate them all I would like to discuss in greater detail one set of papers that originated from a single German institution. Josef Beuth, MD, and his colleagues at the Institute of Medical Microbiology and Hygiene, University of Cologne, have intensively investigated the full range of mistletoe's activity. For reasons of scientific precision, they studied the effects of the galactoside-specific lectin found in mistletoe, ML-1.

First of all, they repeated many of the promising results suggested in other test tube experiments. They found that ML-1 "upregulated" various immune functions, while "downregulating" tumor cell proliferation. This preparation also killed cancer cells: they found a "pronounced dose-dependent cytotoxicity" in various cell lines (38).

In mice, a regular injection of a very small amount of ML-1 caused an enhanced proliferation, maturation and emigration of certain white blood cells (thymocytes) (37). The immune cell counts and activities were all enhanced (40). There was restoration of the immune system after steroid treatments and significant effects against metastases as well as bacteria (41, 372).

"Proof of an immune-modulating effect of the lectin ML-I on mononuclear blood cells does not automatically verify its clinical efficacy against cancer," according to skeptics at the Swiss Society for Oncology (169).

And so it became very important to look at the actual effects of these compounds on human cancers. At first, ML-1 was given in a non-controlled way to some cancer patients, twice per week over a four to five week period. In such patients, there was also "significantly increased counts and activities of peripheral blood lymphocytes and natural killer cells. Increased serum levels of ß-endorphin could point to the pain-relieving potential of this compound. There was also demonstrable improvement in quality of life.

These preclinical data became the basis for more advanced prospectively randomized clinical trials. The cancers involved were advanced brain cancer (glioblastoma multiforme), breast and colon-rectal carcinoma. The primary aims of these studies were an improvement in quality of life and protection of the immune system. They also looked at any influence on side effects of chemotherapy, the rate of relapse and metastases, and overall survival. Let us look at each of these in turn.

Thirty-five patients with stages III and IV brain tumors were enrolled in a study. They had all previously undergone immune-suppressive conventional treatments. The white blood cells of ML-1 treated patients returned to normal, after chemotherapy, much faster than did those of the patients who did not receive the mistletoe treatment (250). At six months, treated patients were also found to have an improved quality of life compared to the untreated controls.

In breast cancer, immunomodulation with ML-1 standardized mistletoe extract was also tried. The aim of this initial study was to assess whether this complementary treatment could favorably affect immunological and neuroendocrine measurements.

There were 36 patients in the treatment group, 32 in the control group. All had verified stages III and IV breast cancer. All were receiving chemotherapy. The 25 patients who responded to ML-1 were found to have an improved quality of life. They also had an enhanced activity of most immune parameters (176).

In colorectal cancer, a total of 79 patients were enrolled after surgery, and treated with either a standard chemotherapy regimen or no further treatment at all. The primary aim of the study was to measure changes in quality of life, and, in fact, a significant improvement was shown in the group that received ML-1. There was an "evident benefit for complementary ML-1 treated patients."

However, one problem with this study was that the control group did not receive an inert placebo, and so there might have been some psychological factors to account for the apparent effects of ML-1.

However, the same scientists were careful to point out that "no significant effect of ML-1 administration could be verified on frequency and length of remission, relapse-free interval and overall survival" (178).

New studies are being planned by Dr. Beuth's group at the University of Cologne, for patients suffering from head and neck, breast, and bladder cancer. So far, the Cologne scientists state, no definite conclusions can be drawn from these studies because follow-up is still ongoing. However, the promising data discovered through these prospectively randomized clinical trials "suggest that ML-1 standardized mistletoe extract can be recommended for the tumor entities tested so far" (39).

Another randomized clinical trial was performed with breast cancer patients to determine what happens to their immune systems after they are given a standardized extract of mistletoe lectins.

Subcutaneous injections of ML-1 twice a week caused increases in beta-endorphins, natural killer cells, and T-lymphocytes, all of which should benefit cancer patients. They cautiously noted that this "obvious correlation" between the immune system and the neuroendocrine system could have therapeutical relevance (177).

Reports on the clinical effects of Iscador or other mistletoe products seems to depend on who is doing the reporting, where the report is presented, and how the study is arranged. Thus, there are some highly positive clinical reports in the literature.

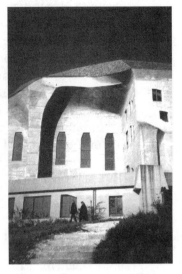

*Goetheanum
Dornach, Switzerland*

In addition to cautious and skeptical findings, there are also some highly encouraging reports. Some German doctors who use Iscador in their practice studied all the cases of ovarian cancer treated between 1969 and 1979 in the Gynecological Ward of an Anthroposophically Extended hospital in Herdecke.

There were 25 patients with primary neoplasms of the ovary who after surgery received treatment with Iscador. Twenty were in advanced FIGO stages III and IV. Five-year survival rates were 100% in stages I and II, 23% in stage III and 0% in stage IV. The records of these patients were matched with 22 other ovarian cancer patients who had received post-operative treatment with Cytoval.

Although the Iscador patients in general were more advanced, they had an average survival rate of 16.2 months as compared to 5.2 months in the group treated with Cytoval. In the stage III patients, survival was 4.2 times longer, and in stage IV it was 1.6 times longer. The differences were statistically significant. They concluded that Iscador was "a useful and effective treatment" of ovarian cancer, without serious side effects.

On the other hand, a report from a more conventional oncologist found no advantage in stage IV renal cancer with lung metastases (230).

Toxicity

Mistletoe has a historic reputation for toxicity. Even Shakespeare mentions "the baleful mistletoe," although he may be alluding to the Balder myth. The American Herbal Products Association classifies *Viscum album* as a class 2d herb, with certain restrictions on its use. Thus it is contraindicated in protein hypersensitivity and in chronic progressive infections such as tuberculosis and AIDS. Patients are advised never to exceed the recommended dose.

The standard dose of the herb taken orally is 2.5 grams, infused in cold water for 10 to 12 hours, up to two times per day. It is also advised that blood pressure be checked regularly by those consuming the tea.

A standard textbook reports that the majority of people taking the tea have no toxic symptoms. Despite that, this source also advises against self-medication (255). Occasional side effects seen with injections of Iscador include chills, fever, headache, angina-like symptoms, circulatory problems, and allergic reactions. It is not uncommon for patients to experience redness or swelling around the site of injection. Although this might be uncomfortable, it is considered a sign that the medicine is having a beneficial, immune-stimulating effect.

In Australia, the following labeling has been proposed for mistletoe-containing products: "Do not take with medications prescribed for high or low blood pressure except on professional advice" (69). In general, while Iscador or the other mistletoe preparations might make perfect sense as adjuvant treatments, they are not recommended for either self-help or self-administration. Patients would be well advised to seek out doctors who are knowledgeable about such treatments. Canadian regulations do not allow European mistletoe in foods. However, in Germany "Mistel" is a common ingredient in teas found in "Reformhausen" (health food stores).

From time to time, opponents of alternative medicine have claimed that Iscador is contaminated with bacteria. However, Iscador is carefully filtered to eliminate bacteria. Routine testing is conducted for microbial contamination, as required by the Swiss International Office for Drug Control. Iscador preparations are also tested for endotoxin contamination. I saw such testing being done on my visit to the Weleda factory. The OTA report concluded that "no cases of serious infection have been reported in the literature as a result of subcutaneous injection of Iscador."

Overall, Iscador seems to be a well studied and reasonably safe product being manufactured and used in an ethical fashion. In some ways, what has happened with mistletoe can be taken as a sterling model for the scientific evaluation of other non-conventional treatments.

Chapter 10 ❧ Chemotherapy's Herbal Roots

"Natural products chemists and phytochemists have always been impressed by the fact that compounds found in nature display an almost unbelievable range of diversity in terms of their structures and physical and biological properties."
—*Monroe E. Wall and Mansukh C. Wani*
Research Triangle Institute, prime discoverers of
camptothecin's anticancer activity (272)

ONE OF THE STRONGEST PROOFS THAT HERBS USED AGAINST CANCER ARE NOT MERELY "SNAKE OIL" IS DERIVED FROM A STUDY of the role that they have played in the development of chemotherapy. At first sight, nothing would seem further from the realm of medical herbalism. Yet about half a dozen of the most important chemotherapeutic agents were first discovered in medicinal herbs. Some of these were being used as folk remedies when they were developed as cytotoxic agents.

The key questions in finding new anticancer agents are: (a) What screening system is going to be used? and (b) What compounds are going to be tested? We shall leave the question of screening systems in abeyance. But broadly speaking, there are two ways of finding new anticancer drugs. The first is the process of rational selection.

A scientist has an idea, a specific biological goal or target, in mind, and devises a chemical agent to perform some specific role in that theory. "Even in its earliest days," it is said in a leading textbook, "cancer drug discovery

159

attracted scientists who had a theoretic basis for testing certain types of compounds." A few outstanding drugs such as methotrexate and 5-FU were created by rational design. And today, there are very sophisticated computer modeling techniques available to help create new agents; however, the same textbook states that "no effective cancer drugs have actually resulted from these efforts" (104).

It is for that reason that the empirical search for compounds in the natural world is still very important. The forests, fields, and swamps have all been scrutinized, in the search for potential cancer cures.

The Search for Plant Drugs

The NCI alone tested over 117,000 compounds of plant origin. About 30 percent of the anticancer compounds currently in use come from natural products or derivatives of these. Despite many difficulties and false starts, "the overall contribution of these complex chemical entities to the management of patients has been extremely worthwhile" (150).

One way of seeing how worthwhile is this: in my book *Questioning Chemotherapy*, I list 32 of the most common multidrug protocols used in cancer treatment today. Of these, only four do not contain some natural product ingredient. The majority contain either one of the herb-derived products discussed in this chapter, an agent derived from a micro-organism or, in one case, a drug derived from a sponge.

We shall briefly mention one large category of natural products used against cancer. These are the microbial antibiotics, which some consider the "most important source of cytotoxic agents" in the natural world. These include potent agents that were derived in the 1940s and 1950s from fermentation broths obtained from soil microbes, such as bacteria, fungi, and related organisms—many of them single cell plants.

Historically, the most important class of anticancer antibiotics has been the anthracyclines. The first was daunorubicin (Cerubidine), which was isolated from a colony of the Streptomyces in 1957, and which became a standby for the treatment of leukemia. Scientists then created a mutant version of Streptomyces and isolated a new drug, doxorubicin (Adriamycin). Unfortunately, these powerful agents can have serious long-term toxicity problems in their ability to damage the heart muscle. Mitoxantrone (Novantrone), a third such drug, may be less toxic in this regard.

However, promising new drugs do not just come from the theoretician's workbench or the medicinal chemist's vat. Many of the most effective drugs in cancer chemotherapy are derived from higher plants. Some of these were discovered as part of the NCI's massive plant screening program. Some of these turned out to be folk remedies for cancer-like conditions. Only too rarely did scientists follow the lead of pioneers Jonathan Hartwell, PhD and James Duke, PhD and systematically investigate those plants that were already in use around the world for the treatment of cancer. And, today, when scientists are more prone to appreciate the uses of exotic plants, there is still a tendency to think that plants used against cancer in the Amazon basin are "ethnobotany," while those used in Topeka, Kansas or Beverly Hills are de facto quackery.

Colchicum Autumnale—Autumn Crocus

It is generally believed that cancer chemotherapy began during World War II, as an outgrowth of poison gas experiments at Yale University. It is true that this work with nitrogen mustard was a turning point. But years earlier, Belgian scientists had begun to experiment with a plant-derived chemical called colchicine in the treatment of both external and internal malignancy. Leading medical botanists have contended that "the modern era [of chemotherapy] began in 1938 when it was learned that colchicine was cytotoxic" (256, 115). Yet its role in cancer has dropped out of the history books. I would like to explore it briefly here.

The common names of *Colchicum autumnale* are autumn crocus, meadow saffron or (inexplicably) naked ladies. Despite these names, "autumn crocus" is neither a crocus nor a form of saffron (nor an aphrodisiac). For example, if you try to use it in place of culinary saffron, you will be in for a nasty surprise. Ingesting any part of this plant can kill you.

Autumn crocus is a European native that was introduced as a garden plant by colonists in North America. It also grows as an escapee in meadows and woodlands. A perennial of the lily (Liliaceae) family, it grows from a solid bulb called a corm. Autumn crocus is sometimes mistaken for wild

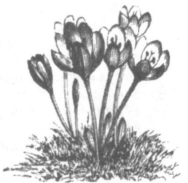

Colchicum autumnale
(autumn crocus)

onion or its leaves are mistaken for a broad-leaved garlic called "ransom" (*Allium ursinum*). The results of such misidentifications are sometimes tragic (368).

In the fall the autumn crocus's corm produces two to six lovely white to purplish-pink flowers. As the name suggests, the flowers resemble the crocus, but there the resemblance stops.

Colchicum was named for the city of Colchis on the Black Sea, where it was first observed flourishing. (Today, commercial sources of seeds and corms are Italy and the former Yugoslavia.) "Autumnale" refers of course to the season in which it blooms. The ancient Greco-Roman physician

Dioscorides knew this plant to be toxic. He is also the first to mention its use in cancer, for he wrote that the leaves of autumn crocus could be "soaked in wine and administered [topically] to dissolve lumps and growths...."

Fast forward half a millennium: a 5th century AD Byzantine doctor named Jacob Psychristus discovered that autumn crocus could be used to treat rheumatism, arthritis, and "podagra." Medical historians now believe that podagra was gout (245). Learning from the Greeks, Arab physicians popularized the use of autumn crocus for gout, but it appears to have been abandoned because of concerns over toxicity. We can speculate that some of their patients were relieved of gout—and then of their lives as well.

But autumn crocus is very effective against this extremely painful disease and so, not surprisingly, it came into use again. In Europe, in 1763 it was reintroduced by Baron von Storck (the same adventurous spirit who also introduced hemlock as a treatment for cancer) and it soon became incorporated into a number of "gout mixtures." Soon these were popularized on the street by enterprising and unscrupulous charlatans. No less a personage than Benjamin Franklin, who himself suffered from gout, is said to have introduced colchicum therapy into the United States (147).

A scientific landmark was the isolation from autumn crocus of the alkaloid colchicine by Pelleiter and Caventou in 1820. And colchicine is still FDA-approved for the treatment of gout. It is one of the most effective medicines known, with dramatically positive results in about 95 percent of cases. It also can have significant toxicity. One problem is that it also causes nausea and vomiting past a certain dose level. However no one know what that dose level will be for any individual. And so, gout sufferers who want to use colchicine usually have to suffer through a bout of stomach upset before they can establish their own effective dose.

Colchicine can suppress the immune system. And worst of all, it can on rare occasions be fatal. Although the fatal dose of acute colchicine poisoning is estimated at about 0.9 mg/kg, deaths have occurred at doses of as little as seven milligrams total. This is just a few multiples of the effective dose and so, as wonderfully effective as colchicine is, it is also a potentially dangerous agent, which most doctors are loathe to employ, but which desperate patients sometimes demand.

Anticancer Properties

Colchicine has an equally remarkable effect on the behavior of cells (332). It was noticed as early as 1889 that colchicine stopped cell division in both plant and animal cells. The details of this were worked out in 1934 by Prof. A.P. Dustin, Sr. of Brussels, Belgium. This was followed by a demonstration at the Second International Cancer Congress, held by coincidence in Brussels two years later. Colchicum is what is called a "spindle poison." Normally, a cell uses its spindle fibers to line up the chromosomes, make a copy of them, and then divide into two new cells. Each so-called daughter cell then has a single set of chromosomes.

When colchicine is present, the spindle fibers can't form, and the cell can't move its chromosomes around. "The affected cell may end up copying some or all of the chromosomes anyway," writes one author, "but it can't parcel them out into new cells, and so it never divides."

For this reason, colchicine is still used in all sorts of experiments in plants and animals. In fact, Medline lists 11,670 scientific papers on colchicine. And cancer research is still going on with this compound (258).

The first clinical experiments with colchicine took place in the early 1940s. Their importance, historically, is that they "helped greatly in convincing research men [sic] of the possibility of cancer chemotherapy" (119).

Folk Usage

The folk use of autumn crocus in cancer goes back at least to the time of the Emperor Nero. Dominici, a great French hematologist and radiotherapist, who died in 1919, is said to have observed favorable effects of colchicine in cancer patients who were receiving x-ray therapy while also undergoing treatment for gout. Other clinicians were making the same observation as well.

People who happened to be on colchicine seemed to respond better to radiotherapy. Doctors quickly rushed to try the latest "cancer cure" without adequately understanding the biological basis of the treatment. This "led to a neglect of the fundamental problem which is at the base of any cancer chemotherapy: Are malignant cells more severely damaged than normal ones? This is of great importance with a chemical like colchicine which affects all types of mitoses" (119).

In some ways, colchicine had biological effects that were similar to Coley's toxins. It was found that the polysaccharide isolated from one component of Coley's toxins, *Serratia marcescens*, also produces hemorrhages in tumors, as colchicine does, and also interferes with cell division (351).

In 1940, a report was published in a US journal on the treatment of human carcinoma with colchicine. Four patients were treated and, although some favorable effects were noted, one patient suffered severe depletion of the bone marrow (leukopenia) and another lost almost all his hair (347).

In another series that year, two out of three patients died of bone marrow damage (55). In 1941, colchicine was applied as a paste or injected as an oily solution to metastatic nodules of epithelial cancers (350).

"The volume of the treated metastases clearly decreased." This experiment was published as a thesis of the University of Montpellier, France, during wartime. And so it is no surprise that it has been ignored by most historians of the field.

Worried by the extreme toxicity they sometimes encountered when giving colchicine as systemic therapy, scientists turned their attention to the external treatment of benign skin lesions, such as venereal papillomas or warts. This may seem odd, but actually warts have many points of similarity with tumors: they are both examples of unregulated growth, and may have a common viral origin.

So it is not a bad model (and in fact Hartwell included wart treatments in his search for antineoplastic agents of folk origin.) A paste made of colchicine and lanolin was applied twice daily to six individuals. "Remarkable regressions [of warts] were observed after several weeks of treatment" (119).

Although the benign growths became increasingly resistant to colchicine, they could then be removed surgically, which was facilitated by the regression of size and extension. A microscopic analysis showed that the cells in question had had their divisions arrested by this unique poison. Also, normal cells seemed much less affected by this treatment than did tumor cells, because there was no skin ulceration with the treatment, and, after the tumor had disappeared, the skin regained its normal aspect. This work was reported in a German journal in 1943 (54).

And here we see the important role that folk medicine has played, and continues to play, in the search for effective antineoplastic medicines. Colchicine is not the only agent of natural origin that has been widely used for the treatment of warts and papillomas. In fact, in the 1950s it was largely replaced by another such agent, podophyllin (containing podophyllotoxins and peltatin). But podophyllin is itself extracted from a folk remedy that we shall meet again—*Podophyllum peltatum*, or mayapple. Podophyllin also acts in an identical way to colchicine, i.e., as a spindle poison.

Finally, what makes this story really "remarkable" is that the third most prominent folk remedy for warts and papillomas, *Chelidonium majus,* or greater celandine, contains an alkaloid, cheliodine, which has also been demonstrated to inhibit spindle formation in tissue cultures (119, 252). At the end of the 19th century, another compound, chelidonine, was advocated as a treatment for cancer (101). And, as this book shall make clear, the use of the celandine-derived agent, Ukrain®, is alive and well in many countries, including the United States (see chapter 22).

Imagine how much time and effort could have been saved had prominent scientists taken the folk reputations of meadow saffron, mayapple, and celandine seriously, instead of allowing their profound importance to be rediscovered by chance. What other fascinating chemicals are present in folk remedies that are still being overlooked because of a resistance to exploring common Western herbs?

This is not to say that colchicine is a "cure for cancer." Far from it. The few clinical trials that were performed were "quite disappointing" (119). However, work continues. As late as 1995, urologists showed that colchicine combined with the drug estramustine suppressed the growth of prostate cancer cells (126). Since there is no effective form of chemotherapy for advanced prostate cancer, this could be an important finding. The scientists declared that "the use of oral colchicine in the treatment of hormone-refractory prostate cancer requires further investigation"—a statement that could have been made with equal justification a half a century earlier (258).

The Vinca Alkaloids

For various reasons, World War Two era experiences with colchicine were largely ignored by subsequent students of the field. The first anticancer drugs in current use found among the higher plants were the vinca alkaloids, vincristine and vinblastine, derived from the Madagascar periwinkle. They were developed in the late 1950s and early 1960s by Canadian scientists and the Eli Lilly company of Indianapolis, who named them "Velban" and "Oncovin." They are now standbys in treating a variety of cancer types.

Vincristine sulfate (Oncovin) and vinblastine sulfate (Velban) are chemicals whose precursor molecule was first discovered in a tropical shrub *Catharanthus roseus*. The "Vin..." in their name alludes to the plant's former scientific designation, *Vinca rosea*.

In a sense, Vincristine and Vinblastine were also a product of research into folk medicine. *Catharanthus roseus* was a good candidate for testing. It is a member of the botanical family (Apocynaceae) that also yielded the historically important mood-altering drug reserpine. This was derived

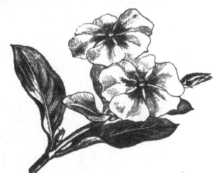

Catharanthus roseus
(Madagascar periwinkle)

from the Ayurvedic herb, *Rauwolfia serpentina,* whose root was chewed by millions of Indians and Africans for mood elevation for 30 centuries. It wasn't until 1931, however, that Western scientists finally "discovered" this plant and not until 1952 that they uncovered the potent chemical in the root, reserpine. This became the basis of the modern tranquilizer industry. A drug company executive said at the time, "We finally figured out that one million Indians couldn't be wrong" (267). (Its rediscovery ushered in a new era of respect of herb-derived treatments, and for Ayurvedic ones, in particular.)

Navelbine

Another drug derived from the periwinkle is vinorelbine. Phase II clinical trials are underway using this as a treatment for ovarian cancer. It is marketed as Navelbine by Glaxo Wellcome, Inc. Thus far, it seems to have a wider range of antitumor activity than the other vinca alkaloids. It has showed some promise in treating patients with epithelial ovarian cancers and, in combination with the drug cisplatin, in treating patients with non-small-cell lung cancers as well. Side effects of this drug include diarrhea, nausea, and hair loss.

Etoposide

Etoposide (VePesid) is an extract of a North American medicinal herb called mayapple. Its proper botanical name is *Podophyllum peltatum*. It also has many common names, such as ground lemon, wild jalap, raccoon-berry and Indian apple, attesting to its widespread use.

One traditional American Indian usage of podophyllum was to treat warts. In China and Japan, the rhizomes of a related plant, P. pleianthum are still used to make a compound called Hakkakuren, which is used to treat tumors of the genitals (113b).

By 1949, a 25 percent solution of podophyllin suspension in oil was considered a standard treatment against a kind of venereal wart called condylomata acuminata (191). This is intriguing, since warts share some similarities, as we have said, with tumors. Other strains of this type of virus are believed to cause some forms of cancer, particularly of the cervix (193).

So how did this become a conventional anticancer agent? In the 1940s, scientists began studying this folk remedy and found that some of the constituents (called lignans) stopped cellular growth. For a while, a podophyllin extract was administered to patients right after their radiation treatment for cancer.

One fraction of the plant was given the name etoposide (VP-16); later, another was called teniposide (VM-26). Together these were found to contain a complex chemical called epipodophyllotoxin, which was naturally linked to a sugar (called glucopyranoside).

The two drugs are only slightly different. They are classified as semisynthetic toxins from mayapple. This means that the raw material for their manufacture must be supplied from the plant itself. It was found to be difficult to cultivate the plants, which required a long dormancy period. (This delicate plant would not grow where the average January temperature falls below 20° F). And so herbalists gathered the herb in the wild and sent it to Abbott Laboratories in North Chicago, where 300,000 pounds a year were used to produce enough medicine to supply the need in oncology.

Etoposide is used in combination with other anticancer drugs in the treatment of lung cancer, non-Hodgkin's lymphomas and refractory testicular tumors. It has also been used in the treatment of leukemias, Kaposi's sarcoma, and neuroblastoma. It is one of the three components in a highly toxic troika of drugs called "ICE."

The parent compound podophyllotoxin binds to tubulin in the cell and inhibits the assembly of the invisible little tubules in the cell. Oddly, the "daughter" compound seems to act in a different manner entirely. It produces DNA strand breaks, and interferes with an enzyme that is involved in unzipping the DNA so that it can reproduce itself. But the exact mechanism of action is unknown (104).

Not surprisingly, given its provenance, this drug is very toxic. It depletes white blood cells and causes nausea and vomiting in many patients who receive it. Like mayapple, it can also cause severe allergic reactions. There has also been critical, but reversible, nerve damage in patients receiving very high doses. Particularly disturbing is the fact that the use of epipodophyllotoxin (either Etoposide or Teniposide) is associated with an increased risk of leukemia.

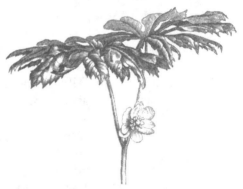

Podophyllum peltatum
(mayapple)

Thus, some patients who are successfully treated with these drugs for acute leukemia or Hodgkin's lymphoma have developed a second acute myeloid leukemia (AML), usually within six years of their initial treatment. In one large retrospective study, 163 cases of second leukemias were found, two thirds of which were AML. The risk is proportional to the dose intensity of the drug, rather than the cumulative dose. Highest risk was associated with weekly or twice weekly administration (218).

Teniposide

Teniposide (Vumon, VM-26) is another semisynthetic derivative of the same plant and is closely related to Etoposide. It is used as a component of various regimens. It is used to treat both Hodgkin's and non-Hodgkin's lymphoma, germ cell malignancies, leukemias, bladder, and small-cell lung cancers. Oddly, it has never been fully approved by the FDA, although it is widely used in other countries (see also chapter 2).

Paclitaxel (Taxol)

In 1971, a complex plant alkaloid, dubbed paclitaxel or Taxol, was isolated as an active ingredient in the bark of the Pacific yew tree (*Taxus brevifolia*). By 1979 it was shown to stop the division of cells by interfering with the shape and functionality of tiny intracellular structures called microtubules. Technically speaking, Taxol increases the stabilization of these microtubules, making them rigid. This increased rigidity interferes with normal cell division. By enhancing the polymerization of tubulin, in effect Taxol makes the cell's inner "skeleton" rigid and nonfunctional. It blocks two phases of the cell's growth cycle, thus inhibiting replication.

Although the craze for this plant has died down, Taxol is still considered one of the most promising of the anticancer plant agents that emerged from the massive drug screening program of the National Cancer Institute. It is exciting to scientists because of the wide range of tumors it can help treat, and also because of some interesting biological properties. At first, Taxol was mainly of interest to scientists investigating the structure of microtubules. Then, in the mid–1980s, scientists began to seriously look at its interaction with cancer. It was first found to have a marked cytotoxic effect on prostate cancer cells.

Taxol is considered the most important new chemotherapeutic agent to be approved in the last decade and a half. Excitement derives from its unusual mechanism of action and its ability to contribute to remissions in some tumors that are no longer responding to more conventional drugs. Response rates in refractory ovarian cancer range from 21 to 40 percent. Phase III studies are underway to assess its role in that disease. "Significant activity" has also been seen in metastatic breast cancer patients (190).

Initially, it was believed that Taxol could only be isolated from the bark of *Taxus brevifolia*. This threatened an environmental crisis, since Pacific yew trees grow slowly and could quickly be driven to near extinction by accelerating demand. However, more recently, methods have been developed to produce the drug semisynthetically. The chemical bacatin III occurs abundantly in the leaves (needles) of various yew species, not just the West Coast variety, but even in *Taxus baccata,* the common English yew. This chemical can then be modified to form Taxol, which occurs in its natural form only in the bark of the scarce Pacific yew (332).

Taxol was subject to a media-fed enthusiasm in the 1980s and early 1990s that sometimes verged on hysteria: cancer patients feared that because of production problems they might not be able to get this "miracle drug." However, the drug turned out to be neither so effective nor difficult to produce as was initially thought. Questions have also been raised about the manner in which Bristol-Myers Squibb, the world's largest producer of chemotherapeutic agents, gained an effective monopoly on the harvesting and distribution of this natural product.

Taxol can also cause serious allergic reactions. In one study, 40 percent of patients suffered nerve damage, with numbness and abnormal sensations in the hands and feet. Many patients also showed a significant depletion of their neutrophils (usually for a short duration). Total hair loss is common. Other toxic effects include nausea and vomiting; inflammation of the mucous membranes; muscle pains; and inflammation of the veins. Heart and lung toxicity can be ameliorated by prolonging the infusions and by pretreating patients with other drugs, such as corticosteroids and antihistamines (292). Rapid heart beat and even more serious heart disturbances also occur. Some patients have died of septic infections after taking this drug (120).

Camptothecin

Camptothecin, another alkaloid, is derived from the wood and bark of a Chinese tree. It was first isolated in 1966 from the stem of *Camptotheca acuminata* (Nyssaceae), the so-called "happy tree" native to the relatively warm areas of such Southeastern Chinese provinces as Szechwan, Yunnan, and Kwangsi (402). This plant had been introduced several times into the USA, and the sample that the USDA tested had come from its Plant Introduction Garden in Chico, California (317).

The USDA's Phytochemical Database says that camptothecin is present as 100 parts per million (ppm) in the stem and 300 ppm in the seed of this tree. The USDA's online Ethnobotanical Database lists anticancer activity as one of the folk usages of this wood, although it is unclear if such usage pre- or post-dated the scientific exploration of the plant.

The story of how camptothecin's properties were identified is a fascinating piece of medical detective work. In the 1950s, a huge number of plants were meticulously collected and identified by the Plant Introduction Division of the US Department of Agriculture, and then shipped to the Eastern Regional Research Laboratory of the USDA in Philadelphia. At that time scientists were mainly searching for plant steroids, which could serve as cortisone precursors. After analyzing the plants for sterols, alkaloids, tannins, and flavonoids, they stored most of the unusual plant extracts.

One of these thousands of extracts was from the leaves of *Camptotheca acuminata*. In 1957, after a visit from Dr. Jonathan Hartwell of the Cancer Chemotherapy National Service Center, Dr. Monroe E. Wall agreed to send him 1,000 plant extracts to test for antitumor activity. Almost a year later Hartwell came back with astonishing news: the only plant extract that had high activity in the CA-755 assay was from this obscure Chinese tree.

Because of Hartwell's efforts, Wall became intensely interested in discovering the exact nature of the compound or compounds responsible for this antitumor activity. However, USDA could not accommodate this search and so "for administrative reasons" in 1960 Wall left USDA and established a natural products group at the Research Triangle Institute in North Carolina. By 1963, he had procured about 50 pounds of wood and bark of the tree and in 1964 he was joined by Dr. Mansukh C. Wani, his long-time collaborator in this work. By 1966, they had isolated the plant-chemical camptothecin from the wood.

What was unusual about this effort was that Wall and Wani used a "bio-directed isolation." This meant that every step of the way they let their search for chemicals be directed by results in antitumor assays. This was the same process that was later used to isolate Taxol. By this time it had been discovered that crude extracts of the tree were very active in a mouse leukemia (L1210) life prolongation test. Since few plant extracts had this sort of activity it generated a great deal of interest in the scientific community. The doses required to prolong the mice's lives were relatively small, between 0.5 and 4.0 milligrams per kilogram of body weight.

A very important test involved "nude mice," a special breed without the ability to reject transplanted tissues. Human tumor tissue of various types were implanted into these mice, which were then given tiny doses of camptothecin. Imagine the excitement of scientists when they saw this drug cure 36 out of 36 samples, covering the majority of human neoplasms (365).

Some people leaped to the conclusion that the cure for cancer was at hand. In 1971, NCI decided to go to clinical trials with a sodium salt of camptothecin, which was water soluble and was therefore easily formulated for intravenous administration to patients. In the dose-establishing Phase I trial, the drug was given to 18 patients and there was a partial response in five of them. These were mainly of gastrointestinal tumors and were of short duration.

The toxicity was blood marrow depression, along with some vomiting and diarrhea. (In another Phase I study of 10 patients there were two partial responses.) Because scientists were not ready to give up, they undertook a Phase II study of 61 patients with adenocarcinomas of the GI tract. But only two patients showed objective partial responses (280). (The Chinese reported somewhat better results, in patients who had not been previously treated with chemotherapy.)

"Unfortunately," wrote John S. Stehlin, MD, of the Stehlin Foundation, which has fostered work on camptothecin, "it started on the wrong leg because, as we now know, the sodium salt used then for patient administration is inactive as far as anticancer activity is concerned, and highly toxic for the patient..." (365).

What is more, some early clinical trials had to be called off when patients experienced "severe, unacceptable bladder toxicity." The reason was that the drug turned particularly toxic when it hit the acidic urine in the patient's bladder (170). Given the high hopes that had been generated by the animal studies, these results were greeted with dismay and shock.

Between 1972 and 1985, there was little interest in camptothecin. During this time, Drs. Wall and Wani were unwilling to give up the dream that this chemical, which had worked so marvelously well in animal models, might still someday have another chance. They developed some 50 look-alike compounds (analogs) of camptothecin. Then in 1985 the story took another odd twist which elevated camptothecin once again to premier status in the world of cancer research.

It was discovered that this drug, by a unique mechanism, inhibited an enzyme called DNA topoisomerase I (or T-I) located in the cell nucleus. This enzyme was found to be extremely important in cell replication, transcription, and recombination. It was the first agent discovered that could inhibit this critical cell enzyme. An exploration of this property opened up a new world not just of camptothecin studies but of basic cellular research. To date, there are over 5,700 articles on topoisomerase in the standard scientific literature, most of this unleashed since 1985 because of the unusual biological activity of this unlikely Chinese tree.

Thus, camptothecin (CPT) reentered medicine through the back door of basic research. "With the mechanism now understood," said Wall, "there opened the possibility for clinical use of camptothecin by virtue of its inhibition of T-I..."

It is not necessary to review here all the clinical work that has been done. At the present time, camptothecin-derived drugs, Topotecan, from SmithKline Beecham, and CPT-11, from Daiichi (Japan) and Upjohn-Pharmacia, have been approved by the FDA for use in ovarian and breast cancer. GG211 is another water-soluble drug derived from Camptotheca. Developed by Glaxo, it is in clinical trials. There are yet others which are entering the pipeline, such as 9-NC.

One of the reasons that scientists find 9-NC exciting is that it causes cancer cells to die by apoptosis, or programmed cell death (76). The lead paper at the plenary session of the 1998 American Society of Clinical Oncology (ASCO) meeting in Los Angeles was on a study of CPT-11 in the treatment of metastatic colorectal cancer (91). So camptothecin is back—big time, and one is likely to hear more about the various forms of this drug in the future.

None of this adds up to the "cure for cancer" which was anticipated by the spectacular animal tests. In fact, the story of camptothecin is a cautionary tale, that what works in mice may not work as well in humans, and therefore it is irresponsible to ballyhoo "cancer cures" based on animal data alone.

But certainly the camptothecin analogs are taking their place as a very useful and interesting class of compounds that, although toxic, work by a mechanism that is different than most other chemotherapeutic agents. And all this came from an obscure tree from southeastern China growing on a plantation in Chico, California.

Maytansine

In the 1970s and early 1980s there was also a great deal of excitement over a new drug called Maytansine. The manner in which this drug was discovered is most interesting. Starting around 1945, a man named Davis began to use an herbal formula for cancer in South Africa. This "Davis Remedy" was eventually patented. In time, "quite extravagant claims were made for this herbal remedy." This was particularly controversial, since it was illegal in South Africa at the time for non-medical personnel to try curing cancer with herbs (175). Davis's formula consisted of several crushed and dried herbs that were used in infusion form. At one time, its popularity in South Africa was similar to that of the Hoxsey, Essiac or Jason Winters formulas in the United States. It consisted of the following:

The Davis Herbal Remedy

Scientific Name	Common Name	Part Used
Maytenus heterophyllus	Maytens	leaves
Scutia martina	—	leaves, roots
Sanseviera spp.	Sanseviera	root

Note: This formula should only be used under a physician's direction. Please see the warning in the front of the book.

Several other herbs were included, but in such low concentrations their identification was never possible.

Maytenus is a genus that consists of about 200 species of trees and shrubs that are native to the tropics and subtropics of both the New and the Old Worlds, some of which have medical uses. Davis said that some of the uses of the formula were to prevent secondary infections near the area of complaint. Scutia leaves and roots were added for their astringent qualities. And Sanseviera was added for its high potassium content.

The Soviet scientist S.M. Kupchan did some early work on the nature of Maytenus and isolated the drug Maytansine from *Maytenus ovatus* (Celastraceae). In the early 1970s he received a patent for this work.

Maytansine was found to be what is called an "ansa macrolide," a kind of anticancer agent that had previously only been isolated from microorganisms. Jonathan Hartwell and Dr. John D. Douros, both of the Natural Products Branch of the Division of Cancer Treatment of the NCI, started to experiment with this nonconventional formula and discovered that Maytenus species were in fact extremely active in the laboratory against some forms of cancer, including lymphoma, melanoma, carcinosarcoma, and leukemia.

The drug was commercially isolated from M. buchananii of Kenya and also from the oddly named *Putterlickia verricosa,* a scruffy little shrub that grows in South Africa. "American scientists have been visiting South Africa quite a bit in the last few years," writer John Heinerman reported in 1980, "bringing back a lot of samples with them to test at NCI laboratories in Maryland." In addition to Maytansine-containing plants, some of the other species they were looking at included *Kigelia pinnata* (sausage tree) and *Sutherlandia frutescens* (kankerhos).

Additional antitumor constituents called phenoldienone triterpenes were also isolated from *Maytenus laevis.* The whole plant of a related species, *Maytenus ilicifolis,* has been used in Brazil as a wash for skin cancers (361).

One problem was that isolated Maytansine was so toxic. The LD50 in rats (or dose that killed 50 percent of test animals, a standard measure) was just 0.48 mg delivered subcutaneously. At one time, Maytansine was the great hope of chemotherapy. There was a great deal of publicity about its promise. Yet it has now dropped from sight and is only mentioned in passing, if at all, in the major cancer textbooks.

The reasons for this were that clinical studies in general were very disappointing. In a number of studies on patients with soft tissue sarcoma there were no responses (shrinkages) at all (104). What is curious about this whole affair is that the cancer claims were being made before scientists discovered Maytansine in the plant. Yet isolated Maytansine had no effect in clinical trials. Perhaps this is just a coincidence. Or perhaps the particular combination of herbs that Davis used had effects that went beyond the effects of a single chemical from a single plant.

The history of chemotherapy thus demonstrates that there are indeed active anticancer agents present in plants, some of which are used in various folk traditions for cancer or other growths. This has been confirmed beyond a doubt by the efforts of scientists such as Jonathan Hartwell, James Duke, and Monroe E. Wall. No amount of propaganda for or against popular herbal "cures" should be allowed to obscure that fundamental fact.

CONTROVERSIES
AROUND THE WORLD

Chapter 11 🌹 HANSI (Argentina)

H ANSI IS A SPANISH ACRONYM FOR "HOMOEOPATHIC ACTIVATORS OF THE NATURAL IMMUNE SYSTEM." OF ARGENTINIAN ORIGIN, IT is currently manufactured in the Bahamas, and imported in the United States by cancer patients under the compassionate use doctrine of the Food and Drug Administration. "Hansi" (i.e., little Hans) is also the nickname of Juan Jose Hirschmann, an Argentinian horticulturist with a special interest in cacti.

Mr. Hirschmann was born in 1942 to Hungarian refugee parents. He developed an interest in cacti during his adolescence and is said to have "worked his way through undergraduate botany at the University of Buenos Aires, experimenting in cacti." After college he developed greenhouses to hold his cacti. According to a company brochure, he financed his activities by selling cacti on the weekend, and quickly learned "that the more grotesque the cactus (due to cancer), the higher the price received."

Because of this experience, he embarked on a project to induce the deformations of "cancer" in cacti. "A wonderful result of this work was his success in reversing the process and eliminating cancer from the cacti."

By a circuitous route, over a 16-year period, he developed homoeopathic solutions that, he said, could fantastically promote or retard growth in plants. His solution was a kind of "energized water." His first patient was his own dog that had cancer. Giving the dog his "water," her tumors gradually disappeared. Then another eight years of experimenting with animals ensued. "Horses were cured," it is said, "and two lions with tumors on their

174

heads were cured."

Following this, a man asked for the "healing water" to treat his dog, but took it himself and "recovered from lung cancer." A pharmacist "gave it to his wife and tumors on her breasts and liver went away." When she stopped her injections, the cancer developed again and she died (14).

The basic HANSI formula is made up of about 10 constituents, which are adjusted depending on the route of administration. At one time the formula was as secret as Coca-Cola (33). However, according to the so-called *Definitive Guide to Cancer,* the basic formula contains various rain forest or desert plants such as *Cactus grandiflora* (cactus), aloe, arnica, lachesis, lycopodium, all in a two to eight percent base of alcohol (107). Since these are present in homoeopathic doses I see little reason to discuss the medical properties of these herbs.

There are also variations on HANSI, which include all of the above ingredients plus extracts of Colocinthis, *Pulmonaria reticulosa, Berberis vulgaris,* and silica (107). Most of these plants are very obscure and not found listed in standard American, British, or German reference books (310).

One frequently hears big claims for HANSI. An unsigned article in the *Townsend Letter for Doctors & Patients* referred to "HANSI: Argentina's Medical Miracle." It claimed that HANSI is effective in treating a wide range of diseases, including "cancer, AIDS, chronic fatigue syndrome, arthritis, asthma and hepatitis." It is said that Hirschmann's early experiments in the 1970s led to "successful treatments for animal cancers."

There has been a study by Darryl M. See, MD of the University of California, Irvine, which established that the preparation is non-toxic in adolescent male mice. But since this product is ultra-diluted (like any homoeopathic product), this should come as no surprise. Almost any substance diluted to an almost infinitesimal degree (4x to 11X, in homoeopathic terms) would predictably be nontoxic.

Perhaps Dr. See is also the "eminent researcher at a major university," mentioned in publicity material, who has demonstrated that HANSI greatly increases the Natural Killer cell activity in the blood of both AIDS and chronic fatigue syndrome patients. These results have supposedly been confirmed in mice. But while I found publications by Dr. See on the enhancement of Natural Killer cells with the herbs Echinacea and Ginseng, I did not find any standard Medline references to such work with HANSI (346).

Many other claims are made for HANSI in both the Townsend Letter article and another anonymous article circulated by the American distributor (9). There has been little research so far on HANSI. I could find no articles on the topic of HANSI out of nine million citations in Medline.

In July, 1990, Hirschmann opened his first clinic in Buenos Aires and hired doctors to begin treating human cancer patients with his products.

HANSI was supposedly so effective that "his first clinic was mobbed by cancer patients." Even with 40 physicians on his staff, it is said, the clinic reached operating capacity in its first week. At its peak it registered 1,200 patients per day.

"Lines formed for blocks, necessitating bringing in police for crowd control," according to a company handout. "The Minister of Health moved to close the clinic. He withdrew his order when thousands of people surrounded the Presidential Palace in a non-violent HANSI-supporting protest" (14).

Needless to say, such riots are not a proof of efficacy. Cancer patients may be whipped into a frenzy for another reason—excessive and premature publicity. The United States saw the latest such frenzy in May, 1998, when the *New York Times* reported promising animal studies on antiangiogenic agents (e.g., Angiostatin and Endostatin) on its front page. Americans may not yet be rioting in the streets, but at the peak of the furor, Judah Folkman, MD, developer of these drugs, was receiving over 1,000 telephone calls per day from patients demanding the purported "cure." (Dr. Folkman himself did nothing to encourage these reports.) Such events have been repeated dozens of times over the years. It proves nothing, except the susceptibility of cancer patients to any offer of hope.

The distributor has said that about 125,000 people have been treated in Buenos Aires. It is said that HANSI "has produced successes with every kind of cancer." The medical evidence from Argentina is "largely derived from retrospective chart reviews and testimonials," and it is "massive, more than enough to justify trials in the US" (8).

Well, perhaps. But company spokespersons do not provide any of these "retrospective chart reviews," nor do they include them with their information packet.

The American managing director of HANSI is David C. Christner. Mr. Christner is an American businessman, entrepreneur, and art collector. He is also himself a cancer patient, who learned about Juan Hirschmann and HANSI while on an art buying trip to Argentina (14). He has pledged that he is committed to performing the "hard science" to provide physicians with "incontrovertible evidence" that HANSI gets results. Like many developers of herbal cancer products, he seems quite sincere.

The company circulates what it calls a "landmark" 1992 study on the treatment of pancreatic cancer by Cesar Bertacchini, MD of the Instituto de Medicina Intergracion in Buenos Aires. This states that HANSI was associated with "a significant increase in the survival of patients."

Of 87 patients enrolled in this study, 60 were still alive at the end of one year. It is said also that after two years, more than 50 percent of the patients were still alive and well. Appetite is said to have remained stable in 57 percent, to have increased in seven percent, while 73 percent had no pain or only mild pain, 56 percent experienced no nausea or vomiting, and 36 percent experienced a reduction in these symptoms.

However, this study is unpublished in any medical journal nor has it undergone peer review. This is inexplicable, seeing that there are now a number of fine, peer-reviewed journals devoted to the study of complementary and alternative medicine (CAM). Generally speaking, these journals are hungry for good clinical studies.

In addition, there are gross inadequacies in the paper. For example, the length of survival is not mentioned in the paper itself. The above figures are derived from company handouts.

Even if we accept the data as given, many questions remain. Even though pancreatic cancer has a reputation for having a very bad prognosis, we still need to know the exact type of cancer, by whom the diagnosis was made, the stage and condition of each patient. Although reports state that none of these patients received chemotherapy or radiation therapy, it is unclear what other nonconventional treatments they might have taken (107).

It is said that there was significant pain relief, etc. But since there was no control group, it is difficult to compare the reported results to the norm, although on the face of it, it could be significant.

I find several aspects of the company's presentation confusing. In a company brochure, they state that "over 1,200 cancer victims have been treated in the United States with a high rate of remission" (14). It is amazing that so few patients have come forward.

After many years there does not appear to be a single clinical trial published in a regular journal on the effects of HANSI in cancer. The sum total of clinical documentation I received from the company was an article from *The Florida Woman Magazine* by a single satisfied patient, Bud German.

Mr. German reports that he was diagnosed with prostate cancer in December, 1992. Instead of having radical prostatectomy (RP), as suggested by three doctors, he started on HANSI on April 1, 1993. By September, 30, 1993 he had a follow-up biopsy at Memorial Hospital and "the cancer was gone." A number of subsequent biopsies were also negative for cancer. Mr. German also reports that he kept a positive attitude and also asked for God's help. "Was it HANSI? Was it prayer?" he asked. "How can I answer those questions?" I called Mr. German, but never received a call back. If confirmed, his would be an impressive case. But one wonders about the 125,000 other people treated with HANSI. Where are their stories?

I need to say a word about the nature of HANSI's manufacture. It is said that HANSI is "homoeopathically prepared." The "H" in HANSI refers to this aspect of its nature. Patients are instructed to shake the medicine vigorously. This sounds like the process of activation called "succussion" in homoeopathic terms. It is then taken by mouth, as an inhalant, and by intramuscular injection into the fleshy part of the upper arm or buttocks.

But this is not a classical homoeopathic preparation, by a long shot. A fundamental basis of homoeopathy is "let like cure like." Homoeopathic drugs are supposed to cause the very symptoms in healthy people that they cure in sick people. This is called a "proving." There is no indication that the HANSI mixture was proven in this manner.

Also, the vast majority of homoeopathic preparations are taken orally. But HANSI is generally taken by injection. In fact, in Sri Lanka, they are even using it as part of "HANSI-puncture," or injection into acupuncture points. This is all very interesting, but seems far afield of classical homoeopathy.

There has at times been an aura of secrecy surrounding HANSI. In 1995, for instance, I was unable to get the ingredient list from the manufacturer. Reporters from the Tampa *Tribune* ran into similar problems. A recent book on alternative cancer treatments published an ingredient list and this has been reported in a number of articles.

On May 12, 1998, a spokesperson for the company refused to reveal the owners of the company to me or even to reveal her own last name. (I later had a friendly encounter with the American distributor, who apologized for this behavior.) But perhaps the most disturbing thing about HANSI is the price. A 90-day supply of HANSI costs $1,500, to be paid by cashier's check to HANSI International, Ltd. in Sarasota, Florida. For a 90-day clinical treatment with lung involvement, the charge is $1,800. There is an additional charge for shipping and handling and the Personal Use Exemption Form states that there are "NO RETURNS. NO REFUNDS."

One is supposed to take HANSI for up to two years, bringing the basic charge to about $12,000. One of the things I find disturbing about this is that HANSI is a homoeopathic preparation. In other words, there are virtually no raw material costs, since the basic plant ingredients have been so diluted as to be practically non-existent.

It is for that reason that most homoeopathic drugs cost in the neighborhood of $5.00 for 100 pellets, which works out to about a dollar a day. On the other hand, no other homoeopathic preparations in America to my knowledge are prepared as injectibles. Certainly, $6,000 per year is a lot of money to pay for an essentially untested, unproven treatment that is lacking in scientific, clinical or even anecdotal data.

I am trying to remain open-minded towards HANSI. Perhaps with so many patients, more compelling evidence for its effectiveness may yet emerge. (The distributor assures me that it will.) I am also sympathetic to anyone struggling with the gargantuan task of getting FDA approval for a new drug. You would think that with over 125,000 patients, the manufacturer could do a lot better than a few articles in popular magazines.

Chapter 12 ❧ Curaderm (Australia)

URADERM IS A NON-TOXIC AND RELATIVELY INEXPENSIVE CREAM
THAT IS MARKETED IN AUSTRALIA AND SOME OTHER COUNTRIES AS
a treatment for malignant human skin cancers. It is available by mail
to North Americans.

Curaderm is not an escharotic black, yellow, or red salve, in the manner
of Harry Hoxsey (see Chapter 5). Nor is it a "secret remedy," like most
cancer salves. It is derived from *Solanum sodomaeum,* a weed that is native
to the southern Mediterranean area. In Australia, it is known as Devil's
apple, kangaroo apple, or Sodom's apple.

Curaderm was discovered in Australia as a folk remedy for skin cancer in
cattle. But although it is exclusively marketed as a treatment for external
cancer, we know from laboratory work that it also kills some internal cancer cells as well. Some of the test tube and experimental animal tumors that
it did kill were sarcomas, melanomas and ovarian cancer cells. However,
there is no internal preparation currently available.

Of all the non-toxic herbal preparations, Curaderm is among the best
understood and designed. It contains solasodine glycosides, which are found
in plants of the nightshade family, including tomato, potato and eggplant
(aubergine). In fact, there are more of these chemicals in a serving of eggplant than in an application of Curaderm. The main difference is that these
chemicals are purified and concentrated in the medicinal formula (66).

The inventor and main proponent is Australian biochemist Dr. B.E. (Bill)
Cham, who was until recently affiliated with the Department of Medicine,

University of Queensland, Royal Brisbane Hospital, Australia. He is a genuine scientist and author of over 80 scientific papers. At least three dozen of these are listed in Medline, mainly on lipid metabolism. Dr. Cham has written about a dozen papers on Curaderm. This preparation is therefore relatively well documented in the peer reviewed literature (66-70).

History

Solanum species were among the 250 herbs employed by Assyrian botanists in the 7th century BC (407). They were mentioned by Hippocrates. The great German historian of cancer, Jacob Wolff, tells us that Galen prescribed the use of "nightshade juice" (succus solani) in the treatment of external cancers (413).

Another species, *Solanum dulcamara,* has long been used as a remedy for skin diseases. In 1825, a prominent physician named Dr. Everard Home (1756-1832) recommended "an infusion of the solanum, or nightshade, in cancers of the breast." This had quite a vogue in Europe and the United States.

The glycoalkaloids from various Solanum species have been identified as having anticancer potential: these include beta-solamarine and solaplumbin. All of these compounds contain rhamnose, a plant sugar that is not usually found in mammalian tissues (66).

Unlike many herbal or escharotic salves, Curaderm is a scientifically based preparation. It contains a standard mixture of solasodine glycosides called BEC (named for Bill Cham's initials). The glycosides in BEC consist of equal amounts of (1) solamargine, (2) solasonine and (3) di- and monoglycosides.

The alkaloid solasodine on its own does not appear to have anticancer activity. It must be joined to specific sugars in order to possess such properties. Equally important, cancer cells must have sugar receptors on their surfaces (called endogenous endocytic lectins, or EELs) in order for them to link up with these solasodine glycosides.

When a cell with EELs on its surface comes in contact with these solasodine glycosides, the two link up. This joining results in a chain of events in which deadly compounds are delivered to the interior of the cell. Solamargine travels by way of the desmosomes (which are part of the supporting structure of the cell) to lysosomes in the interior of the cell. Lysosomes are particles inside cells that contain enzymes. These enzymes would destroy the cell constituents if they were not kept separate.

Any damage to the lysosomal membrane can endanger the life of the cell. Once inside, however, solamargine ruptures the lysosome, effectively killing the cell through a process known as autolysis. The ability of Curaderm (and especially solamargine) to kill cancer cells thus depends on the "fit" of its sugary key to the "lock" of the cell-surface lectins (EELs). It is an elegant treatment.

It was previously known that a preparation containing very high (10 percent) BEC was effective against both malignant and benign human skin tumors. However, astonishingly, a very low concentration of BEC (0.005%) also seems to show effectiveness in the treatment of these diseases.

We know a considerable amount from the scientific record about why and how this compound works against basal cell carcinoma (BCC) and squamous cell carcinoma (SCC) as well as two benign conditions, keratoses and keratoacanthomas.

There is also a possibility (unproven at the moment) that Curaderm could be effective against malignant melanomas and possibly some other cancers that have externalized to the skin.

In an open study with Curaderm, both clinical and histological observations indicated that all lesions (56 keratoses, 39 BCCs and 29 SCCs) that were treated with Curaderm regressed. Meanwhile, a placebo formulation had no effect on a smaller number of treated lesions. In addition, Curaderm had no adverse effect on the liver, kidneys or blood-forming system. Some patients have been followed for over 10 years and have not had a recurrence of their tumors (70).

I am impressed by the evidence presented for Curaderm and believe that the chance of a complete and lasting remission of superficial skin cancer using this product are good. Since SCC and BCC are generally slow-growing, minimally malignant, and rarely life-threatening, they offer a unique opportunity to try such topical agents for several months to see if it eradicates the tumor.

Some people feel strongly that Curaderm is an ideal agent for self-medication, and that any opposition to its use must stem from the greed of dermatologists. I regard skin cancer as a true cancer, and one which should be taken seriously. Patients should not try to self-diagnose and self-medicate, but should consult with a competent dermatologist.

Patients should first have a diagnosis. They could then explain that they would like to try this experimental Australian treatment, and would like the doctor to supervise their use of this. If the doctor agrees, then the patient can return to make sure that the growth is entirely gone and can continue to return periodically just to make sure there is no recurrence.

One danger of unsupervised self-medication is that you can mistake a deadly melanoma for a relatively harmless growth. Then, you might not "get it all" with this still little-understood remedy, or you might miss other lesions on your body that could be just as dangerous. Whenever possible, one should use this agent under the supervision of a doctor. If a doctor refuses to supervise this treatment, perhaps it is time to change doctors.

I realize that it would be tempting to try this preparation on various other malignancies which have manifested themselves on the skin. Again this should only be done under a doctor's supervision. What are some of these?

Malignant melanoma: although Curaderm should NOT be the sole or primary treatment, with the cooperation of one's oncologist you could see what the effect of this cream might be on the lesions.

Sweat gland (eccrine) tumors: There are few usable treatments at the present time. Again, under doctor's supervision, you could try this unique treatment on external lesions of this type.

Kaposi's sarcoma: We know that sarcoma 180 was well controlled in mice using this product. Logically, it might have some beneficial effect against KS lesions as well.

Metastases to the skin from internal cancers: Skin metastases from internal cancers are found in a small percentage of patients. These usually occur if metastases are widespread in other areas at the same time. They occur most frequently as a result of breast cancer, but also from large intestine, lung, ovarian, uterine, pancreatic, and bladder cancer. It is also seen, but rarely, in squamous cell carcinoma of the oral cavity and in sarcomas, etc. Even if Curaderm worked in such instances, it would most likely be used as a palliative.

Curaderm comes in the form of a kit, which contains a small bottle of antiseptic and another of the Curaderm cream. First, you apply the antiseptic to the cancer or the keratosis. Then you apply a small amount of the Curaderm cream and rub it directly into the lesion. You then cover this with a small Band-Aid type bandage. You do this twice daily.

Typically, the lesion and a small area around it will turn red and become slightly inflamed. There may be a burning or stinging sensation. In the days that follow, the growth may ulcerate or even bleed a bit for a week or two. This is the period during which the cancer cells are dying and being sloughed off. The antiseptic is applied prior to the cream to keep the area from becoming infected during this critical period. Also, it helps to remove dead skin cells and allow the cream to reach the cancer cells underneath. You may even be able to see some skin-like material being removed with the antiseptic.

Treatment generally takes three to four weeks. After that it is a good idea to continue applying antiseptic and cream for another week. If the lesions are larger or multiple in nature, then obviously the treatment period may be longer. If a lesion returns after this, one can always repeat the procedure.

Chapter 13 ❦ CoD Tea (Austria)

oD TEA BURST ON THE INTERNATIONAL SCENE IN LATE 1997 WITH A BEAUTIFULLY ILLUSTRATED BOOK TITLED *MIRACLE MEDICINES OF the Rainforest*. This tells the story of an Amazonian herbal mixture that is being used to treat AIDS and cancer (96). In reading this book, and meeting its author, Dr. Thomas David, my overall impression has been a positive one. I think this represents an honest attempt to bring important knowledge to light about the potential healing power of Amazonian herbs.

There are many indications that some herbs from the rain forest could be useful against cancer (see Chapter 19). Dr. David has put together a version of a cancer remedy that is current in one part of the forest. He was certainly not the first white man to penetrate the Amazon in search of new plants, nor was he the first to befriend the much beleaguered Yanamamo Indians. But he is among the first to seriously attempt to market such a mixture, and so it deserves scientific scrutiny.

Dr. David's story began in 1983. While visiting the University of São Paolo, he made friends with a Yanamamo shaman named Katunka, who had accompanied a young patient there. Eventually this shaman invited the "white shaman" to his village or "Maloka." After many adventures, Dr. David was finally given a mixture of herbs for cancer.

Since both David and Katunka were communicating in Portuguese, a language which neither of them spoke very well, it is remarkable that he was able to learn as much as he did. He emerged from the jungle and set up a company to research and develop this indigenous herbal mixture. He also sought out investors to help him develop the product. He called his product CoD Tea, because "CoD" was printed on the burlap bag of the first shipment—and he didn't have time to invent a fancier name.

What's in the tea? We are never told directly, but Dr. David assured me that as soon as his pending patent was approved, the entire world would know. The ingredients are found among a list of twenty different herbs. Dr. David's wife is a Chinese doctor and Dr. David himself is familiar with Japanese Kampo (traditional) medicine.

The formula consists of eight tropical plants, six of these from South America and two from south China. They are thus all tropical or subtropical rain forest plants. The South American portion is, he says, a "very old Indian mixture." Altogether, he and his European colleagues screened a total of 90 plants before they decided on this particular configuration.

The six South American plants are chosen from the following list.
Possible CoD Tea Ingredients

Scientific Name	Common Name	Parts Used
Agrimonia eupatoria	Agrimony	leaves, flowers
Angelica archangelica	Angelica	entire plant
Arctostaphylos uvae ursi	Bearberry	leaves
Artemisia vulgaris	Mugwort	entire plant
Capsella bursa pastoris	Shepherd's purse	(unknown)
Carapa guianensis	Carapa	alcohol extract
Chenopodium ambrosioides	Mexican tea	leaves
Glycyrrhiza glabra	Licorice	root
Hymenaea courbarii	Jatoba	bark
Lamium album	Blind nettle	leaves
Ocimum basilicum	Basil	leaves, flowers
Peumus boldus	Molina boldo	leaves
Plantago major	Plantain	leaves, root
Quassia amara	Pau amago	bark, root
Silybum marianum	Milk thistle	fruit
Smilax aspera	Sarsaparilla	leaves, root
Urtica urens	Dwarf nettle	leaves, flowers
Veronica officinalis	Speedwell	plant

Note: Plants on this list should only be used under a physician's direction. Please see the warning in the front of the book.

He also added several other herbs from Chinese forests. For purposes of evaluation it is essential to know the specific ingredients and their proportion in this mixture and we don't yet know that.

Many books about herbs are entirely lacking in scientific support. But Dr. David presents some impressive evidence that his mixture has beneficial effects on the body's ability to fight cancer: it stimulates leukocytes to release interleukins and other cytokines; stimulates the production of anti-angiogenic factors (he has been in touch with Harvard Professor Judah Folkman, MD, who originated the anti-angiogenic drugs); stimulates the production of endorphins, bringing about pain relief and mood elevation; and finally, stimulates the appetite either directly or through the suppression of chemotherapy-related nausea.

Tests done at the Zytognost Immunobiology Laboratory in Munich in March, 1996 showed a rather dramatic (albeit transient) increase in the levels of the immune functions of white blood cells in cancer patients (96).

Two physicians at Munich's CELLControl Biomedical Laboratories showed that a combination of CoD Tea and the standard chemotherapeutic agent, Epirubicin, had the effect of turning extremely chemo-resistant cells into highly receptive ones. As the two investigators wrote, "It would open up completely new treatment opportunities for those patients who are already resistant to certain chemotherapy drugs" (96).

Since resistance to chemotherapy is one of the major problems in cancer therapy, one would think that this finding would be greeted with universal enthusiasm. So far it has been ignored. The reasons for this are complex. But not long ago, Jerome Kassirer, an editor of the *New England Journal of Medicine* remarked, "In the six-and-a-half years I've been at this journal we haven't published one paper on....herbs. And I must add that we have not even received many papers for consideration. That tells me a lot about the kinds of studies that have been done, because people know we have very high standards."

Yet many medical botanists or new product developers would never consider sending a paper to the *New England Journal,* since its hostility towards the topic is well known. This creates a vicious circle.

Dr. David's book also attempts to summarize the clinical results attained so far with this mixture. In a section titled "Remarkable Results," we are told the outcome of an informal survey of 2,000 patients who have taken the product. According to Dr. David's analysis, 38 percent reported significant improvement, while 46 percent of patients felt "no better/no worse" from taking the tea. (There is no mention of the remaining 16 percent of the patients.) Of the 38 percent who reported significant improvement, nine percent had a complete disappearance of at least one tumor.

One might say that nine percent responses is not bad for patients with advanced cancer (the great majority of those using the tea). But, understand that this is nine percent of 38 percent, which works out to 3.4 percent of the total number of patients. In our conversations, Dr. David affirmed to me that of the 3,500 patients treated so far, three percent had complete and total responses, while 23 percent had partial responses. The most dramatic results were in breast and lung cancer.

One of the things this book could have used was a very detailed report on ten of the 100 or so cases who allegedly had complete responses. This could include a dispassionate description of their case histories, and reprint of their original medical records, including biopsy reports, MRIs, X rays, follow-ups, etc. That we don't get. Instead, there are a series of Patient Reports prepared by an Austrian writer named Werner Stanzl.

Titled "A Journalist on the Trail," it tells how Mr. Stanzl went from total skeptic to true believer in the virtues of CoD Tea. Mr. Stanzl traveled from Austria, where Dr. David lives, to Hungary, where he was born and where most of the CoD patients reside. (There is a Cancer Information Center in Budapest that recommends his tea.)

Here are the cases Mr. Stanzl details:

Auguste O., age 47, lung cancer. She started taking the tea on July 8, 1995. Stanzl visited her on October 12, 1995, just three months after she began the treatment. She tells him, "My tumor has not grown. In fact, it has gotten smaller since my last examination in January." This conveys the impression that the shrinkage is due to CoD tea. However, we learn from the context that she wasn't taking the tea in the spring—so the tumor shrinkage has to be due to some other cause. What could this be? Chemotherapy? Radiation therapy? We aren't told.

Paul M., age 46, lung cancer, metastasis of the liver. He began taking tea in April, 1995. He and his wife both believed that the tea rapidly decreased Paul's need for morphine (and indeed the tea has been shown to increase the production of pain-killing endorphins). In January, 1996, Mr. Stanzl received a letter from Paul's wife stating that he was "doing well, very well." Thus, nine months after starting the tea, he was still alive. This is promising, although a two-year survival would have been more impressive. (The cases were not updated for the American edition.)

Josef Marcali Kiss, age 60, lymph cancer. Began taking the tea in December, 1994. He also had repeated courses of chemotherapy. Mr. Stanzl quoted from his medical report of March, 1995: "Patient has shown a marked improvement in physical and mental condition. He has started to gain weight. One lymph node shows a total remission, ten others show a 50 to 70 percent improvement, and another shows a 40 percent improvement." In September, 1995, his report reads, "Patient is in outstanding physical and emotional condition." In February 1996, he reported that his lymph nodes had not changed. His liver had decreased in size by four centimeters, there was no evidence of further tumor growth, and his condition was stable." This seems impressive. However, what is the exact relationship between these beneficial changes and the four years of chemotherapy the patient has undergone? Was he in remission at the time that he began CoD tea? Was he getting worse? These crucial questions are not even approached in Mr. Stanzl's account.

Elemérné Orban, age 77, bladder cancer. Her tumor was partially removed in a series of laser treatments. In November, 1994, she started CoD tea and felt so much better that she canceled the final laser treatment. In January, 1995, she was told by her doctor that there was no sign of any cancer. There was, however, a scar from the tumor on the bladder wall. But perhaps the tumor was completely removed through the laser treatments? One would like to see the physicians' reports.

"The Nurse." (Declined to give name.) Pancreatic cancer. Had surgery. Began CoD tea one month after the operation. We are told that "by May 1995 her condition had improved," but we haven't been told when she had the operation and when she started the tea. Stanzl visited her over a year later in April, 1996. We have no details on her case. Was this cancer possibly in the head of the pancreas? If so, we should remember that "patients who undergo surgical resection for localized nonmetastatic adenocarcinoma of the pancreatic head have a long-term survival rate of approximately 20 percent and a median survival of 15 to 19 months" (104).

In addition to these, the book contains one-paragraph testimonials. Most report improvements in mood, appetite, energy, and attitude. Some even claim that the tea "saved their lives." However, this is not evidence that CoD objectively extends survival.

There appears to be some scientific support for what Dr. David is trying to do. The book contains very favorable comments from Apostolos Georgopoulos, MD, of the Vienna General Hospital, and some American scientists as well.

Although I was impressed by Dr. David's sincerity, a few elements mitigate this positive impression. This tea is no "miracle," as the title claims. It seems to score a complete remission rate of three percent (with a much higher overall benefit ratio). While some may be disappointed by this, I appreciate Dr. David in admitting this. I suspect that some other herbal "miracles" would yield similar figures if honestly assessed.

The front cover of *Miracle Medicines of the Rainforest* refers to the book as "A Doctor's Revolutionary Work with Cancer and AIDS Patients." We are also told that he was "invited by a Brazilian to give a lecture and demonstration of hip replacement procedure..." (96). The back cover of this book states that "Dr. David runs a clinic in Vienna where he continues his work." It comes as a shock to learn, halfway through the book, that Dr. David is in fact a veterinarian.

Chapter 14 ❧ Aveloz (Brazil)

A VELOZ IS THE COMMON NAME OF *EUPHORBIA TIRUCALLI*. ALSO KNOWN AS SPURGE, AVELOZ IS A SUCCULENT PLANT THAT GROWS TO a height of about thirty feet and is indigenous to tropical areas and rain forests in the Amazon, Madagascar, and South Africa. The main trunk and branches of the plant are woody and brown but the younger branches are green and cylindrical, resembling pencils (hence one of its common names, pencil tree). The leaves are minute and shed early, so they are generally not even noticed. The photosynthetic function of the leaves is taken over by the green branches.

All parts of the plant ooze a milky sap when damaged. Aveloz is often used as a hedge in Brazil. The parts that are used medicinally include the latex sap, the leaves, and (in Chinese medicine) the root. This is a very complex plant, rich in biochemicals.

Some readers might remember that during the energy crisis of the 1970s, Nobel laureate Melvin Calvin vocally advocated the use of this plant as an inexpensive source of petroleum (6). (Hence another popular name, "petroleum bush"). While this idea is not entirely dead, it turned out that the cost of producing such petroleum was higher than Prof. Calvin had initially estimated.

The latex of a related species, *Euphorbia resinifera,* has yielded a powerful new drug, resiniferatoxin. This is an "ultrapotent capsaicin analog," which shows potential as a topical pain killer. Clinical trials to test this hypothesis are underway in Italy (17). So without a doubt there is some potential

188

utility to the genus.

Aveloz has a fantastic folk reputation as a cancer treatment, a reputation, unfortunately, it does not seem to deserve. At least, there is little science to back up the many claims. In two experiments, aveloz proved inactive against cancer cells. The first was an East Indian study of an extract of the aerial parts of the plant against the CA-9KB cell line (106). The second was a study of aveloz stems in Yoshida sarcoma, a form of cancer, of rats, at a relatively high dose of a full gram per kilogram of body weight. This was conducted as part of a survey of Malaysian native plants. Again there was no effect (298).

At the same time, most authorities consider aveloz toxic and dangerous. Canadian regulations do not allow it in foods. Warning labels have to be applied in Australia. One reason is that aveloz's latex produces skin irritation and uveitis (in dogs). It also exhibits tumor-promoting activity in some experiments, to such a degree that African scientists have concluded that "the use of this plant (*Euphorbia bougheii*) as a medicine must be discouraged since the latex extract causes cancer" (158).

Aveloz latex can be extremely irritating to skin and mucous membranes. Redness, swelling, and blisters form after some delay following skin contact. There may also be inflammation, conjunctivitis, as well as burning of the mouth and throat. Any contact of the sap with the eyes can cause temporary blindness for several days.

Taken internally, it can produce nausea, vomiting, and diarrhea.

Such concerns are not new. The herbalist Margaret Grieve notes that in Java it was said

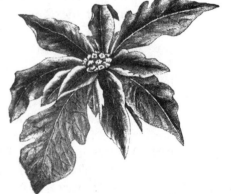

Euphorbia heterophylla
(aveloz, or spurge)

that mere "exhalations from the tree cause the loss of eyesight" (153). Fatalities have also been reported following ingestion of latex for folk healing purposes. According to the American Association of Poison Control Centers, exposure to Euphorbia species constituted the third most likely source of plant poisonings in the United States (239).

Diterpene esters appear to be responsible for these irritating and toxic effects as well as the plant's ability to promote tumor growth. While such esters probably do not cause cancer by themselves, they can interact with subthreshold doses of other carcinogens in laboratory animals. Prof. Varro Tyler states that although its exact chemical constituents are unknown, aveloz has serious potential for harm. Most herbalists would agree with him.

At one time it was said that aveloz had only "very weak tumor-promoting activity" (140). However, a series of scientific articles have suggested that the high incidence of Burkitt's lymphoma (BL) in the so-called "Lymphoma Belt" of tropical Africa coincides with the prevalence of aveloz and its use as a folk remedy. In fact, a plausible mechanism has been suggested: aveloz can induce chromosomal changes characteristic of Epstein-Barr associated Burkitt's Lymphoma (395). Aveloz can also suppress immunity and enhances Epstein-Barr virus (EBV) infections.

"These immunologic findings," Japanese scientists wrote, "strengthen the notion that *Euphorbia tirucalli* [i.e., aveloz] may be an important environmental risk factor for the genesis of African Burkitt's lymphoma" (199). In fact, aveloz and related plants are found more often in the homes of Burkitt's lymphoma patients in Malawi (as folk medicine) than in those of non-infected individuals (395).

Yet, ironically, aveloz has many folk uses, especially as an external treatment for skin cancer. The saps of various Euphorbia species have been used in folk medicine since at least 400 BC for their corrosive properties. The dried latex of *Euphorbia resinifera,* called Euphorbium, was used medicinally at the time of the Roman emperor Augustus (17). In Hartwell, there are eight references to its historical usage against cancer. The earliest of these was attributed to Mir Muhammad Husain, who lived around 1771 AD. *Euphorbia garuana* latex is used in traditional African medicine as a cancer remedy (1).

In many countries aveloz is known as "killwart," because its sap was used by Amazonian Indians and later Dutch, Portuguese, and Galician settlers in northeastern Brazil as a treatment for warts and tumors, particularly of the face. According to Prof. Tyler, a Brazilian physician named Dr. Pamfilio introduced aveloz into conventional medicine in the 1880s or 1890s.

Mrs. Grieve writes that a related species (*Euphorbia amydaloides*) "corrodes and ulcerates the flesh wherever it is applied. Warts and corns anointed with it are said soon to disappear, but great caution is needed in using it, or injury is likely to result to the surrounding skin" (153). In small doses, it has been used in India as an anti-syphilitic medicine. Traditional Chinese Medicine uses a related species, *Euphorbia helioscopia* as a treatment for bone tumors (195).

There is a small amount of scientific data showing that the terpene esters in certain members of the Euphorbia family may have antileukemic effects. Norwegian scientists have isolated triterpenes from *Euphorbia pulcherrima,* which exhibited cell inactivating effects against Ehrlich ascites tumor cells (357). In 1996, scientists at Purdue University isolated six diterpenes from the latex of *Euphorbia poisonii.* Five of them "were selectively cytotoxic for the human kidney carcinoma (A-498) cell line." The potencies of two of these "exceed[ed] that of Adriamycin by ten thousand times" (128). This is quite astonishing, since Adriamycin is itself a very powerful cytotoxic agent.

In sum, there are two sides to the aveloz story—many accounts of harm, as well as some vague accounts of possible benefit. It is, as Varro Tyler says, a two-edged sword, which should be handled with extreme caution.

Several Brazilian species, collectively known as aveloz, have attained local notoriety as cancer "cures." This was picked up by an enterprising US supermarket tabloid, the *Globe,* in the 1970s. American interest in aveloz hit a peak in 1980 when author Alec de Montmorency claimed in a right-wing periodical that aveloz "seemed to literally tear cancer apart" (the *Spotlight,* 7/14/80).

Other tabloid headlines of the time included: "Exotic Shrub may be key to victory in cancer battle! Aveloz now being used for tumor reduction cancer treatment," and "One drop of [aveloz] sap, diluted in a glass of distilled water and taken by the tablespoonful every hour, eliminates cancerous growths in one week."

While it is reasonable to suppose that aveloz could be effective as an external medicine, perhaps acting as an escharotic (see Chapter 6), advocates began talking about using internal doses liberally. This seemed incredible, since as early as the 1930s Mrs. Grieve noted that "the internal use of the drug has been abandoned, owing to the severity of its action."

Aveloz Craze

Although the aveloz craze of the early eighties has largely abated, the Internet has given it new life. Astonishingly, aveloz is being sold as an "underground" cancer treatment. A company called Life Extension, based in Loxahatchee, Florida, advertises aveloz over the Internet. It is important to note that this company is not connected in any way with the well known Life Extension Foundation of Hollywood, Florida, despite the similarity of name and locale.

The small "Life Extension" company claims that aveloz "may hold the key to victory in the battle to destroy cancer...." Supposedly, "the power to eliminate neoplasms, malignant (skin cancers) drew the attention of professors of medicine....Here was an adequate tumor remedy, near at hand," they continue. "Why not try it INTERNALLY to eliminate cancerous tumors? They did and it worked."

This company claims that "five to ten drops of that same solution, depending on size and density, taken every hour, has been known to eliminate cancerous growths in one week. The hard tumor collapses....the cancer has been reduced to an ill-smelling paste by the tissue-tearing (escharotic) properties of the solution. The elimination of the malignancy will cause an irritation of the kidneys, but that's all. You can alleviate that side effect by taking extra vitamin C."

They further recommend using aveloz together with pau d'arco (Taheebo). They claim these "do not cause any serious side effects and they do not interfere with other medications or treatments!" They also claim, without any scientific justification, that the product is "especially effective in cases of leukemia, almost always lowering white cell counts sharply."

In the light of the historic and scientific evidence on toxicity, readers will doubtlessly be startled, as I was, to hear that "aveloz has been proven to have no ill side effects. It can help but can do no harm." The company offers one ounce bottles of aveloz for $35.00 and six bottles for $189.00.

I wrote to the company requesting the name of the "professors of medicine" who had proved the safety and effectiveness of aveloz. I received the following prompt reply from Frances Webster, a customer service representative of Life Extension:

"Dr. Paulo Martin, is the Medical Researcher for the Brazilian Government and an expert on Aveloz and Taheebo, that was referred to. Drs. Augusto da Silva Brito and Lauro Neiva, are others. They were both practicing in Brazil in 1994 when they wrote articles in the Brazilian papers (which were later translated in the English papers) about Aveloz and Taheebo.

"Other Brazilian physicians referred to are Drs. Octavia Lobo and Rube van der Linden. Additionally, the Brazilian Medical Association may be able to point you to yet others. You may also want to contact Dr. Paul Martin; Dr. James Duke at the National Institute Of Health [sic]; Dr. Norman Farnsworth at the University Of Illinois; Dr. Theodoro Myer and/or Dr. Prats Rutiz at the National University of Tucuman; and do some research on your own regarding the effectiveness, uses and results practitioners are having with Aveloz and Taheebo...."

I thereupon sent letters to a variety of Brazilian authorities but received no reply from any of them. I was thus unable to track down any of the Latin American experts who were allegedly supportive of such usage. I did however contact Dr. Duke, who incidentally has never been with the National Institutes of Health. (He recently retired from the US Department of Agriculture.) As I suspected, he was vehemently opposed to cancer patients self-medicating with aveloz and aghast at the exploitation of his name in connection with it. He stated, "I fear aveloz is more likely to cause than cure cancer."

Chapter 15 ❧ Pau d'Arco (Brazil)

PAU D'ARCO IS A POPULAR NAME FOR A GROUP OF TREES OF THE
TABEBUIA AND TECOMA GENERA (145). PAU D'ARCO IS NAMED AFTER
an extinct tribe of Kayapo Indians in northern Brazil who were noted
for their "wonderworkers" (212). (There is still a Pau d'Arco lake in that
area.) The tree and a medicine made from its inner bark are also popularly
known as ipé-roxo ('eepay-rosho') or taheebo, even in the United States.
This has become a very lucrative part of the herbal marketplace.

These trees are found in all parts of continental tropical America, especially Brazil, Argentina, Colombia, Costa Rica, and the Lesser Antilles. A
related plant is found in Africa.

Lapacho colorado is also called "red lapacho" and Lapacho morado is
"purple lapacho," named after the color of their flowers. Both are used to
prepare taheebo tea.

All of the trees are medium-to-large sized with well-formed trunks. The
timber is described as an "axe-breaker," since it has great strength and dura-
bility. Tabebuia species are used throughout Brazil to decorate streets,
boulevards, and parks. Prof. Tyler believes that this tree's fabled "resistance
to decay probably attracted the attention of the natives to the medicinal
potential of the species" (392). In fact, pau d'arco contains powerful chemicals in the bark, which act as protectants against the ravages of decay and
infection.

Tecoma and Tabebuia are among the few plants known to contain the
chemical lapachol (392). This chemical constitutes two to seven percent of

the bark. However, there is a lot of chicanery in the pau d'arco market-place. For example, some unscrupulous marketers have ground up the bit-ter outer bark as well as the valuable inner bark to increase the yield of product. A survey of 12 commercial taheebo products in Canada revealed that only one contained any lapachol at all, and that at a level of 0.0003 to 0.0004 percent, lower than found in any of the Tabebuia species (27).

Unlike some dubious cure-alls, which are more the invention of First World marketeers than Third World shamans, pau d'arco is really used in many tropical and subtropical climates as a folk remedy. Since the 1980s it has also become readily available in many American and European health food stores. It is advocated as an anticancer tea by some holistically orient-ed physicians and sold via the Internet and other outlets (see below).

It is noteworthy that of the eleven species containing lapachol in com-mon use, all have well-established folk usages. Of these, five are related directly to cancer treatment, while two others are related to pain relief. In fact, for some species, cancer treatment is the only usage recorded.

Pau d'Arco and Related Species of Medical Interest

Name	Popular Names	Folk Usage	Country
Tabebuia impetiginosa	Ipe roxo, taheebo	cancer	Brazil
Tabebuia bahamensis	—	anodyne	Bahamas
Tabebuia caraiba	—	cancer	Taiwan
Tabebuia heptaphylla	L. colorado, morado	cancer, leukemia	Brazil
Tabebuia ipe	Ipe roxo	Hodgkin's disease	Brazil
Tabebuia leucoxyla	—	diuretic	Brazil
Tabebuia pallida	—	colds	—
Tabebuia pentaphylla	—	analgesic	—
Tabebuia rosea	Roble colorado	fungicide	S.Amer.
Tabebuia rosea-alba	—	cancer	Brazil
Tecoma spp.	Yellow bells, tekoma	cancer	Brazil

Note: The plants on this list should only be used under a physician's direction. Please see the warning in the front of the book.

Pau d'arco is prepared as follows: two tablespoons of the bark to three cups of hot water. This is allowed to steep or gently simmer for 20 minutes. Patients take one cup in the morning, one at midday, and one before dinner. It can be taken cold, warm or hot without sugar. It should be refrig-erated between servings. It is said that each cup should be drunk without interruption but also not too quickly. Some sources say one can take up to six cups per day. Prof. Valter Accorsi used to regulate the dosage of tea "with a maximum indicated by the appearance of a 'slight rash.'"

Over the years, concerns have been raised about the potential toxicity of pau d'arco tea (391). It is certainly true that one should not just assume that a plant in general use is necessarily safe. In fact, the laborious work of

Dr. Frederick W. Freise has shown that not all pau d'arcos are safe to use as teas (212). Dr. Freise noted some "nasty reactions" to the bark of yellow pau d'arco, *Tabebuia umbellata*. An infusion of this bark, and even more so the wood, caused skin pustules to form. The patients' throats were affected with skin loss and there were bloody wounds. Extreme caution is in order with this and other yellow-flowering pau d'arcos. These include *T. pedicellata* in Brazil and *T. argentea* or *T. aurea* in Paraguay. In addition, *T. aurea* is part of a formula used by indigenous peoples to induce abortion, so it should never be taken by pregnant women.

There are also some toxicity questions about *T. neochrysantha*. Native Tikuna Indians in Colombia have learned to be cautious, and take only an eighth of a cup of this medicine, three times per day.

"Obviously," wrote Kenneth Jones (who has authored an excellent little book on the topic), "one cannot use just any pau d'arco." Yet, astonishingly, the bark of yellow pau d'arco has already been sold in the United States, and in at least one case the reactions were as Dr. Freise forewarned.

That said, most experts affirm that the bulk of pau d'arco sold in stores is safe. The Ministry of Health for the State of São Paulo, Brazil has accepted the safety of this herb. Teodoro Myer, one of the original developers of the product, claimed that "it may be taken in massive doses without fear and it may be combined with other medication, no matter how active the latter is; and it is suitable for children as it is for adults."

Professor Accorsi has noted in regard to alcohol extracts of the bark, "Many people who use too much of the extract (of the inner bark)...will feel a slight irritation, a sort of itchiness, although it is of no consequence. A person can take five grams of extract per kilogram of body weight, daily, with no damage" (212). I have heard reports of this itchiness from American cancer patients.

The American Herbal Products Association lists this as a class 1 herb, which can be safely consumed when used appropriately. It is not mentioned in Brinker's book on adverse reactions (52). James Duke says he wouldn't be afraid to drink one cup containing 10 grams of the herb steeped per day (113). In general, one should stick to the major brands and well-known suppliers.

History

Various species of pau d'arco have been used for a long time in Latin America as cancer treatments. In 1962, the National Cancer Institute central files contained information on its use in Brazil against cancer of the tongue, throat, esophagus, prostate, intestines, lung, head, and leukemia. All of this eventually found its way into Hartwell's book.

In addition, the so-called "active ingredient," lapachol (see below), first isolated from another plant (*Stereospermum suaveolens*) is an old cancer treatment. Preserved in ghee (clarified butter), it is mentioned as an East Indian remedy for abdominal cancer and nasal polyps by several sources dating from the late 19th century (116).

It is interesting that across the Atlantic, in Southern Africa, a similar tree containing the same key ingredient (lapachol) is also widely used as a remedy against cancer. This is *Kigelia pinnata*, the so-called sausage tree (of the same Bignonia family), which has been used in Nigeria as a treatment for malignant tumors, a usage first recorded in 1937. Scientists have now found that extracts of this African tree kill melanoma and ovarian cancer cells and also kill bacteria and fungi (201, 43).

In animal tests at the University of Hawaii, scientists showed that a tea made from a form of pau d'arco, *Tabebuia heptaphylla,* caused a "highly significant inhibition of metastases to the lung" with no further growth of the cancer. It did this, possibly, by stimulating the macrophage cells. Eighty percent of the mice who did not receive pau d'arco died, while 71 percent of those receiving it survived and remained healthy. Hawaiian scientists concluded that "appropriately activated macrophages provide a biological approach to the destruction of the few, but fatal, tumor cells that resist or escape conventional therapies."

The bark of pau d'arco contains numerous catechins, which have a very strong biological activity, even in small doses. Much interest has been stimulated by the presence of catechins in green tea. Japanese scientists found that green tea catechins induce apoptosis in stomach cancer cells. (Apoptosis is programmed cell death, or cell suicide, and is considered a better outcome of treatment than mere cytotoxicity) (179). A similar finding was made at Rockefeller University in regard to breast cancer cells (222). This data can perhaps be extrapolated to the catechins in pau d'arco as well.

Lapachol

As noted, the component of pau d'arco that has generated the greatest amount of scientific interest is a quinone called lapachol. It is structurally related to vitamin K, and has definite anticancer activity. Another key ingredient is a related compound, xyloidone. But lapachol also can cause significant toxicity in people, so that in order to achieve sufficiently high doses one risks considerable toxicity, as well (324a).

Lapachol is normally found as a yellow powder, similar to curry powder, on the surface of the timber of various Tabebuia, Tecoma and Bignonia species. When purified, lapachol has a bright, almost iridescent, yellow color. It was first isolated from the heartwood of various Asian and South American trees in 1857 and was intensively examined at that time. There are 41 citations in Medline relating to lapachol (22).

For example, two scientists at the University of Western Ontario are studying lapachol as a vitamin K1 antagonist. They were inspired to do so by pau d'arco's reputation as a folk treatment (108). In Brazil, the most prominent pau d'arco researcher has been Dr. Oswaldo Goncalves De Lima at the Recife Institute of Antibiotics in Pernambuco (which is now a WHO research center for indigenous plants).

His work has shown that lapachol has activity against herpes, polio, influenza and other viruses in the laboratory. "Naturally," remarks Kenneth Jones, "more work would be necessary in order to learn whether lapachol could be used to treat the diseases these viruses cause" (212).

Pau d'arco's scientific career as a potential anticancer agent is somewhat confusing. A water extract of the bark inhibited by 44 percent the growth of Walker 256 carcinoma in rats. But the doses were relatively high: 200 milligrams (mg) per kilogram (kg) of body weight, administered by intra-peritoneal injection. Pure lapachol did somewhat better—50 percent inhibition in Walker 256 and 82 percent in Yoshida sarcoma. It even had some activity when administered orally (324a).

Based on these results, Hartwell's Natural Products Branch at NCI test-ed pau d'arco extensively for antitumor activity. An odd finding was the antitumor activity observed in the water extracts could *not* in fact be rea-sonably attributed to lapachol or related lapachones. It seemed to be due to some unidentified compounds or a "pro-drug" type compound, which turns into the active ingredient once in the body (247). Due to its activity in the Walker 256 system, however, it was lapachol that was approved for human testing by the NCI in 1976.

Unfortunately, no significant anticancer activity was detected. The reason for this was thought to be that the absorption of lapachol administered by mouth was never great enough to reach the critical antitumor stage (27). The drug was therefore eliminated from the testing program. However, NCI's own finding that lapachol was not the active antitumor constituent throws doubt on the conclusiveness of the entire experiment.

Despite this failure, public (and some scientific) interest in pau d'arco has persisted, as anecdotal accounts of "cures" accumulated. In the 1980s, med-ical botanists still listed this phytochemical as one of the most important antitumor agents found in plants. California oncologist Rowan Chlebowski, MD, PhD, wrote a letter to a medical journal in which he argued that lapa-chol should be reevaluated in the light of modern knowledge of its use and action (78). This has not yet happened in the United States.

There was also one small clinical trial on lapachol in Brazil. It purported to show that three out of eight patients had either complete or partial remis-sions of their cancer after taking an oral dose. The three patients who responded had cancers of the mouth, the intestines, and kidney. It took almost two years for one of the patients to finally respond to the tea. Obviously, this is a very limited study that needs to be repeated. By folk reputation, pau d'arco is also said to have particular activity against leukemia.

Pain Relief

Pau d'arco is sometimes used to relieve pain associated with cancer. One patient wrote to me after taking the tea that she was pain-free from her advanced breast cancer. "I discontinued pau d'arco for one week," she wrote, "and the pain went to around five or six" (on a scale in which 10 is pain-free). When she resumed the tea the pain again vanished.

Although pau d'arco holds some promise as an adjuvant treatment in cancer, it is frustrating to note that it has been heavily and often unethically promoted. This hype originated in Brazil in the spring of 1967. "As hundreds offered testimony before the cameras of São Paulo TV," wrote Kenneth Jones, "people began ripping the bark from the trees wherever they could be found."

A popular news magazine, *O'Cruzeiro,* reported "Cancer has a cure....the news—cure for cancer—is to be taken as being essentially true and honest, or more exactly, strictly scientific." Kenneth Jones is quick to add, "the news was not 'scientific' and contrary to what the story would have had people believe, cancer did not at last have a cure." But this is the way that irresponsible journalists sometimes play with the emotions of cancer patients for their own purposes.

This particular craze had a religious twist, since most stories focused on a cancer-ridden girl in Rio who was reputedly led to pau d'arco tea by a mysterious monk who appeared to her in a vision. Anecdotes of "cures" followed, including one about a nun who was cured of her tongue cancer, a man whose scalp tumors disappeared under topical application, and a patient with stage IV stomach cancer. This man "should have been dead a year earlier," the papers claimed, but now came to a clinic frequently by traveling on foot from outside the city. He appeared to be on the mend. All of these stories led to a near-religious frenzy centered on this tea.

The main champion of pau d'arco was Dr. Valter Accorsi, professor emeritus at the University of São Paulo. Jones describes him as "one of Brazil's most prominent patrons of herbs."

Accorsi was no simple cure monger. He himself later made rather circumspect statements about its effectiveness. He said that after seven years of first-hand observation, he felt it had six main areas of application: as a diuretic, sedative, analgesic, decongestant, antibiotic, and cardiotonic (212).

Just how these properties related to cancer is not clear.

As word spread of a "cancer cure," so did the size of the crowds seeking this miraculous treatment. A news magazine found Prof. Accorsi attending to lines of over 2,000 patients per day, to whom he was distributing the tea free of charge! Multitudes gathered on the lawn in front of the hospital at Santo André, clamoring for the precious bark.

The presence of unruly crowds, and the media circus, caused a backlash among doctors and hospital administrators. They unwisely hung up signs saying that distribution of the bark was henceforth suspended. The populace was not so easily deterred, however. In Campinas, patients and their relatives scaled the walls of the Botanical Gardens to strip the bark from Tabebuia trees. (These had been conveniently identified as "purple pau d'arco" by botanists.) The Garden had to post guards to protect its plants. "Pau d'arco," as Kenneth Jones remarked, "had become a phenomenon."

Reporters later admitted that they had deliberately mischaracterized pau d'arco a "cure" for cancer and diabetes in order to "make it stand out." This they certainly did. The masses were sufficiently aroused and newspapers were flying off the stands. Meanwhile, in the hospital all experiments with pau d'arco were stopped and the entire staff was forbidden to even discuss the matter. They even denied ever having used pau d'arco. "Now it was war," says Jones. *O'Cruzeiro* retaliated by reproducing prescriptions for pau d'arco on the hospital's letterhead.

The suspension of pau d'arco studies reached the legislature, but this political involvement only hardened the doctors' stance. São Paulo Hospital then issued an announcement deriding pau d'arco, announcing that the bark provided "no benefit at all for the treatment of cancer." The Brazilian Cancer Society condemned the use of the tea to treat cancer (247).

Headlines in some newspapers then screamed "Pau d'Arco Doesn't Cure Cancer." They took the doctors' side, calling pau d'arco an "annual cure-all foisted upon an unfortunate and all-too-eager public by the unscrupulous." Meanwhile, to complicate an already murky situation, hucksters began to sell phony "pau d'arcos" for the real thing (212).

Eventually, the whole craze petered out, although a few doctors in South America are still using the tea. A few more animal experiments were done, but the issue was essentially dead. On two occasions (in 1975 and 1979) an open-minded new clinical director of the Hospital of Santo André tried to launch clinical trials, only to be voted down by a majority of the doctors. Even a dozen years after the initial controversy, "they would have nothing to do with such a scheme for fear of being labeled quacks," said Jones (212).

Pau d'arcomania eventually spread to the United States via the tabloid and health press. In the 1980s, phenomenal claims were routinely made for it. A right-wing newspaper, the *Spotlight,* listed 35 diseases which pau d'arco purportedly cured or relieved (6/8/81). *Let's Live* magazine cited reports that pau d'arco "cured terminal leukemia, arthritis, yeast and fungus infections, arrested pain, stopped athlete's foot and cured the common cold." It added that it "has been found to be an effective analgesic, sedative, decongestant, diuretic and hypotensive" (2/85).

Vegetarian Times (7/85) claimed that the bark "is currently being hailed for its effects on cancer and candida...Traditional herbalists agree that it strengthens and balances the immune system" and is a useful remedy for immune system-related problems such as colds, flu, boils, infections, as well as malaria. It "can combat infection, give great vitality, build up immunity to disease, strengthen cellular structure and help eliminate pain and inflammation..."

A Brazilian doctor named Paulo Martin was often quoted in these articles, attesting to the virtues of the miracle tea. A supermarket tabloid, the *Globe,* ran the following statement:

"American herbal medicine experts Dr. James Duke of the National Institutes of Health, and Dr. Norman Farnsworth, of the University of Illinois, confirm Martin's claims. 'Taheebo undoubtedly contains a substance found to be highly effective against cancers...'" (the *Globe,* 98/15/81).

In fact, neither Duke nor Farnsworth believed that pau d'arco was a cure for cancer. Duke was appalled at the way his name was misused and his credentials mistaken. But on the strength of this spurious "recommendation" banner ads quickly appeared: "1,000-year-old Inca cancer cure works." In the public relations material of the promoter, key words were omitted to make it seem that Duke and Farnsworth were behind pau d'arco's promotion.

Once this was established it became part of pau d'arco folklore in the United States. As previously mentioned, when I challenged a distributor of pau d'arco and another Latin American sensation, aveloz, to substantiate her claims of efficacy, she quickly trotted out the alleged endorsement by Norman Farnsworth, and James Duke "of the National Institutes of Health," where he never worked. But this telltale mistake reveals that the original venue of this reference was the *Globe* article. This canard was still making the rounds, and still making money for pau d'arco's promoters nearly 20 years later (113). Alwyn Gentry, author of the most complete scientific monograph on the plant, believes that "while Tabebuia bark clearly includes chemicals with antitumor properties, these are often wildly exaggerated in the herbal medicine literature" (145).

Pau d'arco truly seems to contain some anticancer principles. Its failure in clinical trials is of course disappointing, but the reason may be that lapachol has been overrated as a single "active ingredient." It may be more worthwhile to try the entire tea taken for a longer period of time, perhaps as part of a secondary prevention regimen.

Chapter 16 ❦ Hulda Clark (Canada)

ULDA REGEHR CLARK, PHD, ND, IS A RESEARCH SCIENTIST AND NATUROPATH WITH A STARTLING THEORY ABOUT THE CAUSES AND cure of cancer. Essentially, Dr. Clark believes that cancer is caused by a parasite and can be quickly cured by eliminating that parasite from the body.

Now, parasite theories of cancer are nothing new. Jacob Wolff, in his magisterial history of the disease, devotes an entire section to "Theories of Parasitism" (413). There is no need to review it here, except to say that all prior parasite theories have been rejected by conventional science. But Clark's theory is unique. According to her, cancer is exclusively caused by infection with the human intestinal fluke, whose scientific name is *Fasciolopsis buski*.

Dr. Clark is no amateur dabbler in science. She studied biology at the University of Saskatchewan, where she was awarded both a BA and MA with honors. After two years at McGill University, she received a PhD in biology at the University of Minnesota in 1958 (for a study on the ion balance of crayfish muscle (79, 248, 376). In 1979, she left government-funded research and began private health consulting full time. So, although she was never a major player in the research field, her opinions should carry some weight.

Her theory is influencing many people. In 1990, she says, she first "noticed clues as to the cause of cancer." Her 1993 book, *The Cure for All Cancers,* followed by *The Cure for HIV and AIDS* and *The Cure for All*

Diseases, have become bestsellers in the field of alternative health. Some patients speak with religious zeal about their faith in the Clark method. A Canadian-American bookseller told me that he makes ten times as much money from Hulda Clark's books and products than all other cancer books combined.

The stakes are very high: if Dr. Clark is right, then both a simple cause and cure of cancer have been discovered, and millions of lives can be spared. If she is wrong, however, then thousands of people are being cruelly deceived into following a worthless and possibly harmful regimen. Some might even delay getting treatments that could really help them.

Flukes and Alcohol

"How can the human intestinal fluke cause cancer?" Dr. Clark asks. "This parasite typically lives in the intestine where it might do little harm, causing only colitis, Crohn's disease, or irritable bowel syndrome, or perhaps nothing at all. But if it invades a different organ, like the uterus or kidneys or liver, it does a great deal of harm." In particular, if these flukes establish themselves in the liver, says Dr. Clark, it causes cancer.

She believes that *F. buski* only establishes itself in the liver of some people. These are the people who also have the solvent propyl alcohol in their bodies. Propyl alcohol is responsible for letting the fluke establish itself in the liver. Her central thesis is that "In order to get cancer, you must have both the parasite and propyl alcohol in your body" (80). All cancer patients, she says, have both.

Propyl or isopropyl alcohol is the form most commonly sold in pharmacies, having displaced the once more common ethyl alcohol. It is also present in many industrial products and others, besides Dr. Clark, believe that it is a widespread contaminant in foods and cosmetics. It is nearly ubiquitous.

To get rid of cancer, in her view, is not all that difficult. One has to kill the parasite in all of its stages; second, stop exposure to propyl alcohol; and finally, flush out the metals and common toxins from the body so that the patient can get well. These "common toxins" include many chemicals and heavy metals, including, Dr. Clark says, the mercury-containing amalgam fillings in teeth. (Many alternative doctors believe that mercury-containing fillings are a source of ill health, a position vehemently denied by the American Dental Association.)

Parasite elimination can be performed in one of two ways. One is to utilize a small electrical device called a Zapper, which does the job electronically. Clark gives detailed instructions on how to build a Zapper for under $40 from parts obtainable at Radio Shack. Or one can purchase it for around $100 from advertisements in many health magazines. There is much one could say about the Zapper, but I shall not expound on it in a book about herbs.

Clark says one can also employ a combination of three herbs to kill the parasite and its eggs. These herbs are wormwood (*Artemisia absinthium*); an alcohol tincture of the green rinds of black walnuts (*Juglans nigra*); and whole cloves (*Eugenia caryophyllata*), of the sort one buys whole in the supermarket.

Cloves do have some activity against microbes, viruses and (by reputation) parasites. There is also a history of using cloves unofficially in the treatment of cancer. English herbalist William H. Webb once claimed to have cured a case of recurrent breast cancer with a tea made of cloves, sarsaparilla, burdock, and red clover flower, as well as a suitable diet (343, 154).

Cloves are being actively investigated as a source of an anti-herpes compound, eugeniin (242a). The major component of clove oil, eugenol, has some cancer-inhibiting properties, since papilloma formation decreases by 84 percent when scientists first apply eugenol. Although AHPA considers cloves a class 1 herb, i.e., safe when consumed appropriately, the record is not unmixed: there have been reports of eugenol promoting the growth of tumors (199a).

Herbalist Michael Castleman sensibly remarks that cloves are "one of many healing herbs with both pro- and anti-cancer effects. At this point, scientists aren't sure which way the balance tilts. Until they are, anyone with a history of cancer should not use medicinal amounts of cloves."

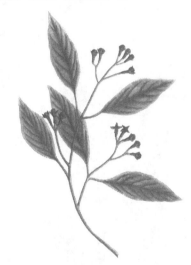

Eugenia caryophyllata
(cloves)

Clark's second herb is a tincture of black walnut rind. This is an old anti-parasite folk medicine. In 1830 Rafinesque wrote that "the green rind rubbed on tetters and ringworm dispels them" (324). According to Lust, "the green rind of the fruit makes a good poultice to get rid of ringworm" (268). Black walnut tincture was a substantial part of the patent medicine business. My guess is that it is an effective dewormer, if worms are indeed one's problem. There is a minor association with cancer: Chinese studies show that an extract of a related species, *Juglans regia*, inhibits various ascites cancers, spontaneous mammary tumors in mice, etc. (47).

In Alabama, Hartwell says, black walnut meat was traditionally combined with milk and apples, to treat leukemia. There is no indication of whether it was at all successful.

Black walnut is a class 2 herb. AHPA warns that prolonged use is not advised due to the presence of significant quantities of juglone, a known mutagen in animals. Carcinogenic effects have been associated with the external use of *Juglans regia* in humans. So like cloves, the record is decidedly mixed.

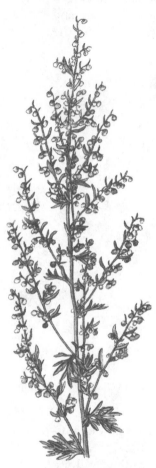

Artemisia absinthium
(wormwood)

Finally, there is wormwood (*Artemisia absinthium*), so named because of its historic use as a vermifuge, i.e., an agent to kill worms. I am unaware of any studies showing that it was ever traditionally used against cancer.

Dr. Clark warns about the toxicity of synthetic drugs. "Drug parasiticides can be extremely toxic," she cautions, "even in the small doses needed" (6). Yet she recommends that patients take 80 capsules of her wormwood combination to cure their cancer, with another 80 capsules to kill the remaining parasites. (This, she says, is the equivalent of half a cup of fresh leaves.) About the toxicity of wormwood, she has this to say:

"The amount you need to cure a cancer is very small, yet you cannot do without it. But the FDA has regulated it as toxic! It is therefore unavailable in concentrated form from herb companies. The evidence for toxicity accepted by the FDA must have been hearsay. I have never seen a case of toxicity, not so much as a headache or nausea. The toxic level must be much higher than is needed to kill these parasites....Of course, the FDA cannot be expected to accept experiences such as mine. We should find out what evidence they did accept" (80).

Here's some evidence: for almost a century it has been well known that wormwood contains very toxic substances. It gained international notoriety as a flavoring agent in absinthe. Vincent Van Gogh, Edgar Degas, and Paul Verlaine could all testify to its harmful effects. "At the end of the 19th century," wrote herbalist Maurice Mességué, who can hardly be accused of anti-botanical prejudice, wormwood was "as great a social menace as the use of hard drugs like heroin is today" (275a).

After an addict killed his family and attempted suicide, most countries banned the drink by 1915.

The volatile oil of wormwood is present in the whole plant in concentrations of 0.25 to 1.32 percent. It contains thujone, a toxic principle present in the volatile oil in concentrations of three to 12 percent (392). How toxic is thujone? Well, the supposedly toxic synthetic treatment for flukes, praziquantel, is deadly to rodents (LD50) when given at a dose of

2500 mg/kg. But the natural substance thujone causes convulsions in rodents when injected at just 40 mg/kg and causes fatalities at 120 mg/kg (a twentieth of the fatal dose of praziquantel).

I do not know how much thujone is in the dose that Clark is recommending and whether this amount could have a detrimental effect. But here is a perfect illustration of the fact that just because a substance is natural does not mean that it is necessarily harmless, or because something is synthetic that it is automatically more dangerous.

The Parasite

Central to Dr. Clark's theory is the parasite itself, *Fasciolopsis buski*. Is there any scientific validity to the idea that *F. buski* is a common parasite of humans and that it causes cancer?

F. buski is a fluke (trematode), a parasitic flatworm whose life cycle involves sexual reproduction in its mammalian hosts, as well as asexual reproduction in its intermediate host, the snail. The life cycle of the hermaphroditic fluke is fascinating. Its first stage is a cercaria. This is a free-swimming larva that emerges from its snail host and encysts on vegetables. The second stage is the metacercaria. This is the encysted stage in the fluke's life history, prior to its transfer to the definitive host, man. They enter humans who eat the raw pods, roots, stems, or bulbs of certain aquatic plants. Finally, there is the mature worm that attaches itself by suckers to an organ and begins to lay eggs. These pass out of the human body, hatch, and begin the cycle all over again.

What happens inside humans is a real medical melodrama. Once in the small intestines, a worm emerges from the ingested cyst, attaches itself by suckers to the inside wall of the intestines (specifically, the mucosal lining of the duodenum and jejunum), and then grows into an inch-long adult, which lives off its human host. It then begins a phase of prodigious egg production. The "purpose" of this egg laying is not to spread eggs around this particular host, however. Huge numbers of eggs are passed out of the host (in the feces, urine or sputum) where—if conditions are sufficiently unsanitary—they find their way again into fresh water. There, they are carried by snails to the roots of aquatic plants.

But how do humans come into contact with aquatic plants? In certain cultures, people eat raw water chestnuts, ingest the cysts, and perpetuate the cycle. It is noteworthy that merely eating raw water chestnuts purchased in the market is probably not enough to become infected. Rather, one must be in the habit of "peeling the metacercaria-infested hull of these vegetables with the teeth before consumption," to quote a standard textbook on the subject (112).

Ingesting raw water chestnuts in the wild might give the victim one or a few parasites to deal with, but never more than the number of cysts that were eaten. To get a raging infection, the patient must be re-infected over and over again. They've got to keep coming back to the rice patty for additional water chestnuts and peeling the hulls with their teeth to become seriously imperiled by *F. buski.*

F. buski infection is usually silent and non-debilitating. True, wherever its suckers grab onto the intestinal wall, it causes ulceration and even some bleeding. But usually that is about all it does. Dr. Barbara L. Doughty has written:

"...Fasciolopsiasis [i.e., infection with *F. buski*]...appears to be associated with few or no disease manifestations in individuals examined in field environments. In a controlled study involving clinical examination, evaluation of growth and development, hematologic studies, and screening tests for intestinal malabsorption, no significant differences between infected and uninfected subjects were found" (32).

Some other sources claim that even in the early stages of infection there may be some abdominal pain, as well as diarrhea and nausea, alternating with constipation (*EB* 4:691). All agree that in a case of a very heavy and untreated infection, there is usually diarrhea, abdominal pain, edema (such as swelling of the face), and passage of undigested food in the feces. General body weakness and fluid retention can have serious consequences, especially in children. But there is no known association with cancer or AIDS—at least none known to people who have spent their professional lives examining this question. (Dr. Doughty, for example, is Professor of Immunoparasitology at Texas A&M University.)

Every standard source says that infection with *F. buski* occurs primarily in East Asia—China, India, Thailand, etc. It is usually contracted after people eat and peel uncooked water chestnuts in the field. The remedy is to stop doing so, and to boil aquatic foods. The disease can also be treated with a number of drugs, such as hexylresorcinol and tetrachlorethylene. If you are an Asian peasant who picks water chestnuts in the wild and then eats them in the traditional manner, you are at moderate risk of developing a symptom-free infection. From a conventional point of view, it is hard to see how others are similarly threatened.

How Common is Fasciolopsis Infection?

Yet Dr. Clark claims that *Fasciolopsis buski* infection is so common that it causes not just some, but *all,* cases of cancer (and, in her other books, of AIDS and other life-threatening diseases as well). By her theory, millions upon millions of people would have to be infected. Consider the numbers.

Between 1990 and 1998 there have been approximately 11 million new cancer cases diagnosed in the United States alone. Over 1.2 million new cases are added each year. And this does not even count the myriad numbers of men with occult prostate cancer, men and women with *in situ* carcinomas, and a vast army of individuals with past, present or future basal and squamous cell carcinomas of the skin, which do not even make it into the record books (5).

For Dr. Clark's theory to be right, every one of these individuals must be harboring egg-laying *F. buski* (as well as traces of propyl alcohol) in their bodies. We are talking about a raging worldwide epidemic of *F. buski* infection! But beyond her own rather mysterious testing procedure, Dr. Clark offers no evidence that this is so.

However, the question of fasciolopsiasis is no stranger to medical science. Public health officials are well aware of its potential for harm and have good reason to be concerned about the possibility of *F. buski* spreading in our societies. They have been trying hard to find out if it is a threat.

Yet every authoritative source says the same thing: that so far, *F. buski* infections "are confined largely to Asia," in particular East Asia. By contrast, Dr. Clark says it is a widespread epidemic all over the world (since cancer exists all over the world) (32). So who is right?

Dr. Clark's method of testing for Fasciolopis is not spelled out in her book, but I suspect that it is not something she learned at the University of Minnesota. In an interview, she stated, "bowel testing... was completely inadequate but I developed an electronic way of testing and that was from my background in physics and biophysics that I was able to do that" (186).

There are, however, standard scientific means of examining stool samples for signs of parasitical infecton. These methods are uniform all over the world and essentially, require demonstrating the presence of *F. buski* eggs in the stool. This Kato-Katz thick smear method provides the clearest proof of all fluke infections.

The most extensive study was a 1987 US government survey of parasite infections among the general population. Among other potential sources of disease, they looked for *F. buski* infections. Those carrying out this huge survey were the Division of Parasitic Diseases of the National Center for Infectious Diseases (NCID), in collaboration with the Association of Directors of the State and Territorial Laboratories. At the end, they issued a 21-page report in the Center for Disease Control's (CDC) *Morbidity and Mortality Weekly Report* (220).

Results were obtained from 49 states (Wyoming, for reasons of its own, did not provide tests for intestinal parasites). A total of 216,275 stool specimens were examined and of these, 43,539 (20.1 percent) were positive for one or more parasites. In other words, one out of five people tested in the

US does have a parasite. Over 15,000 of these were *Giardia lamblia* infection. But how many people had *F. buski* infection? *Only one.* One out of 216,275. We can conclude that it is practically non-existent in the US, which would make it difficult for it to cause 1.2 million cases of cancer per year.

Similar findings have come from other countries, including those where this fluke really is something of a problem. Thus, in Shanghai, Chinese public health scientists tested 5,479 school children and discovered an extraordinarily high 52.2 percent with parasitical infections. Yet the rate of infection specifically with *F. buski* was a mere 0.8 percent (141). And it was found that the rate of fasciolopsiasis was declining in China as a whole (417a).

Ninety-three Thai workers in Israel were also tested. (There are fears that immigrant Asian workers might be spreading the disease to their host populations.) Stool samples revealed that 74 percent of them had parasitical infestations (mainly hookworm). But there were just three cases of *F. buski* infection among such workers (149). In Taiwan, over a thousand Thai workers were tested and not a single case of infection with this fluke was found (314, 262). In Sulawesi, Indonesia, 68.3 percent of the population had hookworm. But no cases of fasciolopsiasis were discovered among stool samples (269). And so forth.

I think we can reasonably conclude that *F. buski* is a nearly non-existent problem in the United States and many other countries. Defenders of Dr. Clark might contend that all these statisticians are covering up *F. buski's* prevalence in order to deny the validity of her theory. However, the majority of these studies were done before Dr. Clark had published a word on her liver fluke theory.

If Dr. Clark's theory were true, then cancer rates should logically parallel parasite infection rates. Yet World Health Organization figures show an opposite trend. Cancer rates are highest in industrialized countries, and lowest in Third World countries. By Clark's theory, you would expect Mexico to have a higher rate of cancer than the US or Canada. In fact, it has half the cancer rate. One would also have to account for the fact that, in general, males have twice the cancer rate of females. I see no reason, according to Dr. Clark's theory, that this should be so.

In *A Cure for All Cancers,* Clark claims that cancer can be totally eradicated in those who follow her treatment program. "This book is not about remission," she writes, defiantly. "It is about cure."

"Give me three weeks," she promises on the back cover, "and your oncologist will cancel your surgery!"

Dr. Clark sets little store in biopsies, pathology reports, X rays, MRI or CT scans, etc. Apparently, she does not employ biochemical tests for any of the known cancer markers. She makes her diagnosis based solely on the presence (or absence) of a single substance: ortho-phospho-tyrosine (which I shall abbreviate OPT). If a person tests positive for OPT, they have cancer. If they don't, they are free of the dread disease.

Dr. Clark states that "although there are no true clinical cancer tests, there are more than two dozen markers. Each can identify a particular cancer with reasonable accuracy. Recently, ortho-phospho-tyrosine has been found to be reliable for many kinds of human malignancies." She cites two articles to support this global statement (197, 419).

Despite her contention, ortho-phospho-tyrosine is not a well-known entity in cancer research. The phrase itself does not occur in any of the major cancer textbooks. It does not occur in this form even once in the nine million articles referenced by the Medline database (nor was it the subject of any abstracts at the 1998 American Society of Clinical Oncology meeting). OPT appears to be a growth factor, or what is known more generally as a protein or tyrosine kinase.

Although this is a promising line of research, nothing indicates that it is a sure-fire test for cancer. It was found to vary considerably in melanoma cell lines (117). It was "inconsistently increased" in ovarian tumor cells (409, 283). It was present in three out of five lymphoma samples and in one out of three human breast cancer samples (409).

To claim that OPT (or related chemicals) have been established as nearly universal markers is to tremendously overstate the case. Nor is it clear how Dr. Clark "tests" for the presence of ortho-phospho-tyrosine. She never says.

Dr. Clark could conceivably be able to cure cancer in isolated instances— "by a fluke," you might say. For example, let us imagine for a moment that although cancer patients do not have *F. buski* infections, they have other parasitical infections (such as giardia). Might not a dose of antiparasite medicine lessen this burden on the immune system, thereby freeing up immunological reserve to fight the cancer? Some people point to the use of levamisole, an immune modulating agent for colon cancer, that doubles as a deworming agent in sheep. No one knows exactly how levamisole works. I have heard it suggested that Dr. Clark's medicines work in the same mysterious way.

Well, perhaps. But before we accept this idea we need proof that Clark's method actually cures cancers as she states. Dr. Clark presents 100 such cases in her book.

To affirm that 100 individuals were cured of cancer requires certain pieces of information. We need to know, obviously, that all of them had cancer. Nowadays, almost everyone agrees that proof of cancer comes through biopsies, which are carefully examined by skilled pathologists. And so the first question is, Did every one of the 100 individuals in Clark's book have biopsy-confirmed cancer? Then, if they did indeed have biopsy-confirmed cancers, did they receive potentially curative treatments (such as surgery) before receiving Clark's treatment? Is there any proof that they were now free of cancer, again by standard tests? How long has this remission lasted? (Five years is a conventional marker of "cure.") Obviously, it would take a book to fully analyze all of Dr. Clark's cases. But, as a sample, let us just examine the first five cases in her book:

Case 1. Lydia Hernandez (all names changed by Dr. Clark herself) consulted Clark for laryngitis. On the basis of her idiosyncratic tests for *F. buski*, propyl alcohol, and OPT, Clark diagnosed Lydia as having breast cancer. Five days later "both breasts are hot and tender with the nipple affected." Ms. Hernandez begins Clarks' program. Four days later she is no longer testing positive for *F. buski* and her "breasts are feeling better." Three weeks later, "Throat feels bad. Head is congested. Breasts OK." Five months later, "she feels much better."

In her summary, Dr. Clark writes, "This was a case where cancer was not suspected until she had the breast symptoms." But obviously heat and tenderness alone are not symptoms specific to breast cancer. There is no independent confirmation that this person ever had cancer, much less was cured of it.

Case 2. Janet Chapman, Thymus Cancer. Clark says Ms. Chapman had recently had a chest X ray and was discovered to have a benign growth in her thymus. Upon surgery, however, they found active cancer in both the thymus gland and local extensions and "a couple of spots" in the right lower lung. Ms. Chapman had 36 radiation treatments over a seven week period. Two months later, she experienced "tightness of chest again." Fluid was taken from her chest. "A tumor is in her left chest cavity," Clark states.

Ms. Chapman tested positive for OPT. After Clark's treatment, one week later she tested negative. Five days after that "she is still coughing and very weak." Three weeks more and "her cough is worse." She is still negative for OPT, however, but is testing positive for formaldehyde and dog heartworm. According to Clark's note: "Dog heartworm also causes coughing." Then comes this amazing statement: "Note: she is simply dying of heartworm and formaldehyde. The cancer was stopped weeks ago." There is, however, no evidence presented that her cancer was in remission.

Case 3. Ida Birdsall, Cervical Cancer. Ms. Birdsall was diagnosed with carcinoma of the uterus (presumably the cervix). She has had a complete hysterectomy, but is still positive for OPT and *F. buski*. After two weeks on Clark's program, she is no longer positive for OPT. The family was "perplexed when the cancer wasn't gone after the surgery....But they carried out the instructions and took on new living habits and became completely free of it." Note that the residual cancer was both "diagnosed" and "cured" by Clark using her own methods. There was no independent confirmation of it, whatsoever.

Case 4. Pamela Charles, Breast Cancer. Ms. Charles was conventionally diagnosed with carcinoma of the breast with metastases to two lymph nodes. She had a lumpectomy and was in the middle of postoperative radiation therapy when she came to Clark. Clark diagnosed her as positive for OPT ("at bone, edge of breast") and for *F. buski* in the liver. Eight weeks later she was negative for both of these by Clark's tests. She agreed to drink three cups of two percent milk, reduce phosphate foods, take a magnesium oxide tablet daily, and continue on the anti-parasite program.

Clark remarks, "Note that Pamela still had the cancer in spite of the recent surgery. In fact, it was spreading to the bone." But confirmation of this comes only from Clark's own "test," not from bone scans.

"Since she was sandwiched into a 15-minute time slot," Clark adds, "I didn't do complete testing." Imagine being able to diagnose local extensions and bone metastases, prescribe or administer a curative regimen, and see the patient out, all in 15 minutes.

Case 5. Brenda Rasmussen, Breast Cancer. Ms. Rasmussen had a "large, malignant lump (size of a hen's egg) over the right breast." She "has not accepted the doctor's diagnosis," Clark writes, "does not wish to talk about cancer." But it is not clear how her conventional doctor made his diagnosis of cancer. Brenda tested positive for OPT as well as various heavy metals. Six months later a friend "called to say she was doing OK but still had her lump. She had not stopped the colonics [which Dr. Clark apparently opposes] nor was she sticking to her new rules of living. We thanked her kindly and wished her well," Clark adds. As a reminder, this is counted as one of the 100 "cured cancer cases" in Dr. Clark's book.

The other cases in the book are of similar quality. Many did not have cancer except by their own self-diagnoses or by the OPT and *F. buski* tests that Dr. Clark devised. Overwhelmingly, those who were diagnosed with cancer by oncologists still had their cancer when they left Dr. Clark's care.

It is doubtful if there is a single patient in her book with a genuine biopsy-diagnosed malignancy who was treated by Dr. Clark and whose full recovery was documented using the standards observed by medical scientists all over the world.

Yet, amazingly, the cult of Hulda Clark continues to grow. Dr. Clark has held seminars for physicians, therapists, and health practitioners, from Africa to Bogota, Colombia, on Nevis Island in the Caribbean. On the Internet you can find dozens of sites promoting her views. One Website, (www.curecancer.com) promises to "Cure Intestinal Cancers in 5 Days, Cure Organ Cancers in 60 days and Cure Brain Cancers in 90 days," all based on Clark's theories. Many companies sell the herbs and electronic gear she recommends. One company ("Specializing in Cutting-Edge Alternative Health Products") sells Zappers for $76. Their Zapper, they report, "is "CERTIFIED and APPROVED by Dr. Clark's son, Geoff Clark." At another site, you can buy Clark's so-called Syncrometer for $189 or a $29.95 video to help you build it yourself (http://www.cris.com/~healthy/).

There is also *The Clark Method* newsletter ($99 for 12 issues), audio and video tapes of Dr. Clark's presentations and an Arizona-based multi-level marketing (MLM) company that sells a parasite cleanse based on her theories (www.healthres.com).

It is understandable that some patients, terrified and confused, would turn towards simplistic solutions. What is more astonishing is that some doctors and authors in the field have uncritically embraced this approach.

In the so-called *Definitive Guide to Cancer,* published by the Burton Goldberg group, Dr. Clark merits two pages of positive discussion. We are told that she "presents 100 case histories illustrating the role of parasites and propyl alcohol in cancer and how an herbal formula...helps to eliminate them." We are also informed that ortho-phospho-tyrosine is "a reliable cancer marker for different kinds of malignancies" (107). Another author states that "since the herbal part of her cure is cheap and not harmful, we can happily do this no matter what else we wish to do" (73).

Such uncritical comments are frequently repeated in health newspapers and magazines. What is lacking in all this is not only logic, but any data to support Hulda Clark's contention that she can cure cancer.

I once requested from a major Clark promoter the names of people who had been cured of cancer by her method. The only reply I got was a fax from a kindly old gentleman who told me that he "knew" he had cancer from the small bore (diameter) of his bowel movements. On his own, he began treatment with Hulda Clark's three-herb program. After taking the treatment, he exulted, "I pooped like a horse!"

This is what passes for proof of "the cure for all cancers."

Chapter 17 ❧ Carnivora (Germany)

CARNIVORA® IS A PATENTED EXTRACT OF PRESS JUICE FROM *DIONAEA MUSCIPULA*, OR VENUS'S-FLYTRAP. THIS A MEMBER OF THE SUNDEW family (Droseraceae). It is used in Germany and some other countries as an immune-modulating and anticancer agent.

The Venus's-flytrap is a low perennial herb with a very restricted range. Found in nature only in the wet boglands and sandy bays of North and South Carolina, this plant is the only member of its genus. It is world-famous as a carnivore, i.e., it eats insects and other small animals. It also does well in terraria, where it can be potted in sphagnum moss, the pots set in about one inch of water. Venus's-flytrap is sometimes grown as a curiosity or for classroom demonstrations. Charles Darwin called it "the most wonderful plant in the world."

The leaves of the plant form an ingenious fly-catching device. The two nearly circular lobes have spiny teeth along their margins and six trigger hairs on each leaf. If these triggers are set off during the daytime they snap shut in about half a second. Glands on the leaf's surface then secrete a red sap that digests the body of the insect, imbuing the entire leaf with a red, flowerlike appearance (*EB* 12:311). The two closed halves with their interlocking teeth prevent the hapless victim from escaping. The acidic, digestive fluid gradually dissolves, and absorbs, the proteins of the prey. After about ten days, the plant opens again, the residual insect debris blows away and the plant is ready for more victims.

Venus's-flytrap is not listed in the standard herbals as a medicinal plant.

Two reasons for this are (a) its limited geographic range and (b) concerns over possible toxicity (although such reports are often exaggerated).

An extract of Venus's-flytrap was introduced into medicine by Helmut Keller, MD, of Germany. Dr. Keller was born in 1940 in Erlangen, and received his medical degree from that city's University in February, 1970. He then served in the Department of Oncology at the Tumor Clinic Oberstaufen, and practiced pediatrics, internal medicine, and surgery from October 1971 to March 1972. From June 1972 till December 1973, he was a researcher at Boston University.

Dr. Keller has been practicing general medicine and treating cancer patients in Germany since 1974. In 1973, while in America, he began testing juices pressed from the Venus's-flytrap, which his wife collected as a hobby. Since Venus's-flytraps are such efficient digesters of protein, Keller had a hunch that they might be useful in digesting the abnormal proteins found in cancer. For the next few months, as a sideline to his work, he applied plant extracts to human cancer cells growing in hamsters. Those animals that received a flytrap extract showed marked reduction in their tumors, he said. Keller dubbed his extract "Carnivora," meaning "meateater," referring to the plant's famous insect-devouring ability.

Since moving back to Germany, Keller has administered Carnivora to about 2,000 patients at his clinic in Germany. Morton Walker, an American medical writer who has written enthusiastically about this treatment, has stated that President Ronald Reagan, Nancy Reagan, and Yul Brynner all received Carnivora treatments.

Keller's company, Carnivora-Forschungs GmbH, has published a chemical analysis of the product. By using a combination of standard techniques (HPLC, etc.) it shows that there are four active ingredients in fresh *Dionaea muscipula*. For the record, these are three naphthoquinones (droserone, plumbagin, and 3-chloroplumbagin) as well as hydroplumbagin-4-0-b glucoside. The last named chemical was newly discovered in Venus's-flytrap by B. Kreher at the Ludwig-Maximillians University of Munich, who has done most of the laboratory work on Carnivora. Plumbagin is a non-toxic substance which has demonstrated antimicrobial and anticancer properties in scientific studies (200, 127, 275, 240, 74).

There are in fact 640 mg of hydroplumbagin-glucoside and 205 mg of plumbagin in each 100 grams of fresh plant. (The other ingredients are only present in minute amounts.) A small amount of these chemicals is found in the finished product. The press juice (extracted from the plant), also contains a mixture of nine amino acids, according to Kreher's analysis (237).

Venus's-flytrap does not appear significantly toxic. Ninety-day studies with rats receiving doses 30-60 times higher than the recommended human dose reported no toxic reactions. There was no significant change in their weight gain, food and water consumption, behavior, blood or urine tests. The only "abnormality" upon autopsy was that their immune systems had been activated. Taken orally undiluted, Carnivora® can sometimes produce mild gastrointestinal disturbances, including nausea or vomiting; when injected, it can also produce a temporary increase in body temperature (up to 38-39° C). Anecdotally, I have heard of inflammatory reactions around the injection site. This should be carefully watched for by clinicians.

The LD50 (the dose at which 50 percent of animals died—a standard measure) by injection was 1550 mg/kg, or 64.82 ml of plant juice per kg in males and slightly higher in females. This is far more than any human patient would ever take. There were no mutations in the Ames or other standard tests, but there was some mutagenic activity in the DNAse and Protease tests. This was ascribed to the much higher dose used, i.e., up to 80 mg/ml. Although all of these were tests conducted for the Carnivora company and were not published in any peer-reviewed journals I see no reason to doubt their accuracy.

Carnivora is often described as an immune-modulating agent. An analysis was carried out on the immune status of 57 patients who underwent Carnivora treatment. A great many parameters of the immune system were looked at. On average, there was overall a beneficial increase in helper cells and a decrease in suppressor cells, leading to an increase in the helper/suppressor ratio. However, it is important to note that no such change was seen in patients who had previously undergone chemotherapy. In fact, there was a slight decrease in total T cells in patients who had previously received chemotherapy.

Dr. Keller has also carried out some laboratory studies of the immune-modulating activity of the whole plant. The first of these was a test of phagocytotis of human granulocytes in vitro against yeast cells. There was a 52.0 percent increase in phagocytosis at a concentration of 2.5 μl (microliters) per ml (milliliters) of the press juice. The active ingredient appeared to be plumbagin.

In two studies of the immune system (phagocytosis by human granulocytes in the test tube), Kreher also found that a very low concentration of plumbagin (and of the related compound, hydroplumbagin-glucoside), markedly stimulated the activity of human white blood cells. In yet another standard test, hydroplumbagin-glucoside was administered to mice followed by an injection of a colloidal suspension of carbon particles. Mice that received the "Carnivora"-derived injection had a much greater ability to clear the carbon particles from their blood (236).

A test was done on cancer in mice. Mice were given Carnivora in three dosage ranges (50, 100 and 200 mg/kg) 24 hours after being transplantated with melanoma cells. As a control, some mice were also given the standard chemotherapeutic drug cyclophosphamide. The tumors were then weighed on the 29th day of the experiment. Not surprisingly, cyclophosphamide had a strong cytotoxic effect on such cells, killing 99 percent of them. However, Carnivora also had a moderate antitumor effect. There was a 59 percent reduction at a dose of 100 mg/kg, a 37 percent reduction at 50 mg/kg, and a 27 percent reduction at 200 mg/kg.

Some support for Keller's thesis has also come from Munich's Technical University. Although scientists there were not looking for a cancer treatment, they observed that plumbagin from Venus's-flytrap produced both superoxides and hydrogen peroxide. In other studies involving interferon, white blood cells were stimulated to produce hydrogen peroxide and thereby kill cancer cells. Together with certain enzymes in the plant, these chemicals were also found to render proteins more digestible for the plant (142).

Some clinical studies with plumbagin have been conducted in India and Brazil (independent of Keller's work). The South American scientists found that plumbagin (isolated from a different local plant, *Plumbago scandens*) was responsible for a complete healing of skin lesions. They concluded that this herb-based remedy could advantageously be substituted for surgery and radiotherapy, mainly for tumors of the external ear and the back of the nose. Radiotherapy, which is normally used in such cases, was judged harmful to cartilage (275).

Soviet studies found plumbagin so harmless that it was recommended as a food preservative (200). While plumbagin is apparently nontoxic, readers should never attempt to produce their own homemade Carnivora. This is because such extracts contain endotoxins, which, if injected, might cause high fevers and other untoward reactions. Keller's Carnivora is said to be purified of all such toxins. There do not appear to be extreme reactions when the drug is administered properly.

The medicine contains one-third press juice; one-third alcohol and one-third purified water. Two milliliters is generally injected into the muscle daily until the doctor observes an increase in the ratio between two kinds of white blood cells. Another two milliliters are then administered to the patient through an intramuscular injection two or three times weekly as a maintenance dose.

By mouth, the patient generally takes 100 milliliters—30 drops of the extract—three to five times a day before meals and diluted in a glass of purified water or tea. Unmixed, it is said to taste like aged whiskey (it contains 60 proof alcohol). It can also be inhaled by means of a cold steam vaporizer.

In 1985, Dr. Keller published a study on the effectiveness of Carnivora in patients with malignant disease. This was published in German, in a non-Medline journal, which may partially account for the fact that it is little known to most scientists outside Germany. There were 210 patients in the study and all had severe malignant disease, including varieties of carcinoma, sarcoma, melanoma, and lymphoma. They were selected for treatment with Carnivora after all conventional therapy had failed, according to the recommended indications of the German Federal Health Office. All 210 had undergone prior treatment with chemotherapy and/or radiotherapy.

The fairly high treatment schedule was 50 to 60 drops five times per day and one ampule of two milliliters intramuscularly per day. In severe cases the parenteral administration was increased to two to three or more ampules per day. Inhalations of the medication were performed in patients who had laryngeal, bronchial, or lung carcinoma. In some cases, other routes of adminstration were also used.

Of the 210 patients, 34 (16.2 percent) showed remission; 84 (40 percent) showed stabilization; 29 (13.8 percent) showed progression; in 63 (30 percent) death could not be prevented, although in 25 of them there was a palliative effect. These palliative effects included not just pain relief but improvements in appetite, vitality, and psychological status.

It is interesting to note that while Venus's-flytrap had no prior medical uses, a related plant was reported to have a marked effect on pain. Millspaugh states that *Drosera rotundifolia*, also called sundew, was a traditional English and American remedy for tuberculosis.

Some 19th century sources claimed that it had a peculiar action upon the lungs and, in fact, the whole respiratory tract, thus leading us to value it deservingly in pertussis, bronchial irritation and even tuberculosis. It was said that it could give a patient a restful night and more peaceful day when the disease was too far advanced for still greater benefit. It is unknown if this property is related to the reported analgesic properties of Carnivora.

Keller says Carnivora is especially effective on primitive tumor tissues, as opposed to highly differentiated ones, which would be a boon, since such primitive tumors are usually more deadly. Carnivora is said to stimulate and modulate the immune system.

For tumors of the brain, and those that have a tendency to spread to the central nervous system, Keller says that Carnivora should be diluted in the sugar Mannitol 20 percent. Mannitol, he says, opens the blood-brain barrier and tends to concentrate the Carnivora in the brain. Keller also says that cancer of the urinary bladder responds very well to Carnivora injected three times per week.

Keller also advocates the simultaneous use of heat therapy (hyperthermia), a procedure that is increasingly popular in Germany.

There are now some imitations on the marketplace, such as "DMP" (*Dionaea muscipula*) or "Venus Fly Trap." Keller considers these dangerous knockoff products.

Dr. Keller claims that Carnivora is effective in treating ulcerative colitis, Crohn's disease, rheumatoid arthritis, multiple sclerosis, neurodermatitis, chronic fatigue syndrome, HIV infection, and certain kinds of herpes.

Carnivora is readily available for application to patients by physicians in Germany and other European countries. (In Germany, such drugs need only to be proven safe, not effective.) It remains unapproved by the US Food and Drug Administration (FDA), however, and cannot be imported or used legally except by people suffering from life-threatening illnesses such as cancer who receive a compassionate use exemption.

The work on Carnivora is impressive compared to most other herbal preparations. However, in the spirit of friendly skepticism, I would point out some deficiencies. The first of these is that most of what we know comes from the Carnivora company itself, of which Keller is apparently the principal owner. Some of these studies were submitted to German government regulatory agencies and formed the basis of its approval for patients with terminal disease. I would feel far more comfortable if these papers were published in peer-reviewed, Medline journals.

While the results reported on clinical effects are promising, we need to know more of what Keller means by responses, remissions, and stabilizations. Is he defining these terms in the same way as the FDA would? Did all the responders have a reduction of measurable tumor by at least fifty percent for 28 days or more? How many had complete responses? Did the stabilizations last six months or more? How did patients with different types of tumors respond? What was the followup on these cases from 1985?

Another criticism might be that almost everything we know about the clinical effects of Carnivora stems from the work of one man, Helmut Keller. While Dr. Keller certainly deserves much credit for having singlehandedly brought a promising new herbal medicine to light, it is more convincing when results are repeated in more than one clinic.

I realize that Dr. Keller has a few collaborators (such as Prof. D.K. Todorov, MD, PhD, DSc, of the National Oncological Center, Sofia, Bulgaria). However, that is for laboratory studies, not clinical work. What has been the experience of other physicians who have used Carnivora? Why have they not published their results? You would think that any agent that could cause 16.2 percent remissions in end-stage patients would generate a great deal of publishable data among Germany's complementary physicians.

Not all of this is Dr. Keller's fault, to be sure. I think the medical establishment has been remiss in not taking up this topic and exploring it vigorously. However, if Carnivora is to pass into the mainstream, it will take more than self-published books, or studies in obscure journals. Carnivora needs to be subjected to a full-scale clinical trial with NCI participation and funding and speedy FDA approval if it turns out to be effective.

Chapter 18 ✿ Alzium (Israel)

THIS IS AN INTERESTING HERBAL TREATMENT FROM ISRAEL. ALTHOUGH THERE IS NO PUBLISHED DATA ON IT, ITS PROVENANCE IS intriguing and its activity has been independently verified in two respectable laboratories. Several years ago, an American-born scribe (i.e., a person who meticulously hand copies the Torah), named Chaim Kass developed a formula for treating colds, flus and other ailments. Using his knowledge of Biblical, Rabbinic, and Arabic sources, Mr. Kass researched and then created a traditional herbal formula which was sold over-the-counter in Israel for five years as "Dalecktex." This is one of those rare instances in which the developer of a new product consciously went to the "ancestors" for answers to modern problems.

Mr Kass's formula is called Alzium in the United States. Since he is a better Talmudic scholar than he is a businessman, Alzium is little known outside the Orthodox Jewish community. Alzium consists of various herbs in a base of water and alcohol. Some herbs in Alzium Formula:

Scientific Name	Common Name	AHPA
Echinacea spp.	Coneflower	1
Commiphora molmol	Myrrh	2b
Scutellaria spp.	Skullcap	1
Crocus sativus	Saffron	2b
Capsicum frutescens	Hot pepper	1

Note: This formula should only be used under a physician's direction. Please see the warning in the front of the book.

There are several other ingredients. I know that he has made the formula available to other researchers on a confidential basis. A patent is pending and I have no reason to doubt that he would also reveal it to regulatory officials, if required.

Saffron is the world's most expensive spice, which costs $25,000 per kilogram! It is most familiar from its use to color and flavor rice dishes. In one experiment, oral administration of a crude extract increased life span of mice with three kinds of cancer by 183 to 212 percent. It inhibited DNA synthesis and was cytotoxic to four different cell lines, and had no harmful effect on normal cells (297).

Saffron is also an emmenagogue, uterine stimulant, and abortifacient. No risk is associated with its consumption in standard food use quantities or in therapeutic doses of less than 1.5 grams per day. However, severe side effects occur on ingestion of 5.0 grams per day and a lethal dose is said to be 20.0 grams (or less than one ounce). It is so expensive that few people are likely to have an ounce on hand at any one time.

Echinacea is hardly a traditional Middle Eastern herb. It is a native of America, west of the Ohio. But over the last 150 years it has become one of the best-known healing herbs around the world and is now universally appreciated. Echinacea contains high molecular weight polysaccharides inulin and echinacin, and is known to stimulate the immune system in five or six different ways (400).

Myrrh and the Bible

Myrrh plays an important role in Judeo-Christian religion. In the Book of Genesis, God instructs Moses to make "an oil of holy ointment, an ointment compounded after the art of apothecary; it shall be an holy anointing oil" (Genesis 30:23-25). In the Christian tradition, myrrh was one of two spices presented to the infant Jesus at the Nativity (Matthew 2:11) and was one of the two herbs that Nicodemus brought as a mixture to be used at the burial of Jesus after the crucifixion (John 19:39). There is even some speculation that the image on the Shroud of Turin was created by a chemical interaction between the ammonia vapors from a dying body and the myrrh-aloe mixture used in ancient funerary rites.

Myrrh, the partner of frankincense in the Bible, is actually an oleo-gum resin that is collected from bushy shrubs in Arabia and Somalia. Its use as a medicine goes back to very ancient times. In fact, according to Egyptian mythology, "the tears that fall from the eyes of Horus turn into the gum ânti," i.e., myrrh. It has long been used as an antifungal, an immune stimulant and detoxifier.

Myrrh is relatively non-toxic, but since it is a uterine stimulant, it is contraindicated in cases of excessive menstrual bleeding. In France, it is permitted for external use only. Doses over 2.0 to 4.0 grams may also cause irritation of the kidneys and diarrhea, but I think that far less than this is contained in Alzium.

Scutellaria (Virginia or Chinese skullcap) is one of the leading herbs for treating nervous disorders, although its value is vigorously disputed by Prof. Varro Tyler. In laboratory work, *Scutellaria baicalensis* inhibits two types of sarcoma and a cervical cancer cell line. *S. barbatae* inhibits sarcoma and Ehrlich ascites (75).

Capsicum, or red cayenne chili, has been used as a circulatory stimulant and nerve tonic. I know of no published work on anticancer activity.

Mr. Kass has worked with a number of laboratories to explore the usefulness of his product as a cancer treatment. The mixture has been studied at the Cancer Pharmacology Laboratory of Children's Mercy Hospital, Kansas City, MO. The principal investigators there were Albert Leyva, PhD and Arnold I. Freeman, MD, who was Chief of Pediatrics at the famed Roswell Park Cancer Institute in Buffalo, New York for 11 years. After leaving Kansas City, Dr. Freeman became an oncologist at Hadassah Hospital in Israel. He has 97 Medline articles to his credit, dating back to 1967. Al Leyva, PhD, is Director of the Cancer Pharmacology Laboratory.

Mr. Kass also comes with a letter of recommendations from the director of gastroenterology at the Shaare Zedek Medical Center in Jerusalem, who writes, "I am familiar with his researches...in the field of ancient medicines. Based on these ancient writings in combination with modern herbal formulas, he has developed several formulas and I find them to have a very substantial scientific basis."

At Mercy Hospital, Kansas, the scientists studied eight of the eleven plant extracts in the formula for their cytotoxic effects on cancer cell lines. The cell lines (in continuous culture) included leukemia, colon, brain (glioma), and lung cancers. Some of these cells were over 100 times more resistant to conventional chemotherapy than standard cell lines. In addition, they tested these herbs against several normal cells. The compounds "showed little toxicity toward normal skin fibroblast cells," according to Dr. Leyva.

One of the herbs in Alzium was extremely cytotoxic to cancer cells. (As I mentioned, saffron is known to have this property, although I do not know if this is the one.) Four others had moderate activity, while two showed little activity (but still could have host-mediated effects). The various plant extracts were not toxic to normal cells at all the tested levels. In a letter on March 27, 1995, Dr. Leyva called the results "very encouraging."

The scientists then tested these herbs against fresh tumor cells derived from individual patients who had a variety of tumors, including three patients with cancer of the ovaries, a patient with cancer of the breast, six patients with cancer of the brain, a patient with cancer of the adrenal glands. There was activity in most cases.

These extracts were able to kill tumor cells that were either dividing rapidly (as happens in cultured cells) or slow growing (as in most patients' actual tumors). It is important to point out that in these experiments the plant extracts were diluted as low as one part per thousand of the plant. Yet they were still effective against cell lines.

The orientation of the Kansas scientists was the isolation of drugs potentially useful in cancer treatment. Mr. Kass's orientation is empirical, i.e., to put together a traditional formula that was non-toxic enough for general use, some of whose components work by killing cancer cells while others support the natural defenses of the body.

Recently, a developmental oncologist of my acquaintance did a similar *in vitro* assay of Alzium with the cancer cells of a patient. The results were also highly positive. Alzium selectively killed the patient's very chemotherapy-resistant cells, even when it was diluted 140 times. Since I knew both the oncologist and the patient, this was for me impressive confirmatory evidence that Alzium contained some highly active components.

And what about human results? Mr. Kass has provided me with brief summaries on twelve patients who have reputedly done well. None of these responses are definitive, as the patients almost always took Alzium in conjunction with some conventional treatment. But about four percent of patients using Alzium alone and about 8-9 percent of patients using Alzium plus some other approach had remissions.

An additional 25 percent reported subjective improvement while taking the mixture. This would add up to a "benefit ratio" of about 40 percent, although obviously much of this improvement is of the subjective kind and could be due to a placebo effect, unless the administration is double-blinded (so neither doctor nor patient knows who is getting the test compound and who is getting a dummy pill).

To people who are accustomed to the exaggerated claims for many of today's cancer "cures," Kass's numbers may be disappointing. But if they stand up to scientific scrutiny, they would be very encouraging. Conventional cancer drugs have been approved for use with no more benefit than this. But proving these effects is another thing. Mr. Kass is not a biotech entrepreneur.

Mr. Kass has provided me the information on what he considers a few of the best responses to Alzium. While cautioning the reader that such undocumented accounts of improvement are generally of little value, I give a few just to convey some of the reason for interest in this product.

Astrocytoma: D.S., a 46-year-old divorced woman had an astrocytoma brain tumor. She had two surgeries as well as radiation and chemotherapy. On the third recurrence she refused chemotherapy, except for steroids. There was extensive paralysis. She started Alzium in November, 1995. After three months, she regained partial use of her right leg, although the right arm remained immobile. It is difficult to know exactly what role Alzium played in this partial improvement and what was possibly due to the steroids.

Glioblastoma: N.E., a 40-year-old married woman, was diagnosed with glioblastoma multiforme (stage IV brain cancer) in November, 1995. A few weeks later she began Alzium. In January, 1996, five weeks after starting Alzium, she underwent neurosurgery to remove the tumor. Her surgeon (whose name is known to me) told her family that "this was the easiest operation I have had in 25 years. Most of the tumor showed gross necrosis and very little blood was lost during the operation." The doctor felt the ease of the operation might have been due to Alzium. Another patient in a coma from a brain stem tumor revived after being fed two bottles of the drops, and has regained some of her functions.

Breast: C.K., a 48-year-old married woman from Brooklyn, NY was diagnosed with breast cancer in 1992. Had chemotherapy and Megace. Cancer metastasized to the spine. By July, 1995 she was paralyzed. She started Alzium in August, 1995. By December 1995, most of the paralysis subsided and she was put on physical therapy. She was still on Alzium almost a year later.

Colon: R.F., was diagnosed with colon cancer metastatic to the lungs. One lung was removed and she had chemotherapy. She started Alzium in June, 1995 in conjunction with another alternative treatment. She had a rapid remission over two months and a CT scan in December, 1995 showed almost complete remission.

Lung, small cell: S.T., a 37-year-old man from Jerusalem, was diagnosed with small cell lung cancer in January, 1996. He took chemotherapy then started on Alzium in March, 1996. By May, 1996 he had an almost 50 percent reduction in the tumor. His doctors were impressed. By June, 1996 he had returned to his normal work schedule. Although doctor and patient are happy, there is no indication that reduction in tumor was due to Alzium rather than to chemotherapy or a combination of the two.

Neuroblastoma: Y. B–D. was a five-and-a-half-year-old child in Jerusalem when he was diagnosed in 1993. His right kidney was removed. He had chemotherapy but, by CT scan, showed little improvement. He started on Alzium in May, 1995. No other alternative treatments were taken. In July, 1995 a CT scan showed shrinkage of the tumor. By September, 1995 most of the tumor had calcified. One year later he was still doing well.

Prostate: B. G., a 55-year-old man from Baltimore, was diagnosed with prostate cancer in 1994. This had spread to his kidneys and his lungs and there were two nodes in his throat. He also experienced a loss of memory. He started Alzium at the beginning of 1996. By September, 1996, his CT scan showed a shrinkage of tumor and he returned to work. The man was also taking other alternative treatments, but the shrinkage of metastatic lesions, if verified, would be encouraging.

Sarcoma: A.L., a 27-year-old man from Spring Valley, NY, was diagnosed with sarcoma in 1994. This was judged inoperable due to its size and location. In September, 1995, he took chemotherapy and shortly afterwards began Alzium as well. Within two months, the tumor had shrunk to an operable size and was removed. The man continued to take Alzium while in remission. The benefit of Alzium in this situation is uncertain, since chemotherapy may well have shrunk the tumor alone. But the patient himself believed in Alzium's contributory value.

Stomach: R.W., a 75-year-old widow, was diagnosed in 1993 with stomach cancer. She had surgery and radiation treatment at that time. She refused to take Alzium because of emotional distress and apathy towards life, but family members gave it to her in secret. After 35 days, she reported feeling much better. An interesting "single-blinded" case. However, in other situations, some patients with stomach cancer have not found Alzium tolerable.

Admittedly these are all preliminary results, lacking in published documentation. They are not submitted as "proof" of anything, except the kind of outcomes that some people find encouraging.

Cancer patients take 26 drops thirteen times per day (or, if pressed for time, 52 drops six times per day). The drops are first diluted in a glass of water and left to stand for 15 minutes in order to dissipate some of the alcohol. Some patients with sensitive digestive systems may find Alzium difficult to digest. One odd finding is that many patients who have taken these drops have developed a tremendous craving for apples and apple juice. No one knows what to make of this, but since apples contain potassium (which may have anticancer activity), Mr. Kass's suggestion is to "go with the flow." Patients naturally might want to take some precautions against constipation, or else there may be no flow to go with.

I have known Chaim Kass for some time and admire his "chutzpah" in developing this unusual formula and attempting to market it against all imaginable odds. He seems to me to be idealistic and giving and I have seen him perform acts of kindness and charity that went beyond what was required of him. However, he is not a scientist and therefore the overall presentation, while honest, lacks sophistication.

Chapter 19 ❧ Cat's Claw (Peru)

Back in the 17th century, the Jesuits made a fortune by monopolizing sale of the bark of the quina-quina tree (Cinchona), a member of the Rubiaceae family. This became the drug quinine, the treatment of choice for malaria. The jungle has also yielded curare, which is derived from the resin of a vine (*Chondrodendron tomentosum*). Used originally as an arrow poison, its alkaloid (tubocurarine) has found its way into medicine as an effective muscle relaxant, used in the treatment of spasms in spastic paralysis and tetanus. It is also used in operations that require the relaxation of muscles, and in fact is considered indispensable to surgeons all over the world (44). Ever since then, people have dreamed of penetrating the Amazonian jungle and bringing back exotic substances of similar utility.

Finding a "cancer cure" is particularly enticing. The search is made plausible by the fact that 70 percent of the plants found to have antitumor activity were found in tropical forests. There have been many contenders. However, no Amazonian plant since quinine has captured the public imagination as another member of the Rubiaceae family, *Uncaria tomentosa*. It is also widely known by its common names, in Spanish uña de gato, and in English, cat's claw.

The "claw" in cat's claw refers to the numerous hook-like thorns of the outer stems. This is a thick, woody vine that winds its way upwards through the Peruvian rain forests and can reach a length of over 100 feet (366).

Cat's claw generally grows in the highlands above 700 to 2,500 meters.

A related species, *Uncaria guianensis,* grows at lower elevations. Both vines are almost identical in appearance and have similar medical uses. The general consensus among Peruvian researchers and physicians is that, medically speaking, *Uncaria tomentosa* provides a "somewhat superior" product.

The parts used in medicine are either a decoction of the inner bark taken as a tea or the powdered inner bark taken as a capsule. The harvesting of roots is also apparently permitted under controlled situations, although there is a debate over whether such a practice is ecologically sound (see below).

Modern exploration of cat's claw dates from the work of a Bavarian immigrant to Peru named Arturo Brell (1896-1974). In the early 1930s, Brell emigrated to a German community about 130 miles east of Lima. There, he set up a school to teach the Indians about modern civilization. He noticed that in the Valley of Entaz, the Indians never seemed to develop cancer. He surmised that this had something to do with the tea they were constantly drinking, made from a woody vine they called "zavenna rozza." The Indian women also said that they used it as a contraceptive. Brell tried it and found that it improved his skin, made his hair grow faster, and "eliminated the painful rheumatism from which he had suffered for years." This vine was cat's claw.

Brell next gave an extract of the vine to a cousin suffering from breast cancer. Her recovery was complete, according to a historical report on Brell that appeared in the newspaper, *El Mundo,* in 1995. Her doctors were said to be astounded. In the early 1960s, Brell teamed up with an American, Prof. Eugene Whitworth of Great Western University, San Francisco, California. Whitworth's professional interest was not in medicine, but actually in recording native dances. But once he and Brell started traveling together, they began to collect unusual plants. Brell sent samples to European laboratories for analysis and even founded a small cancer research center in the jungle. It is said that Brell did a clinical trial in which he compared the outcomes of 100 advanced cancer patients who used the extract with a control group that didn't. After five years he claimed that 64 of the 100 who took the extract were in good health. As Kenneth Jones remarks, "such a study would have to be repeated in more controlled settings" (211).

Brell and Whitworth seem to have made an honest effort to get the vine scientifically tested in the United States. Yet Jones, who closely studied the documentary evidence for his excellent book on the topic titled *Cat's Claw,* reports: "They were blocked at nearly every turn (211). Pharmaceutical companies wouldn't send equipment or staff. People they approached for donations grew reluctant. Members of the Cancer Society made themselves unavailable" (212).

Letters to US Senators went unanswered. Oddly, the only politician who took an interest in this was the Chief Executive himself. At President

Richard M. Nixon's personal request, the US National Cancer Institute became involved in the summer of 1971. Brell sent them samples of *Uncaria guianensis* (the related species). Finally, in 1974, Brell received his answer. It came in the form of a letter from Jonathan L. Hartwell, PhD, the head of NCI's natural products testing division.

"We have found that a sample of the 50 percent aqueous-ethanolic extract of the twigs of *Uncaria guianensis* showed activity in leukemia P388," wrote Hartwell on September 9, 1974. According to Jones, NCI's tests were accurate. However the results were not what NCI had hoped for. Cat's claw clearly did not have the extraordinary power of, say, Camptothecin. However, while cat's claw did have moderate cytotoxic activity, it's real power appeared to lie in its combination of cell-killing with immune-boosting properties, for which NCI did not routinely screen.

There the story might have ended, yet another herb filed away because of mediocre results. No one could have predicted cat's claw's tremendous future in the herbal field.

It happened that one of the many people to whom Brell gave cat's claw was a sawmill owner named Luis Oscar Schuler. In 1967, the story goes, Señor Schuler was dying of lung cancer. After receiving cat's claw tea, along with ten cobalt x-ray treatments, he completely recovered and many years later died at the age of 91. Oscar's case became famous through Peru. Cat's claw was beginning to develop a commercial personality and the man who cured himself of lung cancer became a central part of the story. (His name and occupation varied with the telling.)

Upon Don Oscar's death, it was said, an autopsy revealed no sign of cancer anywhere in his body. People whispered about a "miraculous healing" (270). Lima newspapers and magazines had found a new miracle treatment: "Uña de gato cures cancer."

In few of the popular accounts did readers learn that Oscar had also received radiation treatments. What kind or stage of lung cancer did he have? The five-year relative survival rates in the US for all stages is around 14 percent (328). Some cases of even inoperable lung cancer are "potentially curative" through radiation (189).

In any case, Oscar's granddaughter happened to be a student at the University of Innsbruck, Austria. She told his remarkable story to Klaus Keplinger, a journalist and self-taught ethnologist, who became intrigued, especially since he had recently lost a good friend to cancer. In the period 1979-1981, Keplinger travelled in central Peru, obtaining samples of cat's claw. At personal expense, he had the vine analyzed and the immune-potentiating alkaloids isolated and tested.

Keplinger eventually developed a product called Krallendorn (German for "claw thorn"), which received US patents in July, 1989, July, 1990 and

April, 1994. He first tried Krallendorn against viral infections in animals and then decided to use it against herpes simplex infections in humans. Positive experiences led to a 1987 study in which he gave cat's claw to people with AIDS and observed immunological changes after just 20 days as well as a reduction in AIDS-related symptoms after just 30 days. Eventually, he patented the use of Krallendorn as an immune-modulating agent.

Cat's claw is rich in unusual chemical components. The plant has anti-inflammatory properties, probably due to its steroid-like component, of which the familiar plant constituent beta-sitosterol makes up 60 percent. Stigmasterol and campesterol are also present. In a Lima university dissertation, a root extract was found to reduce the size and number of stomach ulcers in rats, although gastric bleeding was not reduced.

Prof. Hildebert Wagner at the University of Munich has established that there are five or six important oxindole alkaloids in the plant, which are said to enhance the immune system. These alkaloids are active in tiny amounts, whereas large amounts seem to simply shut off the effect (246, 399).

If there is a main ingredient, it is Isomer A (isopteropodine). This has been intensively examined by Wagner and by Keplinger and his associates at Krallendorn. According to their US patent, these alkaloids, particularly isomer A, "are suitable for the unspecific stimulation of the immunologic system."

One standard test for immune stimulation is through a significant increase in the degree of bacteria-engulfing activity, called phagocytosis, by white blood cells in the test tube. This model is used to predict how well a substance could enhance the human body's ability to fight certain kinds of infection—and possibly cancer.

Each of five alkaloids, all the alkaloids together, and a water extract of the root were tested at different doses, and each of them increased phagocytosis from 15.7 to 55.9 percent. The greatest increase came with a medium-strength dose of Isomer A. Oddly enough, increasing the amount of alkaloids 100-fold often did not lead to an important increase in activity, and sometimes led to a decrease. So small amounts might be just as effective, or more effective, than large amounts.

One problem is that the alkaloid content of the roots changes throughout the year, and probably varies from plant to plant, as well. Consequently, the product sold to consumers varies greatly. European samples range from half a milligram to five milligrams alkaloids per gram. Independent analyses have shown that occasionally samples (especially of *Uncaria guianensis*) have no alkaloids, and are probably inert. The same problem has been seen with pau d'arco and many other commercial herbs.

Dr. Rita Aquino at the University of Naples, Italy, has isolated the most active anti-inflammatory parts of cat's claw. These are a dozen glycosides, which were largely overlooked in the isolation of the more dramatically active alkaloids. Some glycosides found in cat's claw were of the rare quinovic acid type, present in both the root and the bark (18, 19, 20, 399).

Are Tannins Dangerous?

Cat's claw also contains at least ten percent tannins, which are chemicals with astringent properties. For maximum effectiveness as medicine, they should not be mixed with milk or cream, should not be drunk very hot, or to excess. Tannins are somewhat contradictory in this context since they have both therapeutic and adverse effects. Very high concentrations of tannins (such as are found in oak galls) have caused gastrointestinal disturbances and kidney damage, as well as severe necrosis of the liver. I am unaware of the actual tannin content of Uncaria tomentosa, but it is unlikely to be in this category. Both carcinogenic and antitumor properties have been reported for tannins in the laboratory. There has been a correlation between increased tannin consumption in tea and cancer, especially esophageal cancer. This is somewhat controversial, however, since there are equal data to recommend tea as an anticancer beverage (6a).

One laboratory test conducted in Spain of a water extract showed no signs of toxicity (336). Scientists looked for signs of toxicity in standard tests. In none of these did cat's claw show any problems. Krallendorn has been used by European patients for over eight years without any obvious toxic effects. Some doctors are giving double and triple the normal dose of 20-60 mg/day of the Krallendorn product without reporting any immediate problems.

In Germany and Austria, Krallendorn is banned for children under three and there is in fact no clinical experience with this. In today's practice, adult cancer patients are generally taking nine 350 mg cat's claw bark or root capsules per day (three capsules 30 minutes after each meal.) Phillip Steinberg has recommended two to six grams daily in divided doses. He says that most people respond with one gram taken three times per day. The well-known complementary physician, Robert Atkins, MD, has recommended even higher doses: three to six grams per day, and up to 20 grams per day in advanced cases (107).

Steinberg also says that if using the tea, one to one-and-a-half quarts per day would probably be most effective. "It should be strong, dark and bitter." Steinberg claims that one-third to one-half the adult dose is effective for infections, with no side effects.. He does state that the herb is *not* recommended for pregnant or lactating women. That is because the herb's traditional usage as a contraceptive suggests that it be avoided in pregnancy.

Kenneth Jones also lists a fairly wide range of contraindications, e.g., in patients undergoing skin grafts and organ transplants; hemophiliacs prescribed fresh blood plasma; simultaneous administration of certain vaccines, hormone therapies, thymus extracts, and insulin; and in children under three. The AHPA lists it as a class 4 herb, which means that it has insufficient data available for classification.

Scientific reputation is just now beginning to catch up with popular usage. In May, 1994 the World Health Organization sponsored the *First International Conference on Uña de Gato*. At this meeting the vine received official recognition for the first time as a medicinal plant (211).

There is some clinical research now underway in Europe using the Krallendorn brand. According to a statement from the Keplinger's company, these clinical studies remain largely unpublished, unfinished, or require larger numbers of patients before the results could be scientifically published. It is for this reason that a Medline search yields nothing convincing about the clinical efficacy of the product, besides the fact of its "moderate anti-inflammatory activity" (349, 331).

According to the company's brochure, 56 patients have been studied over a ten-year period. As expected, those patients whose cancers were in the earliest stages did the best, and some of them have remained in remission for the whole ten years. The best results are said to be in patients with testicular teratomas who also received chemotherapy.

Others who did well included those with adenocarcinomas of the colon who had surgery and in addition used cat's claw. These results have to be viewed with caution, since testicular cancer patients have high survival rates using chemotherapy alone, and 90 percent of patients with early stage colon cancer survive at least five years after surgery, most without the help of herbs (328).

A 1990-1991 study was also conducted on 60 patients with various kinds of brain cancer at the Innsbruck Clinic in Austria. All patients received the standard treatments (surgery, radiation and/or chemotherapy) in addition to receiving root preparations after their discharge from the hospital. The root preparation was not given at the same time as chemotherapy but only between treatments. All patients on the root preparations had increased vitality and suffered fewer side effects from radiation and chemotherapy. However, one year later, only 17 patients remained alive.

There were remissions in five out of six cases of ependymoblastomas grades II and III, and in six out of eight cases of astrocytomas, grade II. It is extremely difficult to sort out the contribution of cat's claw from that of the standard treatments. While short-term remissions are common in many kinds of brain cancer, long-term "cures" are difficult to achieve. We should also reiterate that this information comes from an informational handout for doctors from Krallendorn and, to my knowledge, has never been submitted for peer review.

Cat's claw is a promising herb with potentially beneficial effects on the immune system. The fact that Krallendorn is patented in Europe gives the company an economic incentive to carry out serious research. While we would like to see peer-reviewed studies, what has been done so far is promising. However, that said, there are some aspects of the cat's claw story that I find disturbing.

Part of the popular appeal of cat's claw is the belief that it has been used for hundreds or even thousands of years by the Peruvian Asháninka Indians for the treatment of various health problems. Author Phillip Steinberg (who has made a specialty out of promoting cat's claw) lists these traditional uses as "tumors and other growths, ulcers, gastritis, arthritis, rheumatism, menstrual disorders, prostate problems, asthma, diabetes, viral infections, general debility, gonorrhea and cirrhosis" (366).

As if that weren't sufficient, other articles add bursitis, genital herpes and herpes zoster, allergies, systemic candidiasis, PMS and irregularities of the female cycle, environmental toxin poisoning, a host of bowel and intestinal disorders, organic depression, and HIV infection.

While cat's claw is acclaimed as a potent traditional remedy (including for cancer), it strikes me as odd that there are no mentions of it in any of the standard reference works on herbalism or folk medicine (333).

The AHPA states that "ethnobotanical data are scanty." Dr. Fernando Cabieses of the Peruvian Ministry of Health found Uncaria species missing from the oldest and most important books on Peruvian medicinal plants. There are several possible explanations for this lacuna:

a) Since cat's claw was used as a contraceptive it formed part of "women's medicine," and was hidden from men, including Western ethnobotanists.

b) Explorers shied away from the area in which cat's claw grew because of the fierce reputation of the Asháninkas.

c) Cat's claw was so powerful that it was kept as a jealously guarded secret of the shamans, which few outsiders were ever privileged to learn.

d) A fourth explanation is heretical and is never mentioned by any of the standard sources: that cat's claw may *not* be an authentic Indian remedy, but mainly a modern 20th century commercial invention.

Present-day Indian claims of its ancient ancestry have to be weighed against the fact that almost all cat's claw is harvested on their quarter-million acre habitat in Peru and this has become the Indians' major source of income (214). One can also find street vendors in every Peruvian city selling "uña de gato" on the street. But "the chances of obtaining the correct species are slim, because...there are so many different herbs known by that name," according to a writer on the topic (366).

Few rain forest plants in history have been as heavily promoted as this one. According to *Whole Foods Magazine,* cat's claw was the eleventh top selling herbal supplement in US health food stores in 1995, representing 2.9 percent of all sales. It was listed as the number one "up-and-coming herb for 1996," garnering twice as many points in this category as its nearest rival.

Flyers and pamphlets in health food stores, articles in popular magazines, television and radio reports, newsletters devoted solely to this topic, Websites and books galore proclaim the glories of cat's claw. Almost invariably, the adjectives "curative," "miraculous," "exceptional," "healing," and "amazing" embellish its supposed glories.

I know people who speak glowingly of the product: a doctor of biochemistry of my acquaintance wrote that a few months on cat's claw had cured her of "virtually untreatable intestinal problems," including spastic colon and liver dysfunction.

However, what is disturbing is the degree to which the myth of cat's claw is the creation of advertising promotions. One company, for instance, assured customers that "*Uncaria tomentosa*...far surpasses such well known herbs as pau d'arco, echinacea, goldenseal, astragalus and Siberian ginseng, as well as reishi and shitake [sic!] mushrooms, and other natural products such as citrus seed extract, caprylic acid and shark cartilage" (7a).

Step right up and get your miracle cure straight from the Amazonian jungle!

Nowhere is this breathless hype more evident than on the Internet. Websites offer books on the wonders of this miracle herb in a package deal with capsules of cat's claw itself. You can even buy bottles of cat's claw at the same Website that sells Rubber Renu® for your car's tires (www.horizons-marketing.com). Take care of your immune system and your sidewalls from the comfort of your own home.

Another enterprising company promised to supply customers not with plain old "*Uncaria tomentosa*" but with something special called "*Uncaria tomentosa* [Willd] DC." Readers were asked to pay twice as much for this special version. Of course, "[Willd] DC" is not a special type of cat's claw but is the name of the "species authors" who first identified and name the plant: 19th century botanists Carl Ludwig Willdenow and Augustine Pyramus de Candolle.

Hard evidence of cancer remissions due to cat's claw is difficult to come by. Certainly anecdotes abound. In a health food store flyer, Jolie Martin Root, a Florida nutritionist, reported on the case of a 58-year-old woman named Else who was diagnosed with cancer of the ovaries and uterus. "She was told she had just three months to live," says Ms. Root. The woman tried a number of alternative treatments with little success, then on April 1, 1995, she began treatment with cat's claw. By the end of that May her blood work showed great improvement. By July, 1995, Root reports, the woman was feeling much better "and the tumor had stopped growing." By November she was in a stable condition on a combination of cat's claw and Essiac tea. "She was very much alive one year after having been told she had three months to live! She has returned to a normal life!" (333)

Statements that a patient has "just three months to live" are often subjective on the part of a doctor. Statistics from the SEER Program of the National Cancer Institute show that the five-year survival rate for invasive ovarian cancer even with distant metastases is 16.5 percent in women over the age of 50. For uterine cancer it is 24.8 percent. We would have to know a lot more about this woman's condition in order to know what to make of this anecdote. One-year survival of metastatic cancer is encouraging, but hardly conclusive.

For example, we need to know if the patient underwent any further "orthodox" procedure, such as cytoreductive surgery for advanced-stage ovarian disease. If so, her average expected survival should be in the neighborhood of 16 to 40 months (104). Did she have hormonal treatment? Palliative radiotherapy? These could add to her lifespan. Obviously, too many questions remain before we can accept this anecdote, or similar accounts, as demonstrating real benefit from taking this herb.

Similarly, one online *Cat's Claw Newsletter* reported that "Barbara, age 58, from West Palm Beach, Florida, has had a tumor on one ear and another on the side of her head for approximately 18 years. She began using Cat's Claw in capsule form in June of 1994, taking three 350 mg. capsules three times per day. She reported that both tumors have shrunk by half within approximately two months" (www.realtime.net). This seems questionable. Were these tumors biopsied? If not, how did Barbara know they were malignant?

Patient Feels Better

In another case, reported by a naturopathic physician, a 66-year-old woman was diagnosed with breast cancer. Her tumor was excised, the lymph nodes were negative, and she was in the midst of radiation treatment when she started on 3,000 milligrams per day of cat's claw. She also had weekly acupuncture treatments. The woman experienced no hair loss and her energy level remained stable. The minor burns she received from the radiation therapy healed quickly. Her physicians were said to have been amazed by the speed of her recovery and the woman reported feeling better after the treatment than before she was diagnosed with cancer (366).

But hair loss is not a side effect of radiation therapy, unless the hair follicles themselves are damaged or destroyed by the treatment; there is absolutely no reason they would be in a case of early-stage breast cancer (189). So this purported "benefit" is meaningless.

Things like energy level or speed of recovery are difficult to assess in any single case, although they could be addressed through randomized trials in which one group gets radiation plus cat's claw while the other gets radiation plus a placebo (inert pill).

These are typical of the kinds of uninterpretable results that are employed to convince people to buy this product. They lack the kind of detail that would be necessary to convince any person who was not already predisposed to believe in the value of this "miracle from the Andes."

Even the staunchest defender of cat's claw will admit that there have been shenanigans involved in its marketing. For instance, there has a war of words between advocates of inner bark vs. those promoting the roots. There are disparate claims that one or the other contains a much higher percentage of disease-fighting alkaloids.

Steinberg's Apology

At one time, nutritionist Phillip Steinberg was an inner bark advocate and and publicized the idea that it was illegal in Peru to harvest the root, because of the threat such practices posed to the continued existence of the plant. Now Mr. Steinberg says that he was deceived and that the root is legally harvested in an ecologically sound manner. Starting in April, 1996, a Peruvian company has been legally cutting small enough sections of the root to allow the vine to regenerate itself.

But why did Mr. Steinberg formerly believe that root harvesting was illegal? He had been given copies of three official letters of the Peruvian Ministry of Agriculture stating as much. It turned out that these letters, which even bore the Minister's seal, were either forgeries or disinformation. The letters were provided to Steinberg by—you guessed it—a major supplier of cat's claw bark.

"I...must hereby apologize for unwittingly participating in the spreading of wrong information about cat's claw," Phillip Steinberg wrote, contritely. Consider that he is a long-term worker in the health food industry, who has made this topic his speciality. Imagine how confused the ordinary citizen is likely to become as she hacks her way through the Amazonian jungle of misinformation, attempting to arrive at a realistic estimate of the value of this herb.

Chapter 20 ❧ Noni Juice (Polynesia)

WHAT IS NONI JUICE AND WHY ARE SO MANY PEOPLE DRINKING IT? NONI IS HAWAIIAN FOR A PLANT KNOWN SCIENTIFICALLY AS *Morinda citrifolia*. Also known as Indian mulberry, noni grows as a small evergreen tree at elevations of up to 1,300 feet. It has large oblong leaves, white flowers, and a very distinctive yellow, grenade-shaped fruit.

Unlike cat's claw, there is no question that noni is part of folk medicine. It has been used extensively in both Polynesia and Hawaii as a general health tonic, and specifically for diabetes, heart disease, and high blood pressure. It is also rubbed on wounds, cuts and abrasions of all sorts. One Maori has written that "noni is part of our lives." It is also said that noni is used as a traditional remedy for cancer by Polynesians (182). It is discussed in a number of scholarly works on tropical folk medicine.

In the 1980s some scientists began experimenting with the properties and uses of this plant. What they found was interesting. *Morinda citrifolia* contains some unusual compounds (181). In 1993, scientists at the University of Metz in France found that a freeze-dried extract of noni roots had a "significant, dose-related, central analgesic activity...." The French scientists concluded that "these results are suggestive of sedative properties," which happened to be one of the traditional indications. However, these experiments were conducted with roots, not fruit, which is the main object of present-day attention.

Main Experiment

Most of the interest in noni is focused on a small set of experiments carried out by Professor Annie Hirazumi and colleagues at the Department of Pharmacology, John A. Burns School of Medicine, University of Hawaii, Honolulu. Prof. Hirazumi administered pure noni juice to a pet dog when it was dying. The dog recovered, and she set out to discover more about this fruit. Her group reported that when they injected a relatively large amount (750 mg/kg) of noni juice into animals with cancer every other day, the mean survival time was 33.5 days. This was compared to just 14.8 days in the controls.

While there were no survivors out of 23 control mice, 9 out of 22 treated animals were still alive at the end of the experiment. They also reported that the juice was not cytotoxic to cancerous or normal cells, even at high concentration. This indicates a host-mediated effect.

At a 1995 biology society meeting, they reported in more detail on the use of noni against transplanted tumors. An alcohol precipitation of the fruit juice was shown to give protection against cancer when it was injected into the peritoneal cavity of the mice.

Thirty-four mice were first implanted with Lewis lung carcinoma cells. Treated mice were given a total of five injections. Again, the mean survival was increased to 32.7 days compared to 14.7 days in the controls. Concurrent treatment with immunosuppressive drugs destroyed the anti-cancer effects of noni, "suggesting the antitumor activity acts via activation of host immune system," they wrote. They also reported that noni demonstrated a protective effect against an experimental leukemia that was caused by the inoculation of tumor-causing viruses. It prevented the enlargement of the spleen by 51 percent.

All experiments point to the conclusion that noni juice "...seems to act indirectly by enhancing host immune system involving macrophages and/or lymphocytes' (183).

This is encouraging, even exciting. But several caveats need to be emphatically stated. First, most of these studies were conducted with alcohol extracts of noni, not plain juice. Additionally, the compound was injected into the peritoneal cavities of the animals, whereas humans take this as a drink. The dosage was many times what human patients would take.

So, while suggestive, these studies on transplantable tumors in animals (from a single laboratory) are not necessarily predictive of human anti-cancer effects.

Much of the interest in noni has been stimulated by Ralph Heinicke, PhD. Dr. Heinicke is a graduate of Cornell University and the University of Minnesota. He lived in Hawaii from 1950 to 1986, where he worked for the Dole Pineapple Company, the Pineapple Research Institute, and the University of Hawaii.

Dr. Heinicke discovered and patented an alkaloid he named "xeronine." Xeronine is an enigmatic molecule which rapidly comes and goes in the body. It is formed from "proxeronine," which Dr. Heinicke first isolated from pineapples and then from noni. (He states that it is no longer present in pineapple because of the depletion of the soil.)

Heinicke wrote that "identifying the pharmacologically active ingredient of noni has been difficult —for an understandably good reason. The active ingredient is not present in the plant or fruit! Only after the potion has been drunk does the active ingredient form. Sometimes!" he adds, with some humor.

Heinicke calls xeronine a "relatively small alkaloid...which is physiologically active in the picogram range.' A picogram is a trillionth of a gram.

Although the xeronine thesis is often cited as dogma, there is reason for caution. There are three patents relating to xeronine. But a search of the Medline and CancerLit databases revealed no published peer-reviewed studies on xeronine or proxeronine. The words do not occur, although we found three papers by Dr. Heinicke on other topics. It is difficult to understand why he has not shared this discovery with the scientific community at large.

And while it is well known that alkaloids are highly bioactive substances, they are often present in much larger quantities in plants. Take for instance one of the best known of all alkaloids, nicotine. This can constitute up to 9.0 percent by weight of tobacco leaves! (332) This is astronomical compared to Dr. Heinicke's picogram-range xeronine. Some further explanation of xeronine's mechanism of action is clearly needed.

Crazy About That Plant

In February, 1992, Isabella Abbott, the GP Wilder Professor of Botany at the University of Hawaii, told the Sunday *Star-Bulletin & Advertiser* that in Hawaii "people are crazy about this plant. They use it for diabetes, high blood pressure, cancer," as well as many other illnesses. She herself was receiving ten phones call a week on the topic.

Here was a dream-come-true for enterprising salesmen in the natural health field. But there was a problem. The main obstacle to marketing noni as a food supplement was an esthetic one. According to Prof. Abbott, "It smells like something the dog dragged in." The aforementioned Maori writer put it bluntly: "The traditional juice stinks and tastes terribly bitter—it's almost unbearable." According to another scientist, "If one is dying and all other remedies have failed, then and only then will the average person drink noni juice. The flavor of juice made from ripe Hawaiian noni is terrible. None of my colleagues would touch the untreated juice...."

But a Utah company called Morinda, Inc. was up to the challenge. It mixed noni with water and blueberry and grape juice concentrates and the stuff is now selling briskly through a network marketing pyramid. I have tasted it and found the mixture similar to prune juice. Whatever was offensive about it has now clearly been masked by the other ingredients.

Thanks to the Internet and network marketing, noni has now developed into a craze. Most alternative doctors and many patients have been contacted in one way or another by the company's associates. Some doctors are selling it to their patients, and many other patients have found their way to the juice, with or without an attendant "healthy" diet. So, the question naturally arises, is there anything to noni?

What's In That Noni?

None of the distributors of the product have been completely forthcoming with information. But Morinda, Inc. did send me an analysis of the nutritional value of their product. It shows that noni contains a significant amount of vitamin C, about 6-7 mg of ascorbic acid per ounce, which is about the same as orange juice, at about 25 times the cost. (The price of noni juice is $30 to $35 per bottle, plus $5 shipping and handling.)

Noni also contains 21 other vitamins and minerals, but in minuscule amounts. As the company itself makes clear, noni is "not a significant source" for any other nutrient. And since the product that was analyzed also contained blueberry and grape juice concentrates, as well as natural flavors, it is impossible to tell how much of the value of the final product is due to noni and how much to these well-known ingredients.

Strange Fruit?

Noni juice appears to be non-toxic. All of the animal and cell-line experiments I have seen so far have found no evidence of toxicity. The company has assured me that noni is on the FDA's Generally Regarded as Safe (GRAS) list. They also assure me that noni was listed as an acceptable food for US troops in the Pacific during World War Two.

However, I think some caution and common sense are in order. Just the fact that noni has been consumed in Polynesia in various emergency situations cannot be considered de facto proof that it is without any potential harm, especially for long-term use. Some traditional herbs have proven quite dangerous upon closer inspection.

The main distributor is to be commended for having Corning Hazelton

Laboratories run tests for gamma isotope radiation, heavy metals, pesticide residues, yeasts, and molds. Their product passed its tests with flying colors.

But what piqued my curiosity was the fact that a well established reference work in botany, *Hortus Third,* states that *Morinda citrifolia* fruit "has been reported to be poisonous" (30). Hortus gives no references for its cautionary statement. When I asked the scientific director of the noni company about this, his response was not reassuring.

He proceeded to lambaste me for daring to cite an out-of-date work from 1902. It was futile to point out that the edition I was citing dated from 1976 and that *Hortus Third* is an authoritative work, published by the Liberty Hyde Bailey Hortorium, a division of Cornell University. He failed to send me any more recent data.

One small manufacturer of noni pills gave the most entertaining response. He claimed on the Net that his product was "FDA Approved." Knowing a little about the FDA, I found that hard to swallow. When I wrote to him requesting substantiation for this claim, he sent me this almost unintelligible reply: "About the being toxic, I wouldn't be in business today. Noni is like a apple or orange that you on the fruit stand. Because it has be put in a capsule that don't make a drug." That about settled it.

Testimonials

Noni would just be another health food wannabe if it were not for the intense promotion that comes from multi-level marketing. I have found 271 separate Websites devoted to noni juice. Once again, this demonstrates the power of the Internet as an amplification mechanism for reputed "cancer cures."

Quite a few testimonials are being put forward about nearly miraculous effects from taking the juice. A distributor sent me a four-page tabloid called *Health News* (vol. 3, no. 2), which bore headlines such as "An Ancient Cure from Paradise," "Healing From Across the Seas," and "No More Wheelchair!" On the front page it states that noni is "a healing fruit" that "helps cancer."

And what is *Health News?* It looks like a regular newspaper, but is produced by a company that specializes in "Third Party literature for network marketing distributors." It is sold by the bundle to multilevel marketers who use the mails to recruit new customers, who then themselves become salesmen in an expanding pyramid.

You will not find a single cloud in the blue Polynesian skies of Nonidom. Noni, it appears, cures bowel obstruction, chronic fatigue, severe back pain, menstrual problems, sinus congestion, knee blow-out, water on the knee, and severe arthritis. It can also be useful in incurable cancer, they say.

"In Polynesia," a Utah man just returned from the tropics is quoted as saying, "anytime someone has an 'untreatable' or terminal illness—when it seems that everything else has been tried but nothing has worked—they reach for noni."

He tells how a Polynesian woman "became a believer in noni after her friend's cancer went into remission after only two weeks of using the juice." Such second and third-hand accounts are the stock-in-trade of health "miracles." As the manufacturer instructs its distributors, success in this field depends on telling great stories.

A follow-up issue of the same newsletter (vol. 4, no. 2) contains testimonials from three physicians. One of these, Mona Harrison, MD, is identified as former assistant dean of Boston University School of Medicine and chief medical officer of DC General Hospital. She wrote:

"One of my patients was suffering from kidney cancer with metastases, or the movement of malignant cells, to her lung and brain. She had been given only two weeks to live. Within that two-week period, she took noni juice and it cleared up her lung lesions. That was back in November [1997] and she is still with us." (I received this newsletter in February, 1998.)

Another patient, the doctor writes, "had liver cancer and a swelling of fluid in the abdominal area. After seven days on noni juice this acidic [sic] fluid cleared up completely."

Dr. Harrison concludes, "she and the first case I mentioned were terminally ill cancer patients who no one anticipated would make it, but they are alive today because of noni." If true, this is no small news. The complete remission of lung metastases or ascites within a period of one to two weeks is the medical equivalent of a UFO landing on the front lawn.

I had to learn more. Since there was no address, city or phone number listed for Dr. Harrison, I tried emailing her care of the "newsletter" in which her comments appeared. Several weeks later I received the following reply:

"We apologize for the delay in responding to your request. Unfortunately, we are unable to give out information on how to contact Dr. Harrison from our *Health News* edition on noni juice. But we have passed on your information to her office so that she can contact you. Thank you, Triple R. Publishing, Inc." Unfortunately, that was the last I have heard from or about the elusive Dr. Harrison.

The noni sales force maintains a toll-free telephone hot-line where both company officials and gratified patients tell their stories. I listened to one of these sessions and heard a cancer patient state that he stopped getting chemotherapy-associated infections when he took noni juice for just a few days. Another cancer patient declared that he felt remarkably better. Let's hope these people are not deceiving themselves.

Noni is mainly sold by Morinda, Inc., a multi-level marketing company in Utah. They claimed sales of $1.5 million in October, 1996 and anticipated monthly sales of $2.5 million by the end of that year.

"Do you have a problem with that?" a company spokesperson asked me, aggressively. I replied that I might, because some of the "cured patients" heard on the tape now had a vested interest in the financial success of the product. They therefore might be tempted to exaggerate the benefits they received.

The spokesperson was irate at this response. He accused me of disloyalty to the capitalist system and made me sit through a lecture on the evils of the FDA and the glories of medical freedom of choice.

He also told me that his company "was not interested" in a story about noni and cancer right now. When I said that I didn't need their permission to write such an article, and that I wasn't looking for a relationship of any sort with his company, he was astounded.

"You just made my day. You're the first writer I've spoken to who hasn't wanted money to write about noni." Now there's a fine commentary on the state of medical journalism at the end of the 20th century!

Chapter 21 ❧ Oleander (Turkey)

ERIUM OLEANDER IS A PLANT OF THE APOCYNACEAE ORDER. ITS
COMMON NAME IS ROSE BAY, LAURIER ROSE, DOGBANE, OR JUST
plain oleander. It is native to the Mediterranean region but is
found in the wild as far east as Japan. Oleanders are also commonly grown
outdoors in mild climates, such as California, Arizona, and the US South.
Oleanders are inexpensive and are cherished by gardeners for their drought
resistance. In northern climes, they are sometimes grown as house plants.

The one thing that most people—especially parents—know about oleanders is that they are highly poisonous. When I was a graduate student at
Stanford University, my great fear was that my children would start nibbling
the attractive oleander plants that ringed the married student housing where
we lived.

Most parts of the plant contain the poison, including the leaves (green or
dried), the milky juice, etc. Many domestic animals have died after eating
this plant. A sheep can be killed by eating a mere one to five grams of fresh
leaves. Symptoms of oleander poisoning include nausea and vomiting,
abdominal pain, dizziness, drowsiness, decreased pulse rate, irregular
heart action, diarrhea, unconsciousness, respiratory paralysis, and finally,
death. Not surprisingly, oleander has been used as a means of suicide since
antiquity.

Oleander has been well studied and contains many interesting (and
dangerous) compounds. The chief toxicity seems to come from a cardiac
glycoside, oleandrin. It also contains neriin, as well as rutin and ursolic acid,

as well as many other substances. Oleandrin is similar to digitoxin and the other substances found in the foxglove (*Digitalis purpurea*), which, properly used, have tremendous utility in heart disease. Oleandrin, isolated in 1932, is sometimes used medically as a cardiotonic and diuretic. Through the use of sophisticated techniques (mass spectrometric analysis), French scientists were once able to ascertain the exact blood level of oleandrin that caused symptoms in an emergency room patient. It was 1.1 nanograms per milliliter of blood, an incredibly small amount (388).

Oleander in History

Oleander is mentioned in the *Code of Hammurabi* (c. 1750 BC), which drew on older Sumerian traditions. According to herbal historian Edith Grey Wheelwright, "The Mesopotamians seem to have discovered the properties of the virulent Order to which the oleander belongs" (407). Medical historian Henry Sigerist said that Babylonian physicians used a mixture of oleander, licorice, and other substances as a hangover remedy: it was to be used "if a man has taken strong wine and his head is affected and he forgets his words and his speech becomes confused"(354). Oleander is almost certainly the "rose of the waterbrooks" of the Bible, and the "willow of the brook" used in the Feast of the Tabernacle. It also was probably the rhododendron of the ancient Greeks. Pliny the Elder knew oleander well and described both its roselike appearance and poisonous qualities (319).

In 1807, when the French invaded Spain, 12 soldiers in the French army cut some oleander branches and used them as skewers for shish-ka-bob. All twelve became desperately ill, and seven of them died (407).

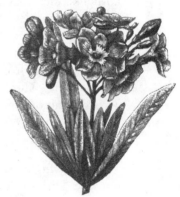

However, opinions differ on whether oleander really deserves all of its frightening reputation. A recent scientific review assures us that "the human mortality associated with oleander ingestion is generally very low, even in cases of intentional consumption (suicide attempts)" (244).

This is not to say that one should start ingesting oleander plant parts for any purpose. Make no mistake: this is a deadly poison! Most Western herbals sensibly leave oleander out entirely, since it is entirely inappropriate for self-medication.

Nerium oleander
(oleander)

Oleander extracts are used in homoeopathic medicine. There, infinitesimally small doses are claimed to have a marked action on the skin, heart, and nervous system, producing and curing paralytic conditions marked by cramp-like contractions of the upper extremities. It is used for a vast number of indications, ranging from weak memory to valvular disease.

But bear in mind that these homoeopathic preparations are from the third to the thirtieth potency. That means that often they have been so incredibly diluted that no actual oleandrin molecules remain in the little white pills (46).

There are at least 15 references from around the world to the use of *Nerium oleander* as a folk remedy for cancer. For example, it is mentioned by various Arabic physicians of the Middle Ages (Masarjawal who flourished in the 8th century AD as well as Rhazes, Abu Mansur, and the celebrated Avicenna).

Its use against cancer is recorded in Puerto Rico, Cuba, North Africa, Venezuela, India, Libya, Antilles, Morocco (where it has been widely used), and Argentina. Duke commented: "With such a fabulous folk repertoire of anticancer activity, oleander will probably be found to contain more proven anticancer agents than just the rutin and ursolic acid reported from *Nerium indicum*" (113). This remark is turning out to be prophetic.

One should no more ignore these important leads than with such plants as *Catharanthus roseus* (Madagascar periwinkle), which yielded Vincristine and Vinblastine. And in fact, oleander is in the same family as the periwinkle (244).

There has been a small amount of conventional scientific work on the anticancer potential of this plant. Italian scientists found "cytotoxic and antileukemic activities of the extracts from oleander plants containing cardiac glycosides" (49).

There are other chemicals present, and these may also have anticancer activity. Scientists at the University of Regensburg in Germany extracted polysaccharides from the crushed leaves, but further animal tests were not encouraging. There were only "some indications for mitogenic activity and a weak macrophage-mediated cytotoxicity" (294).

Anvirzel

All this might have remained an obscure footnote to medical history had not one Turkish doctor decided to follow up on some local folk traditions. The result was a patented and trademarked experimental treatment called Anvirzel.

Anvirzel is a water extract of *Nerium oleander*. The most astonishing thing about it—considering its provenance—is that it appears entirely non-toxic. The chopped leaves, stems, and flowers are treated in various ways to bring out its therapeutic potential and eliminate the toxic principles. Anvirzel was invented more than 25 years ago by a Turkish surgeon, Huseyin Ziya Ozel, MD. In his private clinic he began using this extract as a cancer treatment. Supposedly, Dr. Ozel "was able to compile convincing results and data that demonstrated remarkable efficacy using the drug as a treatment for cancer" (11). In the 1970s, he published two articles on this compound in Turkish medical journals.

Around 1994, I was contacted by a patient advocate who claimed to have seen "miracles" in his clinic. I wrote to Dr. Ozel at that time but received no reply, possibly because of language difficulties.

Originally, Dr. Ozel made the preparation in his kitchen. His one requirement was that the patient had to develop a fever after treatment, which he considered an indispensable sign that the immune system was being activated. In fact, Dr. Ozel would not continue treatment if the patient did not develop a fever. It is interesting that now that the drug is being produced under sterile conditions, there are no more fevers among its recipients. Apparently, patients were developing fevers with the "kitchen table" preparation because of bacterial contamination.

On August 4, 1992, Dr. Ozel received an American patent (#5,135,745) for "Extracts of Nerium species, methods of preparation, and use therefore." According to this patent, the inventor had found "a polysaccharide enriched extract of Nerium species containing an immunologically active polysaccharide useful in treating cell-proliferative disease in mammals."

How can an oleander product, like Anvirzel, not be toxic? According to Joseph Nester, president of Ozelle Pharmaceuticals, an American company trying to get approval for the drug, the toxins in *Nerium oleander* are simply not water soluble. Through Dr. Ozel's patented process the manufacturers are able to eliminate the toxic principles from the final drug.

Although company officials are tightlipped, I was given a copy of a report written in early 1998 that makes very sweeping claims. Dr. Ozel himself is said to have treated 494 cancer patients with this herbal extract. "His high percentage of success was ignored given the fact that the drug was a botanical product, and was an injectable compound that defied traditional medicine's theory of poisoning cancer cells..." Also, Turkey was not considered a "viable testing theater for reliable clinical studies."

One expects promotional statements from purveyors of herbal cancer remedies. By contrast, Mr. Nester was cautious in his statements to me, and made it clear that the company was not seeking to recruit any patients at the present time. He made few claims, and in fact all of those had to be squeezed out of him by persistent questioning.

However, he acknowledged that the summary on Anvirzel that I had received was genuine and had been written by Dr. Masters, an associate of the company, in January, 1998. This summary gives some idea at least of the enthusiasm that the product has generated within the company.

There have been Phase I and Phase II trials in Ireland under the direction of Patrick Kelly, MD of the Johns Medical Center. According to the Masters document, the treatment has demonstrated "unparalleled efficacy in the treatment of cancer, validating much of Dr. Ozel's work." The drug is said to have produced most of, or all, of the following results in patients:

1. *Improvement in quality of life*
2. *Pain reduction or elimination*
3. *Return of energy, appetite and function*
4. *Arrest of metastatic cancers*
5. *Regression of cancer*
6. *Remission of cancer*
7. *Bone regeneration*
8. *No significant side effects*

It also stated that all 46 patients were still alive and "have shown improvement that has surpassed or defied expectations of conventional treatments." According to Mr. Nester, two of the 46 patients have now died, one after quitting the program.

Now obviously, to achieve one or two of these effects in even a significant minority of patients would be a considerable achievement. And we all know that "too-good-to-be-true" results are generally not true. However, I remind you that this document is not being used to sell a product to cancer patients.

Informally I have been told that the best results have been in prostate, lung, and brain cancer, where they have seen objective remissions. In sarcomas they have seen stabilization and possibly remission of as many as nine tumors. The hardest cancer to treat so far has been liver cancer.

I cannot vouch for the accuracy of any of these claims. However, I spoke to a scientist (unconnected to Anvirzel) who was present when they made a presentation at one of America's most famous cancer centers. She said that some of their clinical cases looked "very interesting," and an oncologist present was impressed enough that he agreed to launch a small, unpublicized pilot study of the compound.

Mode of Administration

Basically, 0.5 cc of the product is injected into the muscle on a daily basis. Later the dose and frequency may be adjusted as indicated. The injection can be self-administered or performed by a health professional or family member.

So far, the drug has been provided free of charge by the company to those in the Phase I and Phase II trials in Ireland. In addition, a number of American patients have received it via "compassionate use INDs" (Investigative New Drug applications) from the FDA. Patients have had to be willing to meet the company's stringent requirements:

1. Make a serious commitment to get well.

2. Be willing to give up toxic medications, habits and behaviors which would be counter-productive. Listed under this category were not just heavy smoking, alcohol, and illegal drugs, but "chemotherapy drugs" and "radiation."

3. Eat a diet which promotes health rather than supports disease. Also take supplements, as prescribed.

4. Submit a history of current disease state and up-to-date medical treatment records.

5. Keep a diary of beginning signs and symptoms as well as progressive signs and symptoms and complaints, as directed.

6. Keep a record of administration of Anvirzel and any reactions experienced.

7. Provide reports on an interim basis as requested by the research coordinator either by a once-every-two-week telephone call or personal appearance.

8. Be willing to be re-tested medically at prescribed intervals to determine actual progress.

9. Understand that one can withdraw from the study with a minimum of notice and also that the study subject can be canceled from the program for reasons as follows:

    a. If the monitoring doctor feels that it is in the patient's best interest to stop;

    b. If the company cancels the study;

    c. If the patient is not cooperating with the protocol.

"We strongly feel that the product will ultimately replace some, if not most, of the current toxic methods of treatment that are being prescribed," they wrote. They call it "the first true alternative to accepted toxic therapies for viral related and immunodeficiency related diseases. We feel it is likely that continuing documentation in advanced trials will cause this drug to become a primary treatment rather than an alternative when treating cancer and AIDS."

These are, of course, big claims, and such claims almost always fail to materialize. Nevertheless, although, clearly, published data is lacking, I am impressed by a number of things.

First, the company is not selling the treatment, but has mainly provided it free of charge to test subjects, according to the guidelines of the FDA.

Second, they are seeking FDA approval of marketing along the lines of the standard three-phase clinical trial track. (A new set of clinical trials is scheduled to take place at US medical institutions and they appear to have performed serious preclinical toxicology and animal studies.)

Also, there is a US patent on the drug and the technique of extraction, and a long history of both popular and clinical work with this product in various countries.

Anvirzel is a good illustration of how the folk record of traditional cancer treatments can still be utilized to uncover promising agents from some of the most common plants.

Chapter 22 🌹 Ukrain (Ukraine & Austria)

ONE OF THE MOST COMMON FOLK TREATMENTS FOR CANCER IS THE GREATER CELANDINE (*CHELIDONIUM MAJUS*). THERE ARE NUMER- ous references to it in Hartwell. Mrs. Grieve states that "greater celandine is a very popular medicine in Russia, where it is said to have proved effective in some cases of cancer" (153). And it was used in English cancer remedies, along with comfrey, goldenseal, and other herbs (343).

Greater celandine (so named to distinguish it from an unrelated plant, lesser celandine, which is used to treat hemorrhoids) is an attractive member of the poppy family. In summer, its stem is filled with a bright and acrid orange-colored juice.

Pliny tells us that its name is derived from the Greek chelidon, or swallow, because it flowers when the swallows arrive and fades at their departure. Its acrid juice has been used to remove films from the cornea of the eye. Pliny also says that this property was discovered by swallows, which gave another reason to name the plant after them.

Gerard knew of this usage through Dioscorides (who was Pliny's contemporary). The Renaissance herbalist wrote:

"The juice of the herbe is good to sharpen the sight, for it cleanseth and consumeth away slimie things that cleave about the ball of the eye and hinder the sight and especially being boiled with honey in a brasen vessell, as Dioscorides teacheth."

In the Middle Ages a drink made of celandine was supposed to be good for the blood. According to the Doctrine of Signatures, because of the yellow-orange color of its flower and acrid juice it was also reputed to be good for jaundice. Its use as a treatment against growths probably began when its corrosive juice was used to destroy warts, ringworm, and corns. As noted, it was an ingredient in Mrs. Johnson's 1754 "receipt" for curing cancer (see chapter 2).

Like other active plants, celandine is rich in alkaloids, which are among the most potent compounds known to man. (Only some bacterial toxins are more potent by weight.) These range from 2,500 to 22,000 parts per million of the plant. There are three chemically different groups of alkaloids that have been extracted from the plant. The most prominent of these are chelidonine and chelerythrin, which is narcotic and poisonous.

Chelidonium is on James Duke's short list of folk anticancer species that contains active compounds.

Some patients may be tempted to self-administer greater celandine for cancer or other conditions. In fact, several popular herbals even include concoctions made from the root stock or the green portion of the herb itself. Despite its folk reputation, I know of no scientific studies on the use of the herb as a treatment for cancer.

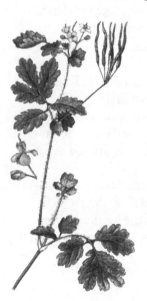

"The whole plant abounds in a bright, orange-colored juice," says Grieve, "which is emitted freely whenever the stems or leaves are broken. This juice stains the hands strongly and has a persistent and nauseous taste and a strong, disagreeable smell. It is acrid and a powerful irritant" (153).

To my knowledge, greater celandine can be toxic and should never be administered in any form except by health care professionals who are both trained and licensed to utilize botanical medicines.

Celandine did not come to prominence until the late 20th century, when it was included as one of two ingredients in an anticancer medicine called Ukrain (NSC 631570). Ukrain is a unique product that acts in at least two ways on cancer (by killing cells and by increasing the immune response).

Technically, Ukrain is a conjugate of an herb and a chemotherapeutic drug. It is obtained by what are called thermal adduction processes from the purified alkaloids of *Chelidonium majus* and a cytotoxic drug called thiotepa (thiophosphoric triaziridine).

Chelidonium majus
(greater celandine)

The result is a semisynthetic product that requires many purification steps, using chloroform and ether, to achieve a final product that is about 90 percent pure. It comes in the form of yellow-orange crystals.

For something that stemmed from folk cancer treatments, Ukrain has a considerable amount of research behind it. In 1996, one European scientific journal published a special edition with 42 articles on this compound, from groups around the world. This is one of the most impressive accumulations of scholarship of any "alternative" cancer treatment.

Ukrain is the brain child of Dr. J. Wassyl Nowicky (pronounced "No-vít-skee"), director of the Ukrain Anti-Cancer Institute of Vienna, Austria. The product is manufactured by the JW Nowicky Pharmaceuticals of Austria. It was developed in 1978 and first unveiled at the 13th International Congress of Chemotherapy, held in Vienna in August 1983 (303). Ukrain is named after Dr. Nowicky's native country (without the final "e").

About Thiotepa

Thiotepa was the first anticancer agent produced by the German pharmaceutical industry. It is an aziridine, which is closely related both chemically and therapeutically to the first American anticancer drugs, the nitrogen mustards. Its major use at the present time is as a part of a drug regimen called VATH, used to treat metastatic breast cancer. It sometimes substituted for cyclophosphamide in patients whose bladders cannot tolerate that drug (168). It is also used in patients who have pleural effusions, and as a treatment for bladder cancer and pediatric solid tumors. Because of its toxicity to the blood-forming cells, thiotepa is being investigated for use in high-dose bone marrow transplant regimens (104).

One of the most intriguing aspects of Ukrain is its relative lack of toxicity. Plant alkaloids by themselves can be highly irritating and toxic. So too is thiotepa. What makes Ukrain so unusual is that this forced marriage of herb and drug yields a compound that is lacking in toxicity to normal cells. Yet it seems to have a strong affinity for killing cancer cells.

The LD50 (amount that will kill 50 percent of experimental animals) is 350-450 mg/kg in rodents, which is several thousand times higher than the therapeutic doses that are used in humans (231).

In hamsters and rats no clinical signs of toxicity could be found. The only problem was a slight decrease in the average hamster litter size (216). Nor does Ukrain induce anaphylactic shock in mice or guinea pigs.

In addition, for three years healthy human volunteers in Poland, Austria, and Germany received repeated courses of the new drug.

Some of the subjects reported slight tiredness, an increase in thirst and urine excretion. There was some slight and short-lived pain at the intramuscular injection site. But there were no other significant changes observed (94).

In cancer patients, a favorable sign is the so-called "typical Ukrain reaction." Dr. Nowicky describes this as an increase in pain, rise in body temperature to 38-39° C (equal to 100.4° to 102.2° F), a feeling of weariness and weakness, swelling in the tumor area, with cold and hot sensations. This is similar to the healing reaction frequently seen with other immunological treatments of cancer.

Investigation of Ukrain is now underway not just in Austria, but in Canada, France, Germany, the Netherlands, Switzerland, and even Thailand and Swaziland. At the present time, Ukrain is only available from Dr. Nowicky's center in Austria; in North America it is only being used at some "alternative" clinics such as the Atkins Center for Complementary Medicine in New York or the American Biologics hospital in Tijuana, Mexico.

Ukrain is patented (US #2,670,347), registered in the Republic of Belarus (#1330-65) and has been the subject of dozens of scientific papers. I shall summarize some of those that support the use of this compound.

First of all, Ukrain was tested against 60 different human cancer cell lines at the US National Cancer Institute (NCI). In all cell lines (at a dose of 10/-4 mM) there was a remarkable 100 percent growth inhibition. One possible mechanism in the test tube, was that Ukrain "seems to change the oxygen consumption of malignant cells in an irreversible manner" (304). While it increased the oxygen consumption of both normal and malignant cells, oxygen consumption normalized in non-cancerous cells within 15 minutes, but decreased irreversibly to zero in cancer cells, effectively killing them.

Ukrain has also been shown to inhibit DNA, RNA, and protein synthesis in malignant cells (301). It is thus highly toxic to cancer, but does little or no damage to non-cancerous cells (e.g., fibroblasts or endothelial cells) in the test-tube. It has also been shown to accumulate at the site of a tumor or its metastases.

In addition, in mice, Ukrain is a powerful biological response modifier (BRM), or stimulator of the immune system. Most scientists believe that cancer is accompanied by a breakdown of the immune system and could therefore be influenced by modulation of that system.

Some BRMs, such as high-dose interleukin, may cause undesirable or even life-threatening adverse effects. But when Ukrain was given intravenously to mice, it was nontoxic, yet had a striking therapeutic effect. By day 15, only one out of five treated mice had developed tumors, while all five control mice had tumors and were already beginning to show signs of cachexia (wasting), according to doctors at the University of Miami. This difference was attributed to the stimulation of macrophages, a critical part of the immune system.

Ukrain is contraindicated in pregnancy, and in patients with high fevers. If patients have "expansive processes" in the central nervous system (e.g., brain tumors or metastases) they should be treated cautiously and only in the clinical setting because of possible (but reversible) tumor swelling. Caution is also advised for children in the growing phase.

It should not be used in conjunction with cortisone derivatives or other immune-suppressive medicines, since these neutralize the immune-stimulating effects of Ukrain. Also, cancer patients in the terminal stages of the disease, who have pronounced cachexia (wasting syndrome) have little prospect of success with Ukrain.

A Phase II clinical study of 70 cancer patients (aged 14 to 80 years) was carried out under contract to the Ministry of Science and Research of Austria. "A high percentage of patients were in very advanced stages and had received chemo-and/or radiation therapy prior to Ukrain treatment" (304).

This study established that the drug was cytostatic or cytotoxic to many types of cancer. The mechanism of action was most interesting. First of all, Ukrain induced apoptosis, or programmed cell death, which is characterized by cell surface "blepping" (blistering), and changes in the permeability of cell surface membranes. This is usually associated with fragmentation of the DNA. However, with Ukrain, there was a significant increase in DNA content (what scientists call ploidy) instead of DNA fragmentation. The second method of inducing cell death occurred when cells displayed one or two large blisters on their cell surfaces, according to Dr. A. Liepends of St. John's, Newfoundland.

These included leukemias, lung cancer, both small and non-small cell, colon cancer, central nervous system cancer, melanoma, ovarian cancer and renal (kidney) cancer. These were among the cell types that were shown by the NCI to be inhibited by Ukrain.

It is noteworthy that while the drug is almost completely non-toxic in people without cancer, many of the treated patients "no matter what stage, experienced subjective and objective adverse effects such as pain in the tumor area, itching, thirst, forced urine excretion, nausea, feeling of warmth, fever, etc., but of short duration.

"These side effects are believed to be reactions to tumor degradation products," said Dr. Nowicky, "and are observed when the patient responds to therapy" (304). No cases exist in which the treatment had to be discontinued because of such adverse effects (295).

Nowicky and his coworkers claim an overall 93 percent "success" rate in early stage tumors, 72 percent in those with minimal (lymph node) spread, and 30 percent in late stage (advanced, metastatic) cancer. Needless to say, different people define "success" in different ways.

In another study, 36 cancer patients in stage III were treated with Ukrain (300 mg over 30 days). Many of the patients (who had rectal, breast, ovarian, liver and skin cancers) showed tumor regression, especially those with liver metastases. The standard tumor markers also declined (302).

Another study looked at nine patients with stage IB cervix cancer (with tumors larger than four centimeters). Two to three weeks after starting Ukrain treatment, a radical hysterectomy and lymphadenectomy was performed on each woman. Three of the nine patients showed partial tumor regression and six remained stable. All patients were still alive after six months (316).

In another study, eight patients in various stages I-III (three with breast, three with uterine, and one each with melanoma or lung cancers) were treated with Ukrain. They also received 1,000 mg of vitamin C. During two series of injections their general condition improved. The stage I and II operated patients had no recurrences for at least 1.5 years. The advanced stage patients remained stable for some time (93).

In another study, nine men with lung cancer (seven with small cell and two with non-small cell lung cancer) who were previously untreated, were given Ukrain. Scientists were interested in looking at their immunological response, which was indeed improved with the treatment. Some of these patients were subsequently given chemotherapy. There was objective tumor regression in four patients. The median survival time was 14 months for the responders, with significant improvement in their general condition (363).

Another test was done on nine patients with stage III or IV cancers of various kinds (four with cholangiosarcoma, four with head-and-neck cancers and one with breast cancer). One patient, whose body temperature rose to 38° to 39° C (100.4° to 102.2° F), had the largest tumor reduction. A partial remission was seen in three patients, a minimal remission in one, three remained stable, and two patients showed progression of their disease. It is noteworthy that there is no standard treatment for stage IV sarcomas. Ukrain induced remission in 25 percent of patients and stabilization in another 25 percent. If confirmed, these would be exceptional results (396).

Ukrain has also had some success with bladder cancer. Five patients with fairly large bladder tumors (T2) were entered into a study in Warsaw. The tumors had invaded through the 'lamina propria' (a layer of connective tissue) into the inner half of the muscle and were palpable by their surgeon.

These patients opted not to have surgery, but to take Ukrain instead. They received an intravenous injection of ten milligrams of Ukrain every second day. In all five patients the tumors are said to have been eliminated by Ukrain without surgical intervention. The amount needed to eliminate the bladder cancer varied from 300 to 600 mg, and the time of treatment varied from three to six months. There was a six to twelve month follow up in each case, showing that they were negative for recurrence (56).

Another study evaluated the effects of Ukrain on patients with advanced colon cancer, who had already received chemotherapy. After recurrences in 18 patients, nine were treated with Ukrain while the other nine received the standard drug 5-FU. Positive immunological changes were seen in the Ukrain-treated patients. In addition, a relative decrease in tumor mass and an increase in tumor necrosis was seen in this group.

Treatment had to be discontinued in some patients in the 5-FU group, whereas it was well tolerated in the Ukrain group. The authors, from the Ukrainian State Medical University, Departments of General Surgery and Oncology, concluded that Ukrain may be used in a complex therapy for locally spread colon cancer. The most recent figures from the Ukrainian Anti Cancer Institute claim that the long-term survival rate in the Ukrain treated patients is 83.3 percent compared to 44.4 percent in the 5-FU treated controls.

Life Style Changes

Although Dr. Nowicky is not an "alternative practitioner," he does make certain lifestyle suggestions as part of the treatment. He advises patients to maintain a quiet manner of life with abstinence from nicotine and alcohol during and after therapy.

He stresses the need for healthy nutrition and possible supplementation with vitamins and minerals for those who are deficient. He says that, if at all possible, patients should take time off from work, at least during the first series of treatments. All physical activities, either at work or in sports, should be avoided during treatment.

In many ways, Ukrain is a model for what can and should be done with other herb-derived products. Dr. Nowicky has carefully worked out the basic pharmacology and biochemistry of the product, defined, patented and registered his product, and then interested many other scientists in using it in both basic and clinical research.

The result has been an impressive body of literature. Ukrain could be a very useful treatment for many kinds of cancer because it both kills cancer cells and simultaneously stimulates the immune system in a beneficial direction. More intensive work is clearly warranted.

The nearly total disinterest of the American cancer community in this agent is inexplicable. Some of this disinterest has to do, of course, with its origin in herbal medicine. (There were only five papers on natural products out of 2,200 given at the 1998 ASCO meeting.) But this alone cannot be a sufficient explanation. After all, it is well known to oncologists that many chemotherapeutic agents are of natural origin. In fact, one manufacturer in the exhibit hall arranged a lovely display of periwinkles, yew trees, and even chaparral to reinforce that point.

I think there have to be other explanations. First of all, Ukrain is relatively non-toxic, while the vast majority of chemotherapeutic agents (including those of natural origin) are highly poisonous. There seems to be an inherent prejudice on the part of some chemotherapists towards "competitive" non-toxic agents. (See my book, *Questioning Chemotherapy*.)

Second, Ukrain may have been "tainted" by association with alternative practitioners who have taken anti-establishment positions. The two main advocates in the US are the outspoken Robert Atkins, MD, and Robert Bradford of American Biologics, Inc. of Tijuana, who promoted the sale and use of laetrile (amygdalin), a substance that most oncologists view with abhorrence.

Although Ukrain is intended for use by physicians, it is also sold directly to patients. Thus, oncologists are likely to hear about it (if they hear about it at all) by way of patient inquiries rather than through the "normal" mechanism of medical journal advertisements and pharmaceutical "detail men." In addition, the price of this substance is high compared to other herbal products, although reasonable when compared to chemotherapy.

Finally, although no herbal product has a better track record of publications, a glance at the references will show that most of them are in relatively obscure European journals, and none in such core publications as *JAMA,* the *New England Journal of Medicine, Cancer,* etc. The scientists doing the work are mainly of Eastern European origin, which may also count against them in some Anglo-American circles.

Many of the publications come from a single journal, *Drugs Under Experimental and Clinical Research* which, although it has a distinguished editorial board (including Dr. George Mathe), has been criticized in the past for publishing special issues on the work of controversial Houston physician, Stanislaw R. Burzynski, MD, PhD.

Most of these reservations seem irrelevant to the question of whether or not Ukrain actually can benefit cancer patients. It is difficult to study the scientific record and not come away convinced that Ukrain is a fascinating and promising new herb-derived agent, which deserves intensive scrutiny at the highest levels. The National Cancer Institute should arrange clinical trials and Ukrain should be widely used in practice if it is effective. The failure of American scientists to adequately investigate this promising herb-derived agent is, in my opinion, unacceptable.

Chapter 23 ❦ Aloe Vera (United States)

*"The public must learn how to cherish the nobler and rare plants,
and to plant the aloe..."* —*Margaret Fuller (1810-1850)*

"Outrageous...a fraudulent promotion." —*FDA compliance officer Roma Egli,
commenting on the Internet sale of aloe vera products (1997)*

ALOE VERA IS A PERENNIAL SUCCULENT WITH A STRONG FIBROUS ROOT AND A ROSETTE OF FLESHY BASAL LEAVES. IT IS A MEMBER OF THE lily family that is native to Eastern and Southern Africa but now cultivated most intensively in the West Indies and other tropical countries. Aloe has many accepted uses in medicine and cosmetics. Its use as a cancer therapy is more controversial.

The functional part of the plant is the gel, a clear, mucilaginous material that is derived from the inner portion of the spiky leaves (also called the parenchyma). Manufacturing aloe vera gel for the market requires, first and foremost, separating it from the inner cellular debris and other specialized cells (392). These other cells contain a bitter yellow juice or latex which can cause intestinal distress unless it is removed. (At one time this was cherished as a cathartic medicine.)

Aloe is complex, with approximately 150 known ingredients. The amount of each constituent is generally very small, since the plant is about 99 percent water. However, there is a rich distribution of important and potentially therapeutic ingredients: vitamins A, C, E, choline, B12, folic acid, etc. 20 of the 22 amino acids, including seven out of the eight essential ones; nine minerals; 12 anthraquinones; eight enzymes; auxins and gibberellins; lignin; salicylic acid; saponins; four plant steroids; lupeol and several sugars.

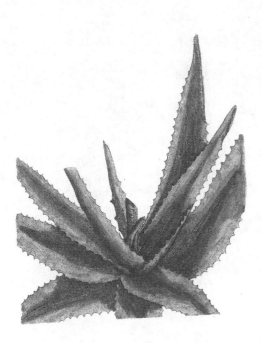

Aloe vera
(aloe)

Aloe has a long history of use as an external remedy for irritations, cuts, and burns—perhaps the most important such item in history. On the day that Christopher Columbus set sail for the Indies he wrote in his diary, "All is well, aloe is on board!" (174)

It has been popular as a folk medicine all over the world, including China, Java, Nepal, and Malaya. Its beneficial effect on skin has been known for millennia. In fact, its production is a multimillion dollar industry, especially since it is a common ingredient in lotions and shampoos for the mass market.

Aloe is a relatively safe plant when the juice (freed of the bitter constituent) is consumed orally. The AHPA rates aloe for internal use as a class 1 herb, i.e., it can be safely consumed when used appropriately. While generally a safe substance, there are some potential adverse effects. There are reports of skin or intestinal irritation from both applying and ingesting extracts of aloe. For external use, the AHPA gives it a 2d rating, since it may delay wound healing following laparotomy or cesarean section.

Aloe has been used medicinally since ancient times. It was known to the ancient Egyptians and is mentioned in the Ebers Papyrus as an effective treatment for infections, skin ailments, and constipation (407). Alexander the Great is said to have fought a war to obtain a supply of this plant for his wounded warriors.

It has also played a small role as a traditional cancer remedy and is mentioned by Hartwell as a treatment for gastric (stomach) cancer in Venezuela. It is also a traditional treatment for warts, a disease that is related in some ways to cancer (174).

Aloe entered cancer management in the 1930s, with the first reports of the successful treatment of x-ray and radium burns using this gel. In the following decades this preliminary practice led to further experimental studies on laboratory animals. Most of these early studies suffered from poor experimental design and/or contained insufficient test samples. Conflicting or inconsistent results were obtained (156).

Aloe vera contains many polysaccharides. While in the past, these chemicals did not excite as much interest among plant chemists as, say, alkaloids, scientists have now shown that polysaccharides can stimulate an immune response in people. This has given aloe vera new importance.

In general, however, test tube and animal studies have not supported a strong anticancer role for *Aloe vera*. Typical is a report from the 1950s that showed no activity in sarcoma 37 of a suspension of powdered plant parts (35). In a Korean test there were only weak effects in the test tube using purified leaf gel injected into the peritoneal cavity of mice (204). More recently, there have been some indication of antitumor activity when aloe juice was injected (also intraperitoneally) into mice with Ehrlich ascites and sarcoma 180 (308).

Russian scientists have experimented with aloe as a possible way of stopping the spread of cancer. They used three types of tumors in rodents and concluded that while aloe did not affect the primary tumor, it appeared to reduce the overall tumor mass as well as the frequency of metastases (152). Aloe juice has also been shown to enhance the antitumor effects of chemotherapy (5-FU and cyclophosphamide) (360).

Most of the recent interest in aloe stems not from government laboratories but from the activities of a single company, Carrington Laboratories Inc., of Irving, Texas, which patented a unique carbohydrate fraction of the leaf gel called acemannan (Carrisyn®) and now dominates the aloe pharmaceutical industry (422).

Acemannan is a potent immunostimulant, but to obtain a gram or so of this compound from the normal aloe vera juice found in stores one would have to drink between two to four glasses. It is therefore impractical (and expensive) for patients to try and get a therapeutic dose in this way.

Acemannan affects the immune system in various ways. It has an effect on macrophages and stimulates those cells' cytokine production. There is a dose-dependent increase in the production of two cytokines, IL-6 and TNF-alpha, when acemannan is ingested by animals (406).

To my knowledge, the efficacy of aloe or acemannan has never been rigorously tested in cancer patients. There are a few intriguing hints, however, that aloe might play a beneficial role in human cancer. Strongest of these is that acemannan has been approved by the Food and Drug Administration (FDA), in an injectable form, for veterinary use against two kinds of animal cancer, fibrosarcomas and feline leukemia.

Feline leukemia is a highly deadly and communicable disease among cats.

(Luckily, there is no evidence that it is communicable to people.) Feline leukemia is caused, like AIDS, by a retrovirus, this one the feline leukemia virus or FeLV. This virus is so deadly that once cats develop clinical symptoms they are usually euthanized (352).

In an experiment, 44 cats with clinically confirmed feline leukemia were given acemannan injections weekly for six weeks. They were then re-examined at the end of another six weeks. At that time, 71 percent of the treated cats were still alive and seemed to be in good health (163). Twenty-nine percent had died. Normally, about 70 percent of such animals would be expected to be dead.

There have been a number of other promising studies in animals. In one, acemannan had favorable effects on pets with spontaneous cancers (228). Eight dogs and five cats with fibrosarcomas were treated with acemannan in combination with surgery and radiation therapy. All had recurrent disease or a poor prognosis for survival. Four of the twelve animals had tumor shrinkages, with a notable increase in necrosis and inflammation at the tumor sites. Complete surgical excision was then performed on all animals and acemannan treatments were continued monthly for one year.

Seven of the thirteen animals remained alive and tumor-free (in a range of 440 to 603+ days), with a median survival time of 372 days. The authors concluded that "acemannan immunostimulant may be an effective adjunct to surgery and radiation therapy in the treatment of canine and feline fibrosarcomas." In another study, there was a decreased mortality in mice with sarcoma that were given acemannan (315).

Scientists also reported that "rapidly growing, highly malignant and invasive sarcoma grew in 100 percent of implanted control animals, resulting in mortality in 20 to 46 days....Approximately 40 percent of animals treated with acemannan at the time of tumor cell implantation... survived." The scientists, who were at Texas A&M University, concluded that "acemannan-stimulated synthesis of monokines resulted in the initiation of immune attack, necrosis, and regression of implanted sarcomas in mice" (259).

Based on such results, during the 1980s and early 1990s, Carrington Laboratories issued many public statements exaggerating the effect and potential of its products. They even suggested at one point that they might have found a cure for AIDS. Such statements were taken up, publicized, and then sometimes exaggerated by AIDS activists.

The company's own executives have now acknowledged that they exaggerated the benefits of the aloe-based drugs the company had under development. In fact, Carrington has since abandoned its AIDS program entirely, chief executive Carleton E. Turner told the *Washington Post* (27).

Aloe has also been a favorite of various multi-level or network marketers, the sort that thrives by door-to-door sales or over the Internet. One such company is Mannatech™ Inc. based in Coppell, Texas. They manufacture and sell "Man-Aloe," and similar products. Mannatech describes itself as "a well established network marketing company with a highly-motivated team." If you think that herbal medicine is still a "fringe" phenomenon, consider this: by May, 1998, this company had 368,507 Independent Associates in their network, and reported annual sales of $150 million.

In April, 1998, Mannatech filed for an Initial Public Offering (IPO) of eight million shares of stock. Mannatech, according to spokespersons, "is perfectly positioned to become the dominant force in the multi-billion dollar health and nutrition industry."

But Mannatech's claims for its products are modest compared to some other companies. I have found Websites proclaiming that "Aloe Vera cures 200 diseases including cancer." Another declared:

"We cannot speak in terms of 'CURES FOR DISEASES.' [But] Aloe Mucilaginous Polysaccharides molecules are among the most potent and versatile weapons known to man, that a person could give their body to enhance it's ability to fight disease. THERE ARE NO DISEASES WHICH YOUR BODY IS NOT CAPABLE OF CONQUERING, and Aloe Vera meets those principles."

The Federal Trade Commission (FTC) became so concerned over the proliferation of such claims that in 1997 it sent warning letters to 400 Websites promoting aloe as a cancer cure.

Another way in which aloe vera has been popularized as a cancer treatment is through audio and video tapes. Such tapes have themselves become a big business. It is not uncommon for physicians, in particular, to receive dozens of such tapes, often in duplicate copies.

For example, a company called Health and Wealth wholesales cassette tapes to network marketers for use in mass mailings. Health and Wealth offers nine separate tapes on aloe alone, including *Cancer & Aloe—Cancer Control* and *Is Aloe Vera a Cure for Cancer?* Many of these are by Dr. Lee Ritter, a well-known promoter of aloe's wonders.

In a video titled *Aloe Vera, Nature's Miracle,* H. Reginald McDaniel, a Texas pathologist and aloe researcher, claims that aloe "will be the most important single step forward in the treatment of diseases in the history of mankind." This tape, which the FDA has tried to remove from the market, discusses how to use aloe to treat AIDS and cancer. At another Website, Joe Glickman Jr., of Whitefish, Montana, sells an aloe-based product called Manapol, which McDaniel helped to develop. Glickman says that aloe "fights cancer aggressively."

Another audio tape in this field is by Allen Hoffman, PhD. Although not a multilevel marketing product, Hoffman's tape has been sent out by the hundreds of thousands. Many cancer patients have received at least one copy, sometimes more. Hoffman has advocated the use of a combination of high-dose aloe, which he calls T-UP, and a mineral called cesium chloride as a cancer treatment. According to him, cesium chloride has an affinity for cancer tissues. When it is combined with vitamin C, it enters cancer cells, alters their acidity, and destroys the tumor.

Dr. Hoffman's audio tape bears the message, "There is hope! You don't have to die!" (An unacknowledged takeoff of the title of Harry Hoxsey's autobiography.) On the tape, Hoffman says that he stumbled upon the cancer treatment while doing research in Baltimore on AIDS patients. He claims that although T-UP can be taken orally, it is more effective if injected. In his tape, he criticized US restrictions on such injections and said that for legal reasons it was necessary to travel outside the country to get such shots.

He himself seems to have organized trips to an undisclosed location for people with cancer and AIDS. Although Hoffman sold T-UP to consumers as an oral preparation, there have been repeated claims that he offered US physicians an injectable solution of *Aloe vera*.

Patients are encouraged to take one to four teaspoons of Hoffman's *Aloe vera* product per day. Hoffman claimed that it takes just three months to "rip" the tumor out of the body. The cost of such treatment is approximately $1,800.

Hoffman has made enormous claims for his treatment. I became concerned when acquaintances repeatedly told me of instances of gastrointestinal distress and of their lips turning blue after taking the cesium chloride portion of this treatment. In March, 1997, I called Hoffman's office to find out more about this treatment and hopefully to document some of the fabulous results. What I heard was not reassuring.

His phone associate, who identified himself as Brett, described Dr. Hoffman to me as a "major researcher" at Johns Hopkins University with degrees in biology, biochemistry and medical technology. When I asked about his publications, Brett told me he presumed there were many. However, I was unable to find a single scientific publication by Allen Hoffman, PhD in Medline.

By definition, you cannot be a "major researcher" in the health field and not have a significant track record in the peer-reviewed literature. Johns Hopkins spokespersons now say that Allen Hoffman has not been affiliated with their university since 1979.

I asked Dr. Hoffman and the T-UP staff to put me in touch with some of the many patients who had allegedly been cured on this treatment. I was referred to a public relations advisor, who assured me they were compiling such data. But they never provided me with any names. Each call was cordial, but led to a dead-end. I inquired again in early 1998, but again received no follow-up. At that time, I was told that a Ms. Mary Johnson was a Hodgkin's disease patient who had benefited. When I asked if she was an employee of their company I was told that "they helped her and now she's helping them."

I called her number and asked to speak to her, but although the person on the other end took my message, Ms. Johnson never called me back. My tentative conclusion was that this aloe-cesium treatment was unsubstantiated, overpriced, and possibly dangerous. My advice to cancer patients who asked was to avoid this treatment entirely until further proof of safety and efficacy was provided. Such proof was not forthcoming.

But I now understand that Dr. Hoffman may have had other things on his mind. On February, 25 1998, his treatment received front-page coverage in the *Washington Post*. Their exposé told the story of Tommy Lowery, a patient with advanced prostate cancer, who chose to be treated with a regimen that included injections of Dr. Hoffman's product. The treatments were given at a Manassas, Virginia medical clinic run by Donald MacNay, DO.

Until recently, Dr. MacNay was practicing as an orthopedic surgeon. Subsequently, he set up a clinic to administer Hoffman's aloe products (356).

For a natural herbal product, such treatments can get rather expensive. One family claimed that the cost of three week's treatment at MacNay's clinic was $16,000, including rent while staying in the area. Some families who went to him complained about revolting conditions at the clinic itself: blood spattered on the floor, bathrooms soiled with excrement, and some IV tubes hooked on clothes hangers attached to the ceiling.

Alternative medicine is supposed to offer a more holistic and humane approach to cancer care. Often it does, but at other times it resembles a caricature of get-rich-quick money mills.

Within two days of beginning the treatments in March 1997, the *Post* reported, "Tommy Lowery's body turned purple and began to swell. The skin on his toes cracked open. He died a painful death." Even prosecutors admit that it is difficult to sort out the effects of end-stage cancer from those of toxic medications. But his hometown doctor believe Lowery's death was hastened, if not caused, by the aloe injections.

The *Washington Post* found other patients whose surviving relatives told similar stories. Richard F. King, 41, of Royal Oak, Michigan, who had kidney cancer, went into cardiac arrest in MacNay's office; Clarence Holland Lander, 83, of Waco, Texas, had lung cancer and died in MacNay's office; and Douglas Crabbe, 48, of Cecil County, Maryland, who suffered from cancer of the esophagus, died a week after treatment in Manassas. Even among advanced cancer patients such a string of sudden deaths is suspicious.

According to the *Post,* "Federal and State consumer and law enforcement agencies from Texas to Maryland are investigating the clinic and its supplier," Allen Hoffman. The Virginia state medical board suspended Dr. MacNay's license in September, concluding that his intravenous injections of aloe "may be a substantial danger to the public health and safety." The clinic was closed.

In February, 1998, MacNay was stripped of his license to practice medicine by the Virginia Board of Medicine, which cited fraud, unprofessional conduct and gross malpractice. On April 6, 1998, he was indicted by a Prince William County grand jury for allegedly defrauding cancer patients and for dispensing prescription drugs to his assistant, Ronald R. Sheetz. Mr. Sheetz is a former auto mechanic with no formal medical training, who is said to have administered many of the treatments given to MacNay's patients. MacNay himself faces a maximum of 160 years in prison (Prince William [Md.] *Journal,* 10/14/97).

Because of this case, and heightened governmental vigilance, there has been a pullback of aloe claims in recent months. Neal Deoul, Allen Hoffman's business partner, told the Associated Press that their promotional tapes have been destroyed and that T-UP, Inc. no longer sends out its brochures. He said the company's new attorney had informed the partners that they were in "technical violation" of FDA regulations and that they have stopped such promotions.

"Accuse us of ignorance," Mr. Deoul is quoted as saying. "We didn't know we couldn't do that." Dr. Hoffman's Website (www.t-up.com) has also been "temporarily removed for updates." Other Websites promoting aloe have also pulled in their horns and removed all references to cancer and AIDS According to the *Post,* Dr. Allen Hoffman is the subject of continuing investigations by the Maryland attorney general's office and the US attorney's office in Baltimore (356).

I am sure that some defenders of alternative medicine will suspect that T-UP is being framed. But I found it significant that federal enforcement agencies told the *Post* that "many offers of alternative treatment are honest or harmless." Such a truthful statement would not have been made in the past. Regulators add that many claims are fraudulent and dangerous, which is also true.

The sheer growth of the industry has made it impossible for investigators to keep up with every instance of abuse. The FTC can also do nothing about enthusiastic messages that are posted in Internet discussion areas (some of which may be commercially motivated). One Imperial Beach, California, man regularly posts messages urging cancer patients to try aloe injections. "Such a simple, direct treatment, next to no side effects, and the damn stuff WORKS," said Roger Jones. "If it caught on, it'd be so effective, it'd put millions of doctors out of work."

The aloe story is in some ways typical of what happens to promising herbal treatments in America. There are preliminary reports of benefit, which the "cancer establishment" is extremely slow to pursue, if they are interested at all. There may even be some very promising work in animals.

As the product picks up steam, various knockoff products appear in the marketplace. These are aggressively sold via network marketing schemes, over the Internet, and with audio and video tapes disseminated by the millions. Finally, a cure frenzy takes hold, whipped up by promoters and enthusiasts.

A few people may truly benefit, but it is nearly impossible to sort out their stories from a welter of claims and counter-claims. The quackbusters now chime in with a total condemnation of the product and its advocates. In the end, some people get hurt or even die. The big media arrive on the scene, sometimes using these abuses to attack the use of non-conventional treatments in general. The government finally takes action...not to seriously research the product, as they should have done, but to prosecute the promoters.

Wouldn't it have been better if the National Cancer Institute had vigorously investigated aloe vera and its various byproducts from the beginning, exploring every possible use for cancer patients? A totally fair and open-minded investigation, with the participation of members of the alternative community itself, was needed. This might have dispelled many of the exaggerated claims for this product, while uncovering something of real benefit to patients. In either case, it might have spared the Tommy Lowerys of the world from falling into the hands of fly-by-night clinics. Don't cancer patients deserve that much?

Chapter 24 ❧ Vitae Elixxir (United States)

VITAE ELIXXIR IS A THICK HERBAL MIXTURE THAT CONTAINS A LARGE NUMBER OF HERBS AND TRACE MINERALS. IT WAS INVENTED by a Casper, Wyoming businessman named Ralph Schauss and although manufactured in the United States, has been marketed by Organic Resources, Ltd. of Hong Kong.

Vitae Elixxir is sometimes depicted as a panacea, which can eliminate cancer and its metastases, reduce arterial plaque, eliminate viruses, cure multiple sclerosis, and so forth.

The name "Vitae Elixxir" seems to mean "the elixir of life." An elixir is a "supposed drug or essence capable of indefinitely prolonging life," or a "strong extract or tincture." (I am not sure why Schauss's "elixxir" is spelled with two x's.)

Vitae Elixxir is popularly called the "purple drops," because of its characteristic color. In my one conversation with him, in March, 1994, Mr. Schauss was rather mysterious. He claimed to have cured himself of cancer using this mixture, but I could not get details out of him. He is in his late 70s, but he did not reveal anything about his background, what kind of cancer he had, or how he selected the particular herbs that went into his product. This is intriguing since some of them are uncommon in herbal cancer formulas. (See ingredient chart on next page.)

We shall pass over any discussion of chlorophyllin and allicin, which are herb-derived chemicals, not herbs. However, I find this list unusual. Some of the ingredients are familiar in traditional cancer formulas: bloodroot, goldenseal and garlic in particular. Others are plausible entries, such as St. John's Wort.

Vitae Elixxir Ingredients

Scientific Name	Common Name	AHPA
Chlorophyllin	(plant component)	—
Sanguinaria canadensis	Bloodroot	2b, 2d
Impatiens pallida	Jewelweed	—
Hydrastis canadensis	Goldenseal	2b
Ferula galbaniflua	Galbanum	2b, 2d+
Hypericum perforatum	St. John's wort	2d
Rubus villosus	American blackberry	1
Fumaria officinalis	Fumitory	—
Frasera carolinensis	American columbo	—
Allicin	(ingredient in garlic)	—
Allium sativum	Garlic	2c

Trace Elements: Zinc, Potassium, Barium, Iron, Sodium, Calcium, Copper.

+This is the rating for Ferula asafetida and related species. F. galbaniflua per se is not rated, nor is it mentioned in Brinker.

Note: This list of plants should only be used under a physician's direction. Please see the warning in the front of the book.

But others are rare. *Ferula galbaniflua* is gum resin from Persia or the Cape of Good Hope. This stimulant, expectorant and anti-spasmodic has the "smell and consistency of Venice turpentine," says Mrs. Grieve. A related plant is used in Beirut as an aphrodisiac. How did this get into an anticancer formula from Wyoming?

The presence of American blackberry may help account for the characteristic purple color of the drops. Blackberry has been used as an astringent (because of the presence of tannic acid). But other than that, it is unknown to cancer medicine. Fumitory is a "weak tonic" which is "slightly diaphoretic, diuretic and aperient" (153). The root of *Frasera carolinensis,* also called American Columbo or Green Gentian, has been used as a tonic, cathartic, emetic, and stimulant. It also is unknown in cancer medicine.

Nor is this formula without potential side effects. According to CancerGuide Webmaster Steve Dunn (and many other patients), "it tastes just horrible!" A purple-colored "information sheet" I received from Mr. Schauss calls Vitae Elixxir "a nutritional adjunct, compatible with other programs you may be following." He suggests that "in those with particularly sensitive stomachs, drink lots of liquids, or eat food, or slowly drink milk and/or other liquids with extract in it over a period of several hours or more. Antacids with calcium carbonate and/or acidophilus may also be taken." He then adds, "if extreme discomfort is felt, discontinue or reduce usage."

I have frequently heard reports of patients becoming intensely nauseated or even vomiting after taking this preparation, especially in the form of a foot bath which contains dimethyl sulfoxide, or DMSO, a carrier molecule.

This nausea may be due to the presence of bloodroot, whose internal consumption is controversial. It is known that powerful emesis (vomiting) may be caused by as little as one gram of this herb (308). The presence of the toxic alkaloid sanguinarine in bloodroot suggests that this plant should never be used in large amounts. The concentration of bloodroot or the other herbs in this formula is not public knowledge.

Canadian regulations do not allow bloodroot in foods and Australian authorities have proposed labeling that will state "May affect glaucoma treatment. Do not exceed the stated dose." Bloodroot is also contraindicated in pregnancy, which is not mentioned in the materials sent to me.

Steve Dunn also reports on a patient taking Vitae Elixxir for AIDS "who developed severe liver toxicity with jaundice and elevations of liver enzymes to ten times the normal levels. This is potentially lethal!" Dunn cautions. "These problems improved when she stopped the Vitae Elixxir, and worsened when she started it again. In addition, she had been worked up for other causes of liver failure. It seems conclusive that these problems were due to the Vitae Elixxir. It is not known whether this patient was taking the low oral dose or the high dose foot soak, but I would recommend special caution with the high dose method. In addition," he adds, "I think that anyone taking this medication should monitor their liver function. This can be done with a simple blood test" (CancerGuide.org).

Vitae Elixxir also contains an unspecified amount of minerals. Schauss claims that it is "desirable" for patients to take various food supplements, one of which is "iron supplements with copper (if you do not eat meat)." Yet most experts believe that iron is contraindicated for cancer patients except in cases of frank anemia. In fact, scientists at Sloan-Kettering Institute and elsewhere have published over a dozen papers linking excess iron to lowered immunity and to cancer.

"Iron impairs several T-cell functions" they have written, impairing immunity. Other studies have shown a link between iron overload and a cancers of the esophagus, bladder, lung, pancreas, etc. (299, 369, 370).

The Vitae Elixxir mixture, Mr. Schauss said, has been in existence for over 20 years. When I spoke to him, he claimed to have sold or given it away to over 10,000 people. I am sure many more have taken it since then. However, I am unaware of any laboratory or clinical studies on the safety or efficacy of this treatment in cancer or any of the other conditions for which it is commonly used.

Generally speaking, Mr. Schauss claims that there is no contraindication with radiation or chemotherapy or other prescription drugs. But hydrogen peroxide and aloe vera are both said to decrease the effectiveness of the mixture.

There are two ways suggested for taking the drops.

Oral administration: the allegedly maximum dose is six drops taken three times per day as drops mixed with food and drink. One starts with just three drops per day and builds up to 12 drops per day over a period of two weeks.

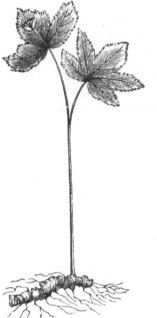

One can increase the dose to 18 drops per day if it is well tolerated. This regimen is recommended for nine months or until the cancer is completely gone. Then one is supposed to continue for one to two years. As mentioned, there is also a foot soak consisting of the purple drops and DMSO.

The drops are prescribed by a number of physicians, such as Michael Schachter, MD, of Suffern, New York. However, he states that "his own experience is still too limited for him to make any compelling statements about the efficacy...." (107).

Mr. Schauss does not advertise and knowledge of the "purple drops" spreads by word of mouth, which can be a powerful marketing tool. Mr. Schauss routinely gives out names and phone numbers of previous customers, which bespeaks confidence in his own product.

Hydrastis canadensis (goldenseal)

Steve Dunn has posted a typical case at his CancerGuide Website. "Mr. G. had kidney cancer. A few months after his kidney was removed, a routine chest X ray showed a two centimeter nodule in one lung, presumed to be metastatic cancer. Mr. G. began taking Vitae Elixxir, and the next chest X ray, a month or so later, showed that the nodule had completely disappeared. Mr. G. remained well for the better part of a year but then relapsed in his bones. He switched to the 'foot soak' which had no effect, and he died about eight months after his relapse."

Dunn, himself a recovered kidney cancer patient, states, "Kidney cancer very rarely does go away by itself (spontaneous remission), and it is possible that this rather than Vitae Elixxir was responsible for the disappearance of Mr. G's lung nodule. I still find this case interesting. Mr. G. did tell me that the foot soak left a bad taste in his mouth and made him a bit nauseous." Mr. G. also called some of the references that Mr. Schauss had given him and while some were unconvincing or ludicrous, others impressed him.

My recommendation would be that cancer patients should avoid Vitae Elixxir purple drops at the present time. I have no confidence in the composition, purity, or consistency of this product, nor do I think clinical testing has been done or is likely to be done. I am also concerned about repeated reports of toxicity and side effects.

The therapeutic claims seem exaggerated. While Mr. Schauss is willing to give potential customers the names and phone numbers of past clients, and some speak highly of the product, most such reports are inconsistent or notoriously difficult to verify. Only scientific tests, retrospective and prospective, could establish the worth of this mixture. Yet Mr. Schauss has expressed an intense dislike for the government and I doubt that an evaluation will take place any time soon.

❦ Conclusions

THE QUALITY OF THE DATA PRESENTED ON BEHALF OF HERBAL CAN-
CER TREATMENTS VARIES CONSIDERABLY. SOME OF THE TREATMENTS
in this book have been shown to significantly benefit cancer
patients. Many represent exciting departures in cancer research and have
provided a good foundation for future work. Others are enticing because
of their long folk history and anecdotal reports. Some others are lacking a
scientific rationale, while a small number come close to classic quackery.

Overall, I consider herbs a useful adjunct to cancer therapy and an exciting area for future research. I would like to make some summary remarks
to three groups who might be reading this book: patients and their loved
ones, oncologists, and botanical researchers.

Patients:

Making a treatment plan for cancer depends on carefully weighing many
factors. Conventional treatments are indispensible in many cases. Most non-
conventional approaches, such as herbs, are helpful adjuncts at the present
time. Many patients find that herbs are beneficial, cause no harm, and generate a feeling of greater hopefulness. But obviously the decisions will
depend on one's own circumstances and state of mind.

Herbs can be used in conjunction with other non-conventional treatment
as well. I discuss 102 such approaches in my book, *Cancer Therapy*. I also
believe that many foods promote well-being and exert a positive effect on

the body's ability to fight cancer. The National Cancer Institute has called on all citizens to consume five portions of fruits and vegetables per day. Especially important are soy, garlic and onions, shiitake mushrooms, broccoli, clover and mung sprouts, and carrot juice.

Most of the herbal treatments deserve serious consideration. However, as a general guideline, I would especially scrutinize those that are heavily hyped, sold through multi-level-marketing or network programs, make too-good-to-be-true claims, or originate from offshore companies operating out of post office boxes in the Third World.

As to price, there is a scale that ranges from virtually free (most of us know where to find unsprayed dandelions or red clover tops) to extremely expensive. Some herbal products are as expensive as standard cancer care.

In any case, be sure to thoroughly research any treatment before you begin. The Internet is an excellent resource, although one must be wary of aggressively promotional or irresponsible sites. In addition to the sites of the conventional agencies, you might also consult Steve Dunn's CancerGuide or my own site, www.ralphmoss.com, which has many useful links.

Physicians

I wish that every cancer patient could be treated by a knowledgeable, sympathetic, and open-minded physician. I think most patients want this as well. Surveys show that a growing number of your patients are using herbal or other complementary treatments. In less than a decade, that number has leaped from 9 percent to between 38 and 60 percent of all cancer patients. The more educated and affluent the patients, the more likely they are to use such adjuvant treatments. We also know that about 70 percent of patients using CAM do not inform their doctors. While that is regrettable, it is not enough that we urge patients to reveal their secrets. We must understand why patients feel the need to hide such usage from their physicians.

I believe that most patients are afraid of being insulted or rejected for sharing this information. Patients need their oncologists to be sensitive and tolerant towards their use of CAM. After all, most herbal treatments are grounded in long historical use, and many have considerable scientific value as well. These methods certainly deserve a fair hearing.

There has been a tendency to dismiss such treatments out-of-hand as "anecdotal" and "unproven." But remember that many practices in oncology are also not grounded in evidence-based medicine. Unfortunately, most patients do not have the luxury of waiting for the completion of conclusive tests on herbs (which may be decades away). They have to make decisions right away.

Oncologists have a responsibility to at least learn about the treatments that are popular with their patients, so that they can discuss them intelligently and help patients make treatment decisions.

I believe in the utility of surgery as well as other conventional treatments that extend survival and improve quality of life. However, I also believe that when used responsibly, many herbs are harmless adjuncts, and others seem to do some notable physiological and psychological good.

I know that many oncologists are also concerned about potential ripoffs. No one wants to add extra costs to their patients' already onerous financial burdens. Indeed, there is reason to be wary of treatments costing thousands of dollars. However, we must realize that some preparations are costly because of the expenses of manufacturing pure and effective remedies or of gaining FDA approval. In general, herbs are remarkably inexpensive, as medical interventions go.

The times in which herbs could benefit your patients include:

(a) during surgery, to bolster the immune system and possibly decrease the possibility of metastatic spread;

(b) during chemotherapy and radiation therapy, to decrease side effects and possibly increase effectiveness;

(c) after definitive conventional treatments, to diminish the possibility of recurrence (secondary prevention); and

(d) after the recurrence of cancer or the failure of all conventional approaches.

I urge you to guide your patients to those herbs that are safe, efficacious, and economical, and to monitor for benefit or adverse events. With the help of this and other educational materials, you can help guide them in the direction of helpful adjuvant treatments.

Researchers:

I think that botanicals and herb-derived products represent one of the most promising avenues for future cancer research. It is well known that many of the most important chemotherapeutic agents emerged from plants and even from the folk tradition. In fact, chemotherapy as we know it today would be inconceivable without the contribution of products of natural origin, such as Vincristine, Vinblastine, Taxol, and Camptothecin.

Some of these were already in use as folk remedies for cancer. Take the case of mayapple, which was widely used by Penobscot medicine men, folk healers, and Eclectic practitioners. Formulas containing mayapple were summarily dismissed as "vegetable soup" by the American Medical Association. But half a century later, this same traditional usage was vindicated, and two important new drugs, Etoposide and Teniposide, emerged into oncologic practice. You have to wonder what other excellent drugs remain hidden in Western herbs, such as the ones discussed in this book.

Many herbs were examined and rejected in the past. But we must remember that there are new ways of evaluating botanical agents, which can more accurately predict whether or not they would benefit patients. Scientists have only begun to investigate apoptotic or various host-mediated effects of botanical agents.

Dozens of herbs can modulate the immune system, inhibit angiogenesis, or exert other positive effects. Some of this work has already begun, especially in Europe or Asia, but remains unknown to most American scientists.

Herbs represent a repository of new research ideas, in a field where new ideas are sometimes lacking. By combining traditional herbal lore with the latest scientific methods, researchers can help create a new era of integrative oncology.

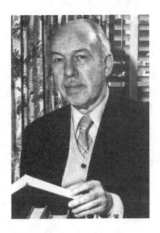

❧ Afterword on Jonathan L. Hartwell

THIS BOOK IS DEDICATED TO TWO OUTSTANDING SCIENTISTS, JAMES A. DUKE, PHD, AND JONATHAN L. HARTWELL, PHD. FOR most readers, Dr. Duke needs no introduction. He is among America's leading herbalists, and is the author of many outstanding works, including the 1997 best-selling book, *The Green Pharmacy*.

By contrast, Jonathan Hartwell will be unknown to all but a few specialists in the field. I would therefore like to summarize his achievements and pay homage to an exemplary career in botanical science.

For many years, Dr. Hartwell was the person at the National Cancer Institute (NCI) who was in charge of the Institute's investigations of natural products.

A native of Boston, he studied chemistry at Harvard University, where he received his bachelor's, master's and doctoral degrees. After working as a research chemist in private industry, he joined NCI in 1938. This was shortly after NCI was established by Congress, but before it moved to its present campus in Bethesda, Maryland. He could therefore be considered one of the founders of the NCI, along with biochemist Dean Burk, PhD, and a few others.

Hartwell pursued two main lines of research. In the first part of his career he concentrated on the discovery of carcinogens in plants and other compounds. In 1941, NCI published his multi-volume work, *Survey of Compounds Which Have Been Tested for Carcinogenic Activity*. This was initially a study of 696 compounds, of which 169 were found to be active. This was expanded in 1951, with a report on 322 carcinogenic compounds. Supplements to this were prepared in 1957 and 1969 with Dr. Philippe Shubik, director of the Eppley Institute at the University of Nebraska, Omaha. The 1971 edition contained 1,667 pages. These books are considered landmarks in the study of chemical carcinogenesis.

In the late 1940s, Dr. Hartwell moved to the Laboratory of Chemical Pharmacology, which was then part of NCI's Drug Research and Development Program. In 1954, he became one of the four assistant chiefs of NCI's new Cancer Chemotherapy National Service Center.

Among other things, Hartwell was in charge of NCI's research communications. He and his staff summarized scientific articles on compounds that were able to destroy cancer cells. This activity gave him an international perspective and brought him into contact with researchers from around the world. The results of his investigations were reported in bimonthly issues of *Chemotherapy Abstracts*. In addition, Dr. Hartwell was founder of the journal, *Cancer Chemotherapy Reports,* which enabled NCI to rapidly communicate its latest research findings to other scientists.

In the next decade, Hartwell became head of the natural products section of the NCI's drug development branch. In this capacity, he began his monumental study of extracts and compounds of natural origin that could be used in chemotherapy. Botanists in his department ranged as far as Kenya and Tanzania in search of plants that might contain anticancer agents. In fact, many of the chemotherapeutic agents of natural origin used today came out of Hartwell's department.

Elsewhere in this book we tell the story of how Dr. Hartwell was instrumental in the development of the drug camptothecin. But he was also fairminded towards non-conventional approaches, such as Cat's Claw tea.

Although he was an organic chemist by training, Dr. Hartwell had humanistic interests that enriched his scientific perspective. He was an avid naturalist with an intense interest in folk medicine. He was especially intrigued when he learned that an herb called mayapple (Podophyllum peltatum) was used by the Penobscot Indians of Maine to treat cancer. In fact, this mayapple cancer treatment was already published in an 1849 medical book as a cancer treatment, and it was also an established part of the Eclectic medical tradition in cancer syrups and formulas. Dr. Hartwell found that the chemical podophyllotoxin, as well as two related compounds, were highly effective in killing sarcoma 37 (see Chapter 10).

"It thus became apparent," he later wrote, "that both the technical literature and the folklore could be sources of information on the use of plants for the treatment of cancer and other growths."

Together with colleagues such as James Duke at the US Department of Agriculture, Hartwell began a survey of plants that had been used around the world to fight cancer. Although some might see this as a mere catalog of thousands of items, it is clear that it was a work of enormous ingenuity, energy, and intelligence, a monumental work of scholarship in the cancer field. Hartwell identified and classified over three thousand plants reputed to be useful against cancer. These citations were derived from (and carefully correlated with) more than 1,000 references on the topic.

Where did Hartwell get his information? He surveyed thousands of old medical texts and histories in many languages to come up with his final selection. His study ranged from the beginnings of written civilization, in Egypt and China to modern scientific articles.

"The history of the herbal treatment of cancer," he later wrote, with no exaggeration, can be identified with "the history of medicine, indeed of civilization." This is a bold claim, but one that is borne out by his research.

As an established government researcher, he had access to some obscure sources as well. For example, he learned that in 1926, the American Cancer Society (ACS) had offered a prize for anyone who could produce a valid method of preventing or curing cancer. They received many entries, 76 of which described putative herbal cures. Although the prize was never awarded, the ACS kept those letters in a dusty bin until the day that Hartwell requested them for his compilation of folk remedies.

Similarly, the NCI itself received scores of letters on reputed cures. Those from the 1950s to the 1970s found their way into Hartwell's compilation, a silent tribute to the many individuals over the years who have attempted to contribute their own ideas to the war on cancer. In addition, the library at his alma mater, Harvard, had compiled a list of medical treatments that were mentioned in its extensive collection of old herbals. From these, Hartwell retrieved 16 more historic cancer remedies. As word of his project spread, correspondents volunteered accounts of many shamanic and folk treatments. Hartwell published his findings in 11 installments between 1967 and 1971 in the scientific journal, *Lloydia*.

Dr. Hartwell retired from the NCI in 1975. His herbal compendium appeared in book form in 1982, under the title *Plants Used Against Cancer,* with a foreword by his friend and coworker, Jim Duke. There was an illustration of the mayapple on the front and a stern warning about toxicity on the back cover. *Plants Used Against Cancer* is now sadly out of print.

In the same year that the book appeared, NCI abruptly canceled its natural products development program. Their focus changed to synthetic chemotherapy and later to the genetic understanding of the disease.

Dr. Hartwell died of pneumonia in Bethesda, Maryland, on March 22, 1991, at the age of eighty-five. Although some new plants could now be added to Hartwell's list, any serious examination of herbs against cancer must begin with his outstanding work.

❧ References

NOTE: Items of exceptional interest are marked with an asterisk and annotated.

1. Abo, KA. Screening extracts of *Euphorbia garuana* N.E.Br. for *in vitro* cytotoxicity. *Afr J Med Sci.* 1988;17:227-230.

2. Adams, J. *Medicinal Plants and their Cultivation in Canada.* Ottawa: Government Printing Bureau, 1915.

★3. *Alternative Medicine: Expanding Medical Horizons.* A Report to the National Institutes of Health on Alternative Medical Systems and Practices in the United States. Washington, DC: US Government Printing Office, NIH Publication No. 94-066, December, 1994. Landmark study for the OAM.

4. Altman, Roberta and Sarg, Michael J, MD. *The Cancer Dictionary.* New York: Facts on File, 1992.

5. American Cancer Society, *Cancer Facts and Figures–1998.* Atlanta: American Cancer Society, 1998.

6. American Herbal Products Association, *Botanical Safety Handbook.* Orlando, FL: CRC Press, 1997.

6a. Anderson, T, et al. Medieval example of metastatic carcinoma: a dry bone, radiological, and SEM study. *Am J Phys Anthropol.* 1992;89:309.

7. Anon. Flor·Essence update. *Health Action* 1992/1993:7.

7a. Anon. Cat's claw. *Townsend Letter for Doctors & Patients.* May, 1994.

8. Anon. HANSI: Argentina's Medical Miracle. *Townsend Letter for Doctors & Patients.* October, 1995.

9. Anon. Homoeopathic herbs for cancer and fatigue: Argentina's HANSI gets remissions. *Alternative Medicine Digest.* 1996;15:63.

10. Anon. Hoxsey Method/Bio-Medical Center. *CA: a Cancer Journal for Clinicians.* 1990;40:51-55.

11. Anon. Information about Anvirzel as a therapeutic product. Statement of Ozelle Pharmaceuticals, Inc., San Antonio, TX, n.d.

12. Anon. Jonathan Hartwell retires but continues writing, anticancer drug work. *The NIH Record.* June 17, 1975.

13. Anon. Jonathan L. Hartwell, NIH Research Chemist [obituary], *Washington Post.* March 23, 1991.

14. Anon. The Healing World of HANSI, Sarasota, FL: Hansi International, Ltd., n.d.

15. Anon. Unproven methods of cancer management: Iscador. *CA: a Cancer Journal for Clinicians.* 1983;33:186-188.

16. Aoki, T. Lentinan. In: *Immune Modulation Agents and Their Mechanisms.* Fenichel, RL and Chirges, MA, eds. *Immunology Studies.* 1984:25:62-77.

17. Appendino, G and Szallasi, A. *Euphorbium:* modern research on its active principle, resiniferatoxin, revives an ancient medicine. *Life Sci.* 1997;60:681.

18. Aquino, R. New polyhydroxylated triterpenes from *Uncaria tomentosa. J Nat Prod.* 1990;53:559.

19. Aquino, R. Plant metabolites. Structure and *in vitro* antiviral activity of quinovic acid glycosides from *Uncaria tomentosa* and *Guettarda platypoda. J Nat Prod.* 1989;52:679.

20. Aquino, R., et al. Plant metabolites. New compounds and anti-inflammatory activity of *Uncaria tomentosa*. *J Nat Prod*. 1991;54:453.

21. Armstrong, David and Armstrong, Elizabeth Metzger. *The Great American Medicine Show*. New York: Prentice Hall. 1991.

22. Arnoudon, A. *Compt. Rend*. 1857;41:1152.

23. Arosa FA, et al. Iron differentially modulates the CD4-lck and CD8-lck complexes in resting peripheral blood T-lymphocytes. *Cell Immunol*. 1995;161:138-142.

24. Austin, S, et. al. Long term follow-up of cancer patients using Contreras, Hoxsey and Gerson therapies. *Journal of Naturopathic Medicine*. 1994;5:74-76.

★25. Ausubel, Kenny and Salveson, Catherine. Hoxsey: *How Healing Becomes a Crime*. 87 minute documentary film. New York: Wellspring Media. 1987. Excellent historical footage on Hoxsey.

26. Awang, DV, et al. Atropine as possible contaminant of comfrey tea. *Lancet*. 1989;2(8653):44.

27. Awang, DV. *Canadian Pharmaceutical Journal* 1988;5:323.

28. Bachelor, J. *The Ainu and their Folklore*. London, 1911.

29. Bader, John P., Chief of Antiviral Evaluations Branch, NCI. Letter to Dr. David Dobbie, June 5, 1993.

30. Bailey, Liberty Hyde, et al. *Hortus Third: A Concise Dictionary of Plants Cultivated in the United States and Canada*. New York: Macmillan Publishing Co. 1976.

31. Baron, Roger. *Bull. de la Soc. Geograph. de Paris*. 1827:8:357.

32. Baron, Samuel [ed.], *Medical Microbiology*, The University of Texas Medical Branch: Galveston, 1995.

33. Barry, Rick. AIDS treatment under investigation: A Florida company markets the produce made in the Bahamas. Tampa (FL.) *Tribune*, Feb. 1, 1995.

34. Beckstrom-Sternberg, Stephen M., and Duke, James A. The Phytochemical Database: http://probe.nalusda.gov:8300/cgi-bin/browse/phytochemdb. (ACEDB version 4.3 - data version July 1994).

35. Belkin, M and Fitzgerald, D. Tumor damaging capacity of plant materials. 1. Plants used as cathartics. *J Natl Cancer Inst*. 1952;13:139-155.

36. Bentley, R and Trimen H. *Medicinal Plants*. London: J&A Churchill. 1880.

37. Beuth, J, et al. Thymocyte proliferation and maturation in response to galactoside-specific mistletoe lectin-1. *In vivo* 1993;7:407-410.

38. Beuth, J, et al.: Einfluß von wäßrigen, auf Mistellektin-1 standardisierten Mistelextrakten auf die *in vitro* (Tumor) Zellproliferation. *Dtsch Zschr Onkol*. 1994;26:1-6.

39. Beuth, J. and Moss, RW. Immunotherapy with mistletoe lectin-1: A scientific approach in complementary oncology. *Zeitschrift für Onkologie/Journal of Oncology*. 1998.

40. Beuth, J. Immunoprotective activity of the galactoside-specific mistletoe lectin in cortisone treated BALB/c-mice. *In vivo* 1994;8:989-992.

41. Beuth, J. Influence of treatment with the immunomodulatory effective dose of the ß-galactoside-specific lectin from mistletoe on tumor colonization in BALB/c-mice for two experimental models. *In vivo*. 1991;5:29-32.

42. Biddle, *Am. Jour. Phar*. 1879:544.

43. Binutu, OA, et al. Antibacterial and antifungal compounds from *Kigelia pinnata*. *Planta Med* 1996;62:352-353.

44. Bissett, NG. Arrow poisons and their role in the development of medicinal agents. In: Schultes, RE and von Reis, Siri (eds.) *Ethnobotany: Evolution of a Discipline*. Portland, OR: Dioscorides Press, 1995.

45. Bjornson, Thorleit. *An old Icelandic medical miscellany*. Oslo, J. Dybwad. Translated and edited by Henning Larsen. Cited in Erichsen-Brown, op. cit..

46. Boericke, W. *Pocket Manual of Homoeopathic Materia Medica and Repertory*. New Delhi, India: Jain, 1994 [1927].

★47. Boik, John, *Cancer and Natural Medicine. A Textbook of Basic Science and Clinical Research*. Princeton, MN: Oregon Medical Press. 1995. Contains many excellent leads and thoughts on this topic. Boik has a particularly good grasp of Traditional Chinese Medicine (TCM) and understands the possible mechanisms through which herbs could exert an anticancer effect. Impressive bibliography. Highly recommended for professionals.

48. Boik, John. Developing a Rational Approach to Complementary Anticancer Therapy. Unpublished article. 1996 [cited in Lerner, et al. 1998].

49. Boisio ML, et al. [Separation and identifying features of the cardiac aglycones and glycosides of *Nerium oleander* L. flowers by thin-layer chromatography]. *Minerva Med*. 1993;84:627.

50. Bott, Victor. *Spiritual Science and the Art of Healing*. Rudolf Steiner's Anthroposophical Medicine. Rochester, VT: Healing Arts Press. 1996 [1984].

51. Brandt, Johanna. *The Grape Cure*. New York: Beneficial Books. 1970 [1928]

52. Brinker, Francis. *Herb Contraindications and Drug Interactions*. Sandy, OR: Eclectic Institute, Inc., 1997.

53. Brinker, Francis. The Hoxsey treatment: cancer quackery or effective physiological adjuvant? *Journal of Naturopathic Medicine*. 1995;6:9-23.

54. Brodersen, H. Mitosegifte und ionisierende Strahlung. *Strahlenther*. 1943;73:196-254.

55. Brown, W.O. Effect of colchicine on human tissues. *Arch Path*. 1940;29:865-866.

56. Brzosko, W, et al. Anti-cancer Studying Group, Warsaw. 20th *International Congress of Chemotherapy*, Sydney, Australia, June, 1997.

57. Buchan, William, *Domestic Medicine, or the Family Physician; Wherein the Prevention and Cure of Diseases, by Regimens and Simple Medicines, are Clearly Laid Down and Considered*. Derby: Thomas Richardson. 1843.

58. Buckman, Notes and Queries, I, iii. 1851.

59. Budge, EA Wallis. *The Divine Origin of the Craft of the Herbalist*. New York: Dover. 1996 [1928].

60. Butler, Francelia. *Cancer Through the Ages*. Fairfax, VA: 1955.

61. Calvin, M. Hydrocarbons from plants: Analytical methods and observations. *Naturwissenschaften* 1980;67:525-533.

62. Canfield, PJ and Hartley WJ. A survey and review of hepatobiliary lesions in Australian macropods. *J Comp Pathol*. 1992;107:147.

63. Carnot, P and Lereboullet, P. *Nouveau Traité de Médecine et de Thérapeutique*. Paris: Librairie J.B. Baillière et Fils. 1927.

64. Cassaday, John M and Douros, John D. [Eds]. *Anticancer Agents Based on Natural Product Models*. New York: Academic Press. 1980.

65. Chabner, BA. Anti-cancer drugs. In: DeVita, VT, et al. [Eds.] *Cancer. 4th Ed.*, 1993:325-417.

66. Cham BE, et al. Solasodine glycosides. Selective cytotoxicity for cancer cells and inhibition of cytotoxicity by rhamnose in mice with sarcoma 180. *Cancer Lett*. 1990; 55: 221-225.

67. Cham BE, et al. Topical treatment of malignant and premalignant skin lesions by very low concentrations of a standard mixture (BEC) of solasodine glycosides. *Cancer Lett*. 1991; 59: 183-192.

68. Cham BE. A semiautomated method for the estimation of ionic calcium activity and concentration in biological solutions. *Clin Chim Acta*. 1972; 37: 5-14.

69. Cham, BE, et al. Antitumour effects of glycoalkaloids isolated from *Solanum sodomaeum*. *Planta Med*. 1987 Feb; 53(1): 34-36.

70. Cham, BE, et al. Glycoalkaloids from *Solanum sodomaeum* are effective in the treatment of skin cancers in man. *Cancer Lett*. 1987;36:111-118.

71. Chambard, R. Revue d'ethnogr. et des traditions populaires. 1926;7:122.

72. Chamberlain AT, et al. Osteochondroma in a British neolithic skeleton. *Br J Hosp Med*. 1992;47:51.

73. Chamberlain, J. *Fighting Cancer: A Survival Guide*. London: Headline. 1997.

74. Chandrasekaran B, et al. New methods for urinary estimation of antitumour compounds echitamine & plumbagin. *Indian J Biochem Biophys*. 1982;19:148-9.

75. Chang, M. *Anticancer Medicinal Herbs*. Hunan. 1992.

76. Chatterjee D, Wyche JH, Pantazis P. Induction of apoptosis in malignant and camptothecin-resistant human cells. *Ann N Y Acad Sci*. 1996;803:143-156.

77. Chihara, G. et al. Inhibition of mouse sarcoma 180 by polysaccharides from *Lentinus edodes* (Berk.) *Sing. Nature.* 1969;222:637-688.

78. Chlebowski, RT, et al. Vitamin K in the treatment of cancer. *Cancer Treat Rev.* 1985;12:49-63.

79. Clark HR, Strickholm A. Evidence for a conformational change in nerve membrane with depolarization. *Nature.* 1971;234:470.

80. Clark, Hulda R. *A Cure for All Cancers.* San Diego, CA: ProMotion Publishing. 1993. There is also an audio tape from Ten Speed Press, narrated by Kitt Weagant.

81. Clark, Hulda R. *A Cure for All Diseases.* San Diego, CA: ProMotion Publishing. 1995.

82. Clark, Hulda R. *A Cure for HIV/AIDS.* San Diego, CA: ProMotion Publishing. 1994.

83. Cohnheim, Julius. *Lectures on General Pathology.* London: New Sydenham Society. 1889.

84. Comac, Linda and Holt, Stephen S. *Miracle Herbs: How Herbs Combine With Modern Medicine to Treat Cancer, Heart Disease, AIDS and More.* Secaucus, NJ: Birch Lane. 1998.

85. Cooke, R. Notes and Queries. I, vii. 1853.

86. Coulter, Harris. *Divided Legacy: The Conflict Between Homoeopathy and the American Medical Association: Science and Ethics in American Medicine 1800-1910, vol. 3.* Berkeley, CA: North Atlantic Books. 1988.

87. Crellin John K. Anton Storck (1731-1803) and British therapeutics. *Clio Med.* 1974;9:103-108.

★88. Crellin, John K and Philpott, Jane. *A Reference Guide to Medicinal Plants: Herbal Medicine Past and Present.* Durham, NC: Duke University Press. 1990. An excellent resource on both folk practices and their scholarly corroboration.

89. Crellin, John K and Philpott, Jane. *Trying to Give Ease: Tommie Bass and the Story of Herbal Medicine.* Raleigh-Durham: Duke University Press. 1989.

90. Culpeper, Nicholas, *The Complete Herbal.* Ware: Wordsworth. 1995.

91. Cunningham, David. A phase III multi-center randomized study of CPT-11 versus supportive care alone in patients with 5-FU-resistant metastatic colorectal cancer. *ASCO Thirty-fourth annual meeting.* Los Angeles, CA, May 16-19, 1998.

92. Daems, Willem F. Ita Wegman, Zürcher Zeit 1906-1920, Basel: *Verlag am Goetheanum.* n.d.

93. Danilos, J, et al. Preliminary studies on the effect of Ukrain on the immunological response in patients with malignant tumors. *Drugs Exp Clin Res.* 1992;18S:55-62.

94. Danysz, A, et al. Clinical studies of Ukrain on healthy volunteers (phase 1). *Drug Exp Clin Res.* 1992;18S:39-43.

95. Daunter B, et al. Solasodine glycosides. *In vitro* preferential cytotoxicity for human cancer cells. *Cancer Lett.*1990;55:209-220.

96. David, Thomas. *Miracle Medicines of the Rainforest: A Doctor's Revolutionary Work with Cancer and AIDS Patients.* Rochester, VT: Healing Arts Press, 1997.

97. Davies, ML and Davies, TA. Hemlock: murder before the Lord. *Med Sci Law.* 1994;34:331-333.

98. Davis, E. Wade. Ethnobotany: An old practice, a new discipline. In: Schultes, RE and von Reis, Siri (eds.) *Ethnobotany: Evolution of a Discipline.* Portland, OR: Dioscorides Press. 1995.

99. Davis, Robert. *Aloe Vera: A Scientific Approach.* New York: Vantage Press. 1997.

100. Debus, Allen G. Science and History: The Birth of a New Field. In: McKnight, Stephen A. [Ed.] *Science, Pseudo-Science, and Utopianism in Early Modern Thought.* Columbia: University of Missouri Press. 1992.

101. Denissenko, P. Traitement de la carcinose par l'usage interne et les applications locales d'extrait de chélidoine. *Semaine Méd.* 1896.

102. Densmore, Frances. Forty-fourth Annual Report of the Bureau of American Ethnology to the Secretary of the Smithsonian Institution, Washington, DC: Government Printing Office, 1928.

103. Dermer, Gerald. *The Immortal Cell: Why Cancer Research Fails.* Garden City Park, NY: Avery Publishing Group, Inc. 1994.

★104. DeVita, Vincent, et al. [Eds.] *Cancer: Principles & Practice of Oncology.* Philadelphia: Lippincott-Raven, 5th Ed. 1997. The bestselling and most influential orthodox textbook on cancer.

105. DeVita, Vincent, et al. [Eds.]. *Cancer: Principles & Practice of Oncology.* Philadelphia: Lippincott, 4th

Ed. 1995.

106. Dhar, ML, et al. Screening of Indian plants for biological activity. Part 1. *Indian J Exp Biol.* 1968;6:232-247.

107. Diamond, W. John, et al. *An Alternative Medicine Definitive Guide to Cancer.* Tiburon, CA: Future Medicine Publishing, Inc., 1997.

108. Dinnen RD and Ebisuzaki K. The search for novel anticancer agents: a differentiation-based assay and analysis of a folklore product. *Anticancer Res.* 1997;17:1027-1033.

109. Dodson, Marcia. Coming into their own. *Los Angeles Times,* Dec. 22, 1997.

110. Dombradi C and Foldeak S. Screening report on the antitumor activity of purified *Arctium lappa* extracts. *Tumori.* 1966;52:173.

111. Dossey, Larry. The right man syndrome: skepticism and alternative medicine. *Alternative Therapies in Health and Medicine.* 1998;4:12.

112. Doughty, Barbara L. Schistosomes and other trematodes. In: Baron, Samuel [Ed.], *Medical Microbiology.* The University of Texas Medical Branch: Galveston, 1995.

★113. Duke, James A. *CRC Handbook of Medicinal Herbs.* Boca Raton: CRC Press. 1985. A classic. Out of the 365 herbs in this book nearly 100 are discussed (at least briefly) for their connection to cancer therapy. As always, "Father Nature Farmacy" is filled with fascinating tidbits, scholarly, amusing and wise.

113a. Duke, James A. The synthetic bullet vs. the herbal shotgun shell. *HerbalGram.* 1988-89.

113b. Duke, James A. and Ayensu, Edward S. *Medicinal Plants of China.* Algonac, MI: Reference Publications, Inc. 1985.

★114. Duke, James A. *The Green Pharmacy.* Emmaus, PA: Rodale, 1997. Entertaining and enlightening work for the general public.

115. Dustin, A.P. Nouvelles applications des poisons caryoclassiques à la cancerologie. *Sang.* 1938;12:677-697.

116. Early R. *Hoxsey therapy.* Unpublished manuscript, 1994. [Cited at University of Texas Website.]

117. Easty DJ, et al. Novel and known protein tyrosine kinases and their abnormal expression in human melanoma. *J Invest Dermatol.* 1993;101:679.

118. Effron, M., et al. Nature and rate of neoplasia found in captive wild mammals, birds, and reptiles at necropsy. *J Natl Cancer Inst.* 1977;59:185.

119. Eigsti, OJ and Dustin, Pierre. *Colchicine–In Agriculture, Medicine, Biology and Chemistry.* Ames, IA: Iowa State College Press. 1955.

120. Einzig, AI, et al. Phase II trial of taxol in patients with metastatic renal cell carcinoma. *Cancer Invest.* 1991;9:133-136.

121. Ellingwood, Finley. *The American Materia Medica, Therapeutics and Pharmacgnosy.* Sandy, OR: Eclectic Medical Publications. 1998 [1919].

★122. Erichsen-Brown, Charlotte. *Medicinal and Other Uses of North American Plants: A Historical Survey with Special Reference to the Eastern Indian Tribes.* New York: Dover. 1989 [1979]. Indispensable for understanding how the appreciation of particular herbs evolved over time. Provides access to many obscure references, especially Canadian ones.

123. Etkin, Nina. *Eating on the Wild Side: The Pharmacologic, Ecologic, and Social Implications of Using Noncultigens.* Tempe: University of Arizona Press. 1994.

124. Evans R, et al. Curaderm. *Med J Aust.* 1989 Mar 20; 150(6): 350-351.

★125. Ewing, James. *Neoplastic Diseases,* 4th Ed. Philadelphia: Saunders. 1942. The outstanding book produced on cancer in America in the first half of the 20th century. Heavy on pathology, light on therapeutics.

126. Fakih, M, et al. Inhibition of prostate cancer growth by estramustine and colchicine. *Prostate.* 1995;26:310.

127. Farr, SB, et al. Toxicity and mutagenicity of plumbagin and the induction of a possible new DNA repair pathway in *Escherichia coli. J Bacteriol.* 1985;164:1309-16.

128. Fatope, MO, et al. Selectively cytotoxic diterpenes from *Euphorbia poisonii*. *J Med Chem*. 1996;39:1005.

129. Fenton, William N. Contacts between Iroquois herbalism and colonial medicine. *Annual Report* of the Board of Regents of the Smithsonian Institution for 1941. Washington, DC: 1942:522.

130. Fields, KK, et al. Maximum tolerated doses of ifosfamide, carboplatin, and etoposide given over 6 days followed by autologous stem-cell rescue: toxicity profile. *J Clin Oncol*. 1995;13:323-332.

131. Fishbein, M. History of cancer quackery. *Perspectives in Biology and Medicine*. 1965;8:140.

132. Fishbein, M. *The New Medical Follies*. New York: Boni and Liveright. 1927.

133. Flint, Vivekan Don and Lerner, Michael. *Herbal Therapies for Cancer:* A Commonweal Working Paper. Research Assistance: Melanie Smith, October, 1997. A chapter scheduled to be added to Michael Lerner's book *Choices in Healing*. Dr. Lerner has posted a draft of this chapter to his Website. It contains detailed discussions of aloe, garlic, mistletoe, laetrile (apricot kernels), Essiac, Hoxsey and ginseng. The discussion is scholarly and pessimistic. Lerner is dubious about most Western herbs sold in the health food market.

134. Foldeak, S and Dombradi G. Tumor-growth inhibiting substances of plant origin. I. Isolation of the active principle of *Arctium lappa*. *Acta Phys Chem*. 1964;10:91-93.

135. Folkard, R. *Plant-lore, Legends and Lyrics*. London, 1884.

136. Fournet, A, et al. Effect of natural naphthoquinones in BALB/c mice infected with *Leishmania amazonensis* and *L. venezuelensis*. *Trop Med Parasit*. 1992;43:219-222.

137. Fratkin, Jake. *Chinese Herbal Patent Formulas: A Practical Guide*. Boulder, CO: Shya Publications. 1986.

138. Frazer, Sir James. *The New Golden Bough*. Edited, and with Notes and Foreword, by Dr. Theodor G. Gaster. New York: New American Library. 1964.

139. Fuller, Robert C. *Alternative Medicine and American Religious Life*. New York: Oxford University Press. 1989.

140. Furstenberger, G and Hecker, E. On the active principles of the Euphorbiaceae, XII. Highly unsaturated irritant diterpene esters from *Euphorbia tirucalli* originating from Madagascar. *J Nat Prod*. 1986;49:386.

141. Gai, L, et al. [Relationship between the rate of parasitic infection and the knowledge of prevention]. Chung Kuo Chi Sheng Chung Hsueh Yu Chi Sheng Chung Ping Tsa Chih 1995;13:269.

142. Galek, H, et al. Oxidative protein modification as predigestive mechanism of the carnivorous plant *Dionaea muscipula*: an hypothesis based on *in vitro* experiments. *Free Radic Biol Med*. 1990;9:427-34.

143. Gathercoal, EN and Wirth, EH, *Pharmacognosy*. 2nd ed., Philadelphia: Lea and Febiger. 1947.

144. Gendron, G. *Enquiries into the Nature, Knowledge and Cure of Cancers*. London: Taylor, 1701.

145. Gentry, Alwyn H. *Flora Neotropica*. Monograph 25 (II). Bignoniaceae—Part II (Tribe Tecomeae). Bronx, NY: New York Botanical Garden. 1992.

146. Glum, Gary. *Calling of an Angel*. Los Angeles: Silent Walker Publishing. 1988. A reverential yet indispensable account of the life of Rene Caisse. For $45, this book promised to "reveal for the first time publicly how to acquire the formula to brew Essiac in your own home" but at the end informed readers they would need to purchase a videotape for an additional $79.95!

147. Goodman-Gilman, Alfred. Goodman and Gilman's *The Pharmacology Basis of Therapeutics*, 6th Ed. New York: Macmillan. 1980.

148. Grazi, Gianfranco. Introducing an unusual plant. *Mercury*. 1997:16:66-70.

149. Greenberg, Z, et al. [Prevalence of intestinal parasites among Thais in Israel]. *Harefuah*. 1994;126:507.

150. Grever, Michael R. and Chabner, Bruce A. Cancer Drug Discovery and Development. In: DeVita, *Cancer*, 5th Ed. 1997.

151. Grevin, G, et al. Metastatic carcinoma of presumed prostatic origin in cremated bones; from the 1st century AD. *Virchows Arch*. 1997;431:211.

152. Gribel, NV and Pashinskii, VG. [Antimetastatic properties of aloe juice.] *Vopr Onkol*. 1986;32:38-40.

★153. Grieve, Mrs. Margaret. *A Modern Herbal. The Medicinal, Culinary, Cosmetic and Economic Properties, Cultivation and Folklore of Herbs, Grasses, Fungi, Shrubs and Trees with All Their Modern Scientific Uses.* Edited and introduced by Mrs. C.F. Leyel. New York: Dorset Press. 1992 [1931, 1973] Unsurpassed as the number one favorite book of American herbalists. A must-own for anyone seriously interested in plants or medicine.

★154. Griggs, Barbara. *Green Pharmacy. The History and Evolution of Western Herbal Medicine.* Rochester, VT: Healing Arts. 1991. History of conflict in England and US between herbalism and orthodox medicine. A groundbreaking exploration of the topic.

155. Grimm, J. Deutsche *Mythologie,* 4th Ed., Berlin, 1875-1878.

156. Grindlay, D and Reynolds, T. The *Aloe vera* phenomenon: a review of the properties and modern uses of the leaf parenchyma gel. *J Ethnopharmacol.* 1986;16:117-151.

157. Gujar, GT. Plumbagin, a naturally occurring naphthoquinone. Its pharmacological and pesticidal activity. *Fitoterapia.* 1990;61:387-394.

158. Gundidza, M and Kufa, A. Skin irritant and tumour promoting extract from the latex of Euphorbia bougheii. *Cent Afr J Med.* 1993;39:56.

159. Guy, Richard. *Practical observations on cancers and disorders of the breast, explaining their different appearances and events, to which are added one hundred cases, successfully treated without cutting.* London, 1762.

160. Hacker, MP, et al. Toxicologic studies of homoharringtonine in humans and rats. *Proc AACR.* 1983;24:325.

161. Hall, Stephen S. *A Commotion in the Blood.* New York: Henry Holt. 1997.

162. Hand, Wayland D. *Magical Medicine. The Folkloric Component of Medicine in the Folk Belief, Custom, and Ritual of the Peoples of Europe and America.* Berkeley, CA: University of California Press. 1980.

162a. Harisch, G., et al. [Effects of lowest levels of drugs–a contribution to homoeopathy research]. *DTW Dtsch Tierartztl Wochenschr.* 1992;99:343-345.

163. Harris, C, et al. Efficacy of acemannan in treatment of canine and feline spontaneous neoplasms. *Mol Biother.* 1991;3:207-213.

164. Hartwell, JL. Plants used against cancer. A survey. *Lloydia* 1970;33:288-392; 1971;34:386-425; 1971;34:"103-160.

165. Hartwell, Jonathan. Plants and cancer. *Cancer Treatment Reports* 1976;60:980.

★166. Hartwell, Jonathan. *Plants Used Against Cancer.* Lawrence, MA: Quarterman Publishing, Inc. 1982. A reprint of the *Lloydia* articles. Still the single most important work published on this topic in the English language, and probably any language. See Afterword for full discussion.

167. Hartzell, Hal, Jr. *The Yew Tree: A Thousand Whispers.* Eugene, OR: Hulogosi Communications, Inc. 1997.

168. Haskell, Charles M. [Ed.] *Cancer Treatment,* 4th Ed., Philadelphia: Saunders, 1995.

169. Hauser, SP. Unproven methods in cancer treatment. *Current Opinion in Oncology.* 1993;5:646-654.

170. Hawkins, Michael J. "Investigational Agents," in DeVita, VJ, et al., eds. *Cancer:* 4th Ed., Philadelphia: Lippincott, 1993:351.

171. Hedrick, U.P. [ed.]. *Sturtevant's Edible Plants of the World.* New York: Dover. 1972 [1919].

172. Heiligtag, Hans-Richard. Anthroposophical viewpoints on mistletoe. *Mercury.* 1997:16:74-76.

173. Heiligtag, Hans-Richard. The practical application of mistletoe therapy with iscador. *Mercury.* 1997:16:77.

174. Heinerman, John. *Heinerman's Encyclopedia of Healing Herbs and Spices.* New York: Prentice-Hall. 1996.

175. Heinerman, John. *Treating Cancer With Herbs.* Orem, UT: Biworld Publishers. 1980. Contains 42 pages on specific herbs for cancer. Heinerman's eclectic sources include interviews with leading scientists as well as "True-UFO's & Outer Space Quarterly."

176. Heiny, BM and Beuth J: Mistletoe extract standardized for the galactoside-specific lectin (ML-1) induces ß-endorphin release and immunopotentiation in breast cancer patients. *Anticancer Res.* 1994;1339-1342.

177. Heiny, BM, et al. Correlation of immune cell activities and beta-endorphin release in breast carcinoma patients treated with galactose-specific lectin standardized mistletoe extract. *Anticancer Res* . 1998;18:583-586.

178. Heiny, BM, et al. Lebensqualitätsstabilisierung durch Mistellektin-1 normierten Extrakt beim fortgeschrittenen kolorekatalen Karzinom. *Onkologe*. 1997; in press.

179. Hibasami, H, et al. Induction of apoptosis in human stomach cancer cells by green tea catechins. *Oncol Rep*. 1998;5:527.

*180. Hildenbrand, GLG, et al. Five-year survival rates of melanoma patients treated by diet therapy after the manner of Gerson: a retrospective review. *Alternative Therapies in Health and Medicine*. 1995;1:29-37. A groundbreaking retrospective analysis.

181. Hiramatsu, T, et al. Induction of normal phenotypes in ras-transformed cells by damnacanthal from *Morinda citrifolia*. *Cancer Lett*. 1993;73:161-166.

182. Hirazumi, A. *Proceedings of the American Association for Cancer Research*. 1992;33:A3078.

183. Hirazumi, A, et al. Anticancer activity of *Morinda citrifolia* (noni) on intraperitoneally implanted Lewis lung carcinoma in syngeneic mice. *Proc. West Pharmacol Soc*. 1994; 37: 145-146.

*184. Hobbs, Christopher, *Medicinal Mushrooms*. 1995. An instant classic.

185. Hobbs, Christopher. *Kombucha: Manchurian Mushroom Tea, The Essential Guide*. Santa Cruz, CA: Botanica Press. 1995.

186. Hodgson, Cathleen. "Cure For All Cancers: An Interview with Dr. Hulda Clark," American Spirit, Sterling Rose Press, Inc., Berkeley, CA, 1995 (www.freeyourself.com/html/ clark.htm).

187. Hoffman, Brian F. and J. Thomas Bigger, Jr., Cardiovascular drugs. In: Goodman-Gilman, et al., *op.cit.* 1980.

188. Holbrook, Stewart H. *The Golden Age of Quackery*. New York: Macmillan. 1959. Very enjoyable if one-sided social history.

*189. Holland, James, et al. [Eds.], *Cancer Medicine*, 4th Ed., Philadelphia: Williams & Wilkins. 1997. Probably the best of all the orthodox textbooks on cancer, despite outdated chapter on alternatives.

190. Holmes, FA, et al. Phase II trial of taxol: an active drug in metaststic breast cancer. *JNCI*. 1991;83:1797-1805.

191. Horbart, FG and Melton, G. *A concise applied pharmacology and therapeutics of the more important drugs*. London, 1949.

192. Houston, Robert G. *Repression and Reform in the Evaluation of Alternative Cancer Therapies*. Washington, DC: Project Cure. 1989.

193. Howley, Peter M. Principles of Carcinogenesis: Viral. In: DeVita, VJ, et al. [Eds.], *Cancer*, 5th Ed., 1997.

*194. Hoxsey, Harry. *You Don't Have to Die*. New York: Milestone Books. 1956. Out-of-print but photocopies available from the Cancer Control Society, Los Angeles, CA.

195. Hsu, Hong-Yen. *Treating Cancer with Chinese Herbs*. Oriental Healing Arts Institute. Long Beach, CA, 1982.

196. Huang, Osawaa, Ho and Rosen [eds.], *Food Phytochemicals for Cancer Prevention*, vols. 1 and 11, 1994.

197. Hunter, T, et al. Protein-tyrosine kinases. *Annu Rev Biochem*. 1985;54: 897-930.

198. Imai, S, et al. African Burkitt's lymphoma: a plant, *Euphorbia tirucalli*, reduces Epstein-Barr virus-specific cellular immunity. *Anticancer Res*. 1994;14:933.

199. Imai, S. et al. Distribution of mouse mammary tumor virus in Asian wild mice. *J Virol*. 1994;68:3437-3442.

199a. Imaida, K. ete al. Effects of naturally occurring antioxidants on combined 1,2-dimethylhydrazine and 1-methyl-1-nitrosourea-initiated carcinogenesis in F344 male rats. *Cancer Lett*. 1990;55:53.

200. Ingre, VG. [Harmlessness of plumbagine in a biological experiment]. *Vopr Pitan*. 1978;4:74-7.

201. Jackson, SJ, *Proc Annual Meet Brit Assoc Ca Res*, Nottingham, UK, 1995.

202. Janssen, WF. Cancer quackery: the past in the present. *Semin Oncol*. 1979;6:526-535.

203. Jastrow, M. The medicine of the Babylonians and Assyrians. *Proc Roy Soc Med, Sect Hist Med*. 1914.

204. Jeong, HY, et al. [Anticancer effects of aloe on sarcoma 180 in ICR mouse and on human cancer cell lines.] *Yakhah Hoe Chi.* 1994;38:311-321.

205. Jiang, TL, et al. [Trends in studies on antineoplastic herbal drugs in China]. *Chung Hsi I Chieh Ho Tsa Chih.* 1986; 6: 698-702.

206. Jisaka, M., et al. Antitumor and antimicrobial activities of bitter sesquiterpene lactones of *Vernonia amygdalina,* a possible medicinal plant used by wild chimpanzee. *Biosci Biotech Biochem.* 1993;57:833.

★207. Johnson, Lois C. Herbal treatment of cancer & herbal support during chemotherapy and radiation therapy. Talk delivered at the 7th annual *American Herbalists Guild Symposium* in Boulder, Co, June 7-9, 1996. Johnson calls herself "recovering oncologist." She sees no "magic bullet" in herbs, but uses them to help her patients get through conventional treatments.

208. Johnson, RK. Screening methods in antineoplastic drug discovery. *JNCI.* 1990;82:1082.

209. Jones, Cindy L.A. Breast cancer: herbs to beat it, treat it. *Herbs for Health.* January/February, 1998.

★210. Jones, Eli G. *Cancer. Its Causes, Symptoms and Treatment.* New Delhi: B. Jain Publishers. 1994 [1912]. The classic work of Eclecticism on the subject.

★211. Jones, Kenneth. *Cat's Claw: Healing Vine of Peru.* Seattle, WA: Sylvan Press. 1995. As always, a non-promotional, balanced account of a controversial herb based on first-hand explorations.

★212. Jones, Kenneth. *Pau d'Arco: Immune Power from the Rain Forest.* Rochester, VT: Healing Arts Press. 1995. The definitive popular account of this intriguing herb.

213. Jones, Kenneth. *Shiitake: The Healing Mushroom.* Rochester, VT: Healing Arts Press. 1995.

214. Jones, Kenneth. *Uña de gato.* American Herb Association. 1994;10:3.

215. Jordan, E. and Wegner, H. Structure and properties of polysaccharides from *Viscum album. Oncology.* 1986;43S:8-15.

216. Juszkiewicz, T, et al. Teratological evaluation of Ukrain in hamsters and rats. *Drugs Under Experimental and Clinical Research.* 1992;17S:23-29.

217. Kaelin, N. Der Kapillar-dynamische Bluttest zur Frühdiagnose der Krebskrankheit. Dornach: *Philosophisch-Anthroposophischer Verlag.* 1969.

218. Kaldor, JM, et al. Leukemia following Hodgkin's disease. *N Engl J Med.* 1990;322:7.

219. Kapadia, GJ, et al. Carcinogenicity of some folk medicinal herbs in rats. *J Natl Cancer Inst.* 1978;60:683-686.

220. Kappus, KK, et al. Results of testing for intestinal parasites by state diagnostic laboratories, United States, 1987. *Mor Mortal Wkly Rep CDC Surveill Summ.* 1991;40:25-45.

★221. Kasad, Kershasp. *Iscador Therapy of Cancer.* Bombay, India: Progressive Writers Combine. 1990. The best survey in English.

222. Katdare, M, et al. Inhibition of aberrant proliferation and induction of apoptosis in pre-neoplastic human mammary epithelial cells by natural phytochemicals. *Oncol Rep.* 1998; 5: 311-315.

223. Keller, H. Carnivora® Immunomodulation & Cytostatis. Basic Medical Brochure. Nordhalben, Germany: May, 1994. In: Keller, Helmut G., *Oncology Beyond the Year 2000,* n.p., 1998.

224. Keller, H. Krebstherapie mit einem pflanzlichen Wirkstoff–erste Erfahrungen mit einem neuen Phyto-Onkologikum. *Acta Medica Empirica.* 1985;34:416-420.

225. Keller, H. Venusfliegenfallen-Extrakt hilft bei Krebs. *Arzliche Praxis.* 1985;36:1626-1628.

226. Keplinger, Klaus, et al. Oxindole alkaloids having properties stimulating the immunologic system & preparation containing the same. *United States patent #5,302,611.* Apr. 12, 1994.

227. Keplinger, Klaus, et al. Process for the production of specific isomer mixtures from oxindole alkaloids. *United States Patent #5,723,625.* Mar. 3, 1998.

228. King, GK, et al. The effect of Acemannan Immunostimulant in combination with surgery and radiation therapy on spontaneous canine and feline fibrosarcomas. *J Am Anim Hosp Assoc.* 1995;31:439-447.

229. Kingsbury, John. *Poisonous Plants of the United States and Canada.* Englewood Cliffs: Prentice-Hall. 1964.

230. Kjaer, M. Misteltoe (Iscador) therapy in stage IV renal adenocarcinoma. A phase II study in patients with measurable lung metastases. *Acta Oncol.* 1989; 28: 489-494.

231. Kleinrok, Z, et al. Basic central pharmacological properties of thiophosphoric acid alkaloid derivatives from *Chelidonium majus* L. *Pol J Pharmacol Pharm*. 1992;44:227-239.

232. Kloss, Jethro and Moffett, Promise K. *Back to Eden: The Classic Guide to Herbal Medicine, Natural Foods, & Home Remedies since 1939*. Lotus Light. 1990.

233. Knekt, P, et al. Body iron stores and risk of cancer. *Int J Cancer*. 1994; 56: 379-382.

*234. Koch, Heinrich P. and Lawson, Larry D. [Eds.]. *Garlic: The Science and Therapeutic Application of Allium Sativum L. and Related Species*. Baltimore: Williams and Wilkins. 1996. A model monograph with 2,240 scientific references.

235. Kramar, C, et al. Presumed calcified leiomyoma of the uterus. Morphologic and chemical studies of a calcified mass dating from the Neolithic period. *Arch Pathol Lab Med* .1983;107:91.

236. Kreher, B, et al. Structure elucidation of plumbagin analogs from *Dionaea muscipula* and their *in vitro* immunological activities *in vitro* and *in vivo*. *Molecular Recognition Int. Symposium*. Sopron, Hungary, August 24-27, 1988.

237. Kreher, B. Chemische und Immunologische Untersuchen der Drogen *Dionaea muscipula*, *Tabebuia avellandedae*, *Euphorbia resinifera* und *Daphne mezereum* sowie Ihrer Praparate. *Dissertation, Ludwig-Maximillians Universität*. Munchen, 1989.

238. Kreher, B. Structure elucidation of plumbagin analogs from *Dionaea muscipula* and their *in vitro* immunological activity on human granulocytes and lymphocytes. *Planta Med*. 1989;55:112.

239. Krenzelok, EP and Jacobsen TD. Plant exposures...a national profile of the most common plant genera. *Vet Hum Toxicol.*. 1997;39:248.

240. Krishnaswamy, M and Purushothaman, KK. Plumbagin: A study of its anticancer, antibacterial & antifungal properties. *Indian J Exp Biol*. 1980;18:876-7.

241. Kufuor-Mensah, E and Watson, GL. Malignant melanomas in a penguin (*Eudyptes chrysolophus*) and a red-tailed hawk (*Buteo jamaicensis*). *Vet Pathol*. 1992;29:354.

242. Kupchan, SM and Karim, A. Tumor inhibitors. Aloe emodin: antileukemic principle isolated from *Rhamnus frangula* L. *Lloydia*. 1976;39:223-4.

242a. Kurokawa, M, et al. Purification and characterization of eugeniin as an anti-herpes virus compound from *Geum japonicum* and *Syzygium aromaticum*. J Pharmacol Exp Ther 1998;284:728.

243. Kuttan, G, et al. Isolation and identification of a tumor reducing component from mistletoe extract (Iscador). *Cancer Lett*. 1988;41:307-314.

244. Langford SD and Boor PJ. Oleander toxicity: an examination of human and animal toxic exposures. *Toxicology*. 1996:3;109:1.

245. Lascaratos, J. 'Arthritis' in Byzantium (AD 324-1453): unknown information from non-medical literary sources. *Ann Rheum Dis*. 1995;54:951.

246. Laus, G. and Keplinger, D. Separation of stereoisomeric oxindole alkaloids from *Uncaria tomentosa* by high performance liquid chromatography. *J Chromatogr*. 1994;662:243-249.

247. Lawrence Review of Natural Products, St. Louis, MO: Facts and Comparisons. 1998.

248. Laws, HF, et al. Letter: "Pseudo-cystathioninuria"—a note of caution about chromatographic diagnosis. *J Pediatr*. 1974;84:925. One of Hulda Clark's few scientific publications.

249. Lazarou, J, et al. Incidence of Adverse Drug Reactions in Hospitalized Patients A Meta-analysis of Prospective Studies *JAMA*. 1998;279:1200-1205.

250. Lenartz, D, et al. Immunoprotective activity of the galactoside-specific lectin from mistletoe after tumor destructive therapy in glioma patients. *Anticancer Res*. 1996; 16: 3799-3802.

251. LeRoi, Rita. An anthroposophical approach to cancer: five lectures given at the Fellowship Community. *Mercury*. 1997:16:30-65.

252. Lettre, H. Einige Beobachtungen über das Wachstum des Mäuse-Ascites-Tumors und seine Beinflussung. *Hope-Seyl Z*. 1941;268:59-75.

253. Lettre, H. Ergebnisse und Probleme der Mitosegiftforschung. *Naturwiss*. 1946;3:75-86.

254. Lettre, H. Über Mitosegifte. *Ergebn Physiol*. 1950:46:379-452.

255. Leung, AY and Foster, Y. *Encyclopedia of Common Natural Ingredients Used in Foods, Drugs and*

Cosmetics, 2nd Ed., New York: John Wiley & Sons. 1996.

★256. Lewis, Walter H. and Elvin-Lewis, Memory P. *Medical Botany: Plants Affecting Man's Health.* New York: John Wiley & Sons. 1982. Although somewhat outdated, still an excellent resource with valuable insights.

257. Li, Shiyou and Adair, Kent. *Camptotheca Acuminata* Decaisne, [Hsi Shu] (Chinese Happytree): A Promising Anti-Tumor and Anti-Viral Tree for the 21st century. Nacogdoches, TX: Stephen F. Austin State Univ., Schl. of Forestry. 1994.

258. Lien, Eric J. and Li, Wen Y. *Structure Activity Relationship Analysis of Anticancer Chinese Drugs and Related Plants.* Oriental Healing Arts Institute, Long Beach, CA. No date.

259. Lipton, Eric and Smith, Leef. Cancer 'cure' a painful lie? *Washington Post,* February 25, 1998:A1.

260. Lithander, A. Intracellular fluid of waybread *(Plantago major)* as a prophylactic for mammary cancer in mice. *Tumour Biol* 1992;13:138-141.

261. Livingston-Wheeler, Virginia. *The Conquest of Cancer: Vaccines and Diet.* New York: Franklin-Watts. 1984.

262. Lo, CT and Lee, KM. Intestinal parasites among the Southeast Asian laborers in Taiwan during 1993-1994. *Chung Hua I Hsueh Tsa Chih.* (Taipei) 1996;57:401-404.

263. Lo, JS, et al. Metastatic basal cell carcinoma: report of twelve cases with a review of the literature. *J Am Acad Dermatol.* 1991;24:715-719.

264. Logan, Patrick. *Irish Country Cures.* New York: Sterling Publishing Co. 1994 [1981].

265. Lorenz, Friedrich. Cancer: a mandate to humanity. Chestnut Ridge, NY: *Mercury.* 1997;16:1-29.

266. Loveland, CJ, et al. Widespread erosive disease with probable nasopharyngeal primary in a prehistoric Great Basin skeleton. *Bull NY Acad Med.* 1992;68:420.

267. Lucas, Richard. *Nature's Medicine.* N. Hollywood, CA: Wilshire, 1968.

268. Lust, John. *The Herb Book.* New York: Bantam, 1974. One of the most complete herbals in existence, with over 2,000 listings.

269. Mangali, A, et al. Intestinal parasitic infections in Campalagian district, south Sulawesi, Indonesia. *Southeast Asian J Trop Med Public Health.* 1993;24:313-320.

270. Maxwell, Nicole. *Witch Doctor's Apprentice:* Hunting for Medicinal Plants in the Amazon. New York: Citadel, 1990.

271. McGowan, Elizabeth. Good medicine or snake oil? The controversy over herbal remedies. *Plants & Gardens News* (Brooklyn Botanic Garden) 1998;13:1.

272. McGrew, Roderick E. *Encyclopedia of Medical History.* London: The Macmillan Press, 1985.

273. McGuffin, M, et al. *American Herbal Products Associations' Botanical Safety Handbook.* Boca Raton, FL: CRC Press, 1997.

274. Meier, Zeitschr. f. Deutsche Mythol. u. Sittenkunde 1853:1:443.

275. Melo, AM, et al. [First observations on the topical use of Primin, Plumbagin and Maytenin in patients with skin cancer]. *Rev Inst Antibiot.*(Recife) 1974;14:9-16.

275a. Mésségué, Maurice. *Health Secrets of Plants and Herbs.* New York: William Morrow. 1979.

276. Mgbonyebi, OP, et al. Antiproliferative effect of synthetic resveratrol on human breast epithelial cells. *Int J Oncol.* 1998;12:865-869.

277. Millspaugh, Charles F. *American Medicinal Plants:* An Illustrated and Descriptive Guide to Plants Indigenous to and Naturalized in the United States Which Are Used in Medicine. New York: Dover Publications. 1974 [1892].

278. Mitchell, H.W., et al. *British Herbal Pharmacopoeia,* 4th Ed. Bournemouth, U.K.: British Herbal Medical Association. 1983.

279. Moerman, Daniel E. *Geraniums for the Iroquois:* A Field Guide to American Indian Medicinal Plants. Algonac, MI: Reference Publications, Inc. 1982.

280. Moertel, CG, et al. Phase II study of camptothecin (NSC-100880) in the treatment of advanced gastrointestinal cancer. *Cancer Chemother Rep* Part 1 1972;56:95.

281. Mohs, FE. Chemosurgery for skin cancer: fixed tissue and fresh tissue techniques. *Arch Dermatol.*

1976;112:211-215.

282. Mohs, FE. Chemosurgery: microscopically controlled surgery for skin cancer—past, present and future. *Arch Dermatol*. 1978;4:41-54.

283. Mok, SC, et al. Overexpression of the protein tyrosine phosphatase, nonreceptor type 6 (PTPN6), in human epithelial ovarian cancer. *Gynecol Oncol*. 1995;57:299.

284. Moore, Michael. *Medicinal Plants of the Mountain West*. Santa Fe: Museum of New Mexico Press. 1979.

★285. Moore, Michael. *Medicinal Plants of the Pacific West*. Santa Fe: Red Crane Books. 1995. Fascinating and funnier than the comedian of the same name.

286. Morant, R, et al. [Why do cancer patients use alternative medicine]? *Schweiz Med Wochenschr*. 1991;121:1029-1034.

287. Morita, H, et al. Cytotoxic and mutagenic effects of emodin on cultured mouse carcinoma FM3A cells. *Mutat Res*. 1988;204:329-32.

288. Morita, K, et al. A desmutagenic factor isolated from burdock (*Arctium lappa* Linne). *Mutat Res*. 1984;129:25-31.

289. Morris, Nat. *The Cancer Blackout*. Los Angeles: Regent House. 1977.

290. Moss, Ralph W. *Alternative Medicine Online*. Brooklyn, New York: Equinox Press. 1997.

291. Moss, Ralph W. *Cancer Therapy: The Independent Consumer's Guide to Non-Toxic Treatment and Prevention*. Brooklyn, New York: Equinox Press. 1996 [1992].

292. Moss, Ralph W. *Questioning Chemotherapy*. Brooklyn, New York: Equinox Press. 1995.

293. Moss, Ralph W. *The Cancer Industry,* revised ed. Brooklyn, New York: Equinox Press. 1996 [1989].

294. Muller BM, et al. [Polysaccharides from *Nerium oleander:* structure and biological activity]. *Pharmazie*. 1991;46:657.

295. Musianowycz, J, et al. Clinical studies of Ukrain in terminal cancer patients (Phase II). *Drug Exp Clin Res* 1992;18S:45.

★296. Naiman, Ingrid. *Cancer Salves: A Botanical Approach to Treatment*. Santa Fe: Seventh Ray Press. 1997. A very thorough and generally well balanced account of the history and use of cancer salves. I have learned much from Dr. Naiman's exposition and from my correspondence with her on the topic.

297. Nair, SC, et al. Antitumour activity of saffron. *Cancer Lett*. 1991;57:109-114.

298. Nakanishi, K, et al. Phytochemical survey of Malaysian palants. Preliminary chemical and pharmacological screening. *Chem Pharm Bull*. 1965;13:882-890.

299. Nelson, RL, et al. The effect of iron on experimental colorectal carcinogenesis. *Anticancer Res*. 1989; 9:1477-1482.

300. Newman, V. et al. Dietary supplement use by women at risk for breast cancer recurrence. The Women's Healthy Eating and Living Study Group. *J Am Diet Assoc*. 1998;98:285.

301. Nowicky, JW, et al. Sensitization of specific lysis in target-effector-system with derivatives of *Chelidonium majus* L. ("Ukrain") alkaloids–Ukrain. *Proc 16th Int Cong Chemother*. Jerusalem, June, 11-16, 1989.

302. Nowicky, JW, et al. Ukrain both as an anticancer and immunoregulatory agent. *Drug Exp Clin Res*. 1992;18S:51-54.

303. Nowicky, JW. New immuno-stimulating anti-cancer preparation 'Ukrain.' *13th Int Cong Chemother*. (Aug 28-Sept 2, Vienna), 1983, Abst PS 12.5.33/A-6.

304. Nowicky, JW. Ukrain. *Drugs of the Future*. 1993;18:1011-1015.

305. O'Dwyer, PJ, et al. Homoharringtonine--perspectives on an active new natural product. *J Clin Oncol*. 1986;4:1563.

306. Olsen, Cynthia, *Essiac: A Native Herbal Cancer Remedy*. With Contribution by Dr. Jim Chan. Pagosa Springs, CO: Kali Press. 1996.

307. Olsnes, S, et al. Isolation and characterization of viscumin, a toxic lectin from *Viscum album* L. (mistletoe). *J Biol Chem*. 1982;257:13263-70.

308. Osol, A. and Farrar, GE. The Dispensatory of the United States of America, 25th Ed., Philadelphia:

J.B. Lippincott Company, 1955.

309. Oztekin-Mat, A. [Plant poisoning cases in Turkey]. *Ann Pharm Fr.* 1994;52:260-265

★310. Pahlow, Apotheker M. *Das Grosse Buch der Heil Pflanzen.* München, Gräfe unde Unzer. 1993. Definitive German herbal with beautiful illustrations.

311. Pantazis, Panayotis. The Camptothecins: From Discovery to the Patient. *Annals of the New York Academy of Sciences,* vol. 803, New York, NY, 1996. An inspiring account of persistence in science.

312. Patterson, James T. *The Dread Disease.* Cambridge, MA: Harvard University Press. 1987.

★313. Payer, Lynn. *Medicine & Culture,* New York: Henry Holt & Co. 1996. Witty and wise cultural commentary.

314. Peng HW, et al. Imported Opisthorchis viverrini and parasite infections from Thai labourers in Taiwan. *J Helminthol.* 1993;67:102-106.

315. Peng, SY, et al. Decreased mortality of Norman murine sarcoma in mice treated with the immunomodulator, Acemannan. *Mol Biother.* 1991;3:79-87.

316. Pengsaa, P, et al. The effects of thiophosphoric acid (Ukrain) on cervical cancer, stage IB bulky. *Drug Exp Clin Res.* 1992;18S:69-72.

317. Perdue, RE, Jr., et al. *Camptotheca acuminata* Decaisne (Nyssaceae). Source of camptothecin, an antileukemic alkaloid. U.S. Department of Agriculture, Agricultural Research Service. *Technical Bulletin,* No. 1415, 1970.

318. Pettit, George R. *Biosynthetic Products for Cancer Chemotherapy.* New York: Plenum Press. 1977.

319. Pliny [the Elder]. *Natural History.* Jones, WHS, et al. (trans.), 10 vols., Cambridge, MA: Harvard University Press (Loeb Classical Library). 1958-1991.

320. Plotkin, Mark. *Tales of a Shaman's Apprentice.* Orlando, FL: Harcourt Brace & Co. 1998.

321. Potmesil, Milan and Pinedo, Herbert. *Camptothecins: New Anticancer Agents.* Boca Raton, FL: 1995.

322. Powell, RG, et al. Antitumor alkaloids from *Cephalotaxus harringtoninia:* structure and activity. *J Pharm Sci.* 1972;61:1227.

323. Raffauf, Robert. *Plant Alkaloids:* A Guide to Their Discovery and Distribution, The Haworth Press. 1996.

324. Rafinesque, CS. *Medical Flora;* or Manual of the Medical Botany of the United States of North America. Vols 1-2. Philadelphia: Atkinson & Alexander. 1828-1830.

324a. Rao, KV, et al. *Cancer Research* 1968;28:1952-1954.

325. Reedy, Jeremiah [trans.]. Galen, *'De Tumoribus Praeter Naturam,'* A Critical Edition with Translation and Indices. The University of Michigan Ph.D. Dissertation. 1968.

326. Reid, Ellen J. and Betts. TJ. Records of Western Australian plants used by aboriginals as medicinal agents. *Planta Medica.* 1979;36:168-169.

327. Richardson, Mary Ann. Report on research at the Center for Alternative Medicine Research, University of Texas. Presented at the *Integrating Complementary & Alternative Therapies conference,* Arlington, VA, June 14, 1998.

328. Ries, LAG, et al. [eds.] SEER Cancer Statistics Review, 1973-1991: Tables and Graphs, National Cancer Institute. *NIH Pub. No. 94-2789.* Bethesda, MD. 1994

329. Risberg ,T, et al. The use of non-proven therapy among patients treated in Norwegian oncological departments. A cross-sectional national multicentre study. *Eur J Cancer.* 1995;31A:1785-1789.

330. Risberg, T, et al. [Use of alternative medicine among Norwegian hospitalized cancer patients]. *Tidsskr Nor Laegeforen.* 1997;117:2458-2463.

331. Rizzi, R., et al. Mutagenic and antimutagenic activities of *Uncaria tomentosa* and its extracts. *J Ethnopharmacol.* 1993;38:63.

332. Robbers, James, et al. *Pharmacognosy and Pharmacobiotechnology.* Baltimore: Williams & Wilkins. 1996.

333. Root, Jolie Martin. "Cat's claw...Miracle from the rain forest." An informational flyer distributed in health food stores in 1998.

★334. Root-Bernstein, Robert and Michèle. *Honey, Mud, Maggots, and Other Medical Marvels.* Boston:

Houghton Mifflin Co. 1997. Popular anthropology with many insights.

335. Rubin, Philip. *Clinical Oncology.* A Multidisciplinary Approach for Physicians and Students. 7th Ed., Philadelphia: Saunders. 1993.

336. Santa Maria A, et al. Evaluation of the toxicity of *Uncaria tomentosa* by bioassays *in vitro. J Ethnopharmacol* 1997;57:183.

337. Sarrazin-Vaillant, Quebec-Paris: Boivin, 1708.

338. Sato, M, et al. Contents of resveratrol, piceid, and their isomers in commercially available wines made from grapes cultivated in Japan. *Biosci Biotechnol Biochem.* 1997;61:1800-1805.

339. Sawyer, DR, et al. An ancient 'tumour' from pre-Columbian Chile. *Craniomaxillofac Surg.* 1990;18:136.

340. Scharff, Paul [Ed.], Compendium of Research Papers on Iscador for Years 1986-1988, Chestnut Ridge, NY: Mercury Press. 1991.

341. Schwartz, W. Indogermanischer Volksglaude, Berlin, 1885.

342. Schweppe, KW, Probst C. [The attempts at drug therapy of cancer by Anton Storck (1731-1803). History of experimental pharmacology in the old Vienna Medical School]. *Wien Med Wochenschr.* 1982 Mar 15;132:107-117.

343. Scott, Cyril. *Victory Over Cancer Without Radium or Surgery:* A Survey of Cancer Causes and Cancer Treatments. London: True Health Publishing Co. 1939. Scott described himself as a "musical composer with a taste for philosophy and therapeutics." Very useful for information on Great Britain between the wars.

344. Scudder, John M. *Specific Diagnosis.* Sandy, OR: Eclectic Medicine Press. 1994 [1874].

345. Scully, Virginia. *A Treasury of American Indian Herbs.* New York: Crown, 1970.

346. See, DM, et al. *In vitro* effects of echinacea and ginseng on natural killer and antibody-dependent cell cytotoxicity in healthy subjects and chronic fatigue syndrome or acquired immunodeficiency syndrome patients. *Immunopharmacology.* 1997;35:229-235.

347. Seed, L., et al. Effect of colchicine on human carcinoma. *Surgery.* 1940;7:696-709.

348. Seligman, AB, et al. Sassafras and herb tea. Potential health hazards. *JAMA.* 1976;236:477.

349. Senatore, A, et al. [Phytochemical and biological study of Uncaria tomentosa]. *Boll Soc Ital Biol Sper.* 1989;6:517-520.

350. Sentein, O. L'action des toxiques sur la cellule en division. Effets de la colchicine et du chloral sur les mitoses et tissus normaux et sur quelques tumeurs malignes. *Thèse.* Montpellier, 1941.

351. Shear, MJ. Chemical treatment of tumors. IX. Reactions of mice with primary subcutaneous tumors to injection of a hemorrhage-producing bacterial polysaccharide. *JCNI* 1944;4:461-476.

352. Sheets, MA, et al. Studies of the effect of acemannan on retrovirus infections: clinical stabilization of feline leukemia virus-infected cats. *Mol Biother.* 1991;3:41-45.

353. Shimkin, MA. *Contrary to Nature.* Washington, DC: US Government Printing Office. *DHEW Publication No. (NIH) 79-720.* 1979.

354. Sigerist, Henry E. *Primitive and Archaic Medicine, A History of Medicine,* vol. 1, New York: Oxford University Press. 1967 [1951].

355. Sigerist, Henry. *A History of Medicine,* vol. 2, Oxford: Oxford University Press. 1951.

356. Smith, Leef. Clinic Head Indicted Over Aloe Therapy. *Washington Post,* April 7, 1998:B1.

357. Smith-Kielland, I, et al. Cytotoxic triterpenoids from the leaves of *Euphorbia pulcherrima. Planta Med* 1996;62:322.

358. Snow, Sheila (Fraser) and Allen, Carroll. Could ESSIAC halt cancer? *Homemaker's Magazine.* June-August, 1977.

359. Snow, Sheila. *The Essence of Essiac.* n.p., 1994.

360. Solar, S, et al. Immunostimulant properties of an extract isolated and partially purified from *Aloe vahombe. Arch Inst Pasteur Madagascar.* 1980;47:9-39.

361. Sommers, Cynthia. Proof: *Herbs Against Cancer.* Denver, CO: Red Wing Publishing House. 1995 (2nd printing). ISBN 0-9640193-0-2. Describes itself as "the only definitive cancer herbal combining

scientific, literature with herbal folk medicine....Nothing short of a miracle." and so forth. Is an alphabetical compendium of brief monographs, with no footnotes. At several points, Ms. Sommers confuses the Hoxsey and Essiac formulas. Strong on carcinogens.

362. Spalding, MG, et al. Chondrosarcoma in a wild great white heron from southern Florida. *J Wildl Dis.* 1992; 28:151-153.

363. Staniszewski, A, et al. Lymphocyte subsets in patients treated with thiophosphoric adic alkaloid derivatives from *Chelidonium majus* L. (Ukrain). *Drug Exp Clin Res.* 1992;18S:63-67.

364. Statutes of the Realm, 34-35 Henry VIII, c.8. Cited in Griggs, B., *op. cit.*

365. Stehlin, John S. Introduction and overview. In: Camptothecins: From Discovery to the Patient. *Annals of the New York Academy of Sciences,* vol. 803, New York, NY, 1996.

366. Steinberg, Phillip N. *Cat's Claw.* New York: Healing Wisdom Publications. 1996.

367. Steiner, R. *Spiritual Science and Medicine.* London: Rudolf Steiner Press. 1975.

368. Stern N, et al. [Follow-up and therapy of acute colchicine poisoning]. *Schweiz Rundsch Med Prax.* 1997;86:952.

369. Stevens, RG, et al. Body iron stores and the risk of cancer. *N Engl J Med.* 1988; 319:1047-1052.

370. Stevens, RG, et al. Moderate elevation of body iron level and increased risk of cancer occurrence and death. *Int J Cancer.* 1994;56:364-369.

371. Stockwell, C. *Nature's Pharmacy.* London: Century. 1988.

372. Stoffel B, et al. Effect of immunomodulation with galactoside-specific mistletoe lectin on experimental listeriosis. *Zbl Bakt.* 1996;284:439-442.

373. Stone, Julie and Matthews, Joan. *Complementary Medicine and the Law.* Oxford: Oxford University Press. 1996.

374. Stone, WS. A review of the history of chemical therapy in cancer. *Medical Record* 1916;90:628-634.

375. Strehlow, Wighard and Hertzka, Gottfried. *Hildegard of Bigen's Medicine.* Santa Fe: Bear & Co. 1988.

376. Strickholm, A and Clark, HR. Ionic permeability of K, Na, and Cl in crayfish nerve. Regulation by membrane fixed charges and pH. *Biophys J.* 1977;19:29.

377. Strouhal, E. Tumors in the remains of ancient Egyptians. *Am J Phys Anthropol.* 1976;45:613.

378. Suffness, M and Pezzuto, JM. Assays related to cancer drug discovery. *Methods in Plant Biochemistry,* Vol. 6. Academic Press Limited. 1991.

379. Suffness, Matthew. *Taxol®: Science and Applications.* Boca Raton, FL: CRC Press. 1995.

380. Suga, T. and Hirata, T. The efficacy of the aloe plants chemical constituents and biological activities. *Cosmet Toiletries.* 1983;98:105-108.

381. Sugiura, M, et al. Cryptic dysfunction of cellular immunity in asymptomatic human immunodeficiency virus (HIV) carriers and its actualization by an environmental immunosuppressive factor. *In Vivo.* 1994;8:1019-1022.

382. Suzuki, T. Paleopathological study on malignant bone tumor in Japan. Differential diagnosis on osteolytic lesions in the skull. *Z Morphol Anthropol.* 1989;78:73.

383. Taylor, Nadine. *Green Tea: The Natural Secret for a Healthier Life.* New York: Kensington. 1998.

384. Tennent, John. *Everyman His Own Doctor.* Fascimile edition, Williamsburg, 1984 [1732].

385. Thomas, Richard. *The Essiac Report:* Los Angeles: The Alternative Treatment Information Network. 1993.

★386. Tierra, Michael. Use of herbs, magnets and other supplements in Cancer Therapies. Talk delivered at the 7th annual *American Herbalists Guild Symposium* in Boulder, Co, June 7-9, 1996 *[audio tape].* Helpful in understanding the relationship of Traditional Chinese Medicine (TCM) to Western herbalism, not to mention magnet therapy.

387. Tozyo, T, et al. Novel antitumor sesquiterpenoids in *Achillea millefolium. Chem Pharm Bull.* (Tokyo) 1994;42:1096-1100.

388. Tracqui A, et al. Confirmation of oleander poisoning by HPLC/MS. *Int J Legal Med.* 1998;111:32.

389. Tubeuf, K. Monographie der Mistel, München-Berlin, 1923,

390. Tyler, Varro E. Plant drugs, healing herbs, and phytomedicines. *HerbalGram.* No. 33, 1995:36.

391. Tyler, Varro T. *Pau d'arco* (taheebo) herbal tea. *California Council Against Health Fraud, Inc. Newsletter* 6, no. 5, 1983.

★392. Tyler, Varro. *The Honest Herbal. A Sensible Guide to the Use of Herbs and Related Remedies.* New York: Pharmaceutical Products Press. 1993. A bracing corrective to many over-enthusiastic accounts. Tyler was Lilly Distinguished Professor of Pharmacognosy at the Purdue University School of Pharmacy and Pharmacal Sciences.

393. Urech, Konrad. Natural scientific experiments on mistletoe. Mercury 1997:16:71-73.

394. US Congress, Office of Technology Assessment. *Unconventional Cancer Treatments.* OTA-H-405, Washington, D.C.: U.S. Government Printing Office, September 1990. Included in Chapter Four were discussions of chaparral, Essiac, Hoxsey, Mistletoe and Pau d'Arco. The OTA discussions came out of a contentious struggle. They are brief, and sometimes biased or inaccurate. I would urge readers to the approach them with care. See *The Cancer Industry,* 1996 Introduction.

395. van den Bosch C, et al. Are plant factors a missing link in the evolution of endemic Burkitt's lymphoma? *Br J Cancer.* 1993;68:1232.

396. Vatanasapt, V, et al. Preliminary report on clinical experience in the use of Ukrain. *Thai Cancer J.* 1991;17:20

397. Vilches, Lida E. Obregon, MD. *Cat's Claw.* "Uña de gato" Institute de Fitoterapia Americano, 3rd Edition. 1995.

★398. Vogel, Virgil. *American Indian Medicine.* Norman: University of Oklahoma Press. 1970. The classic in its field.

399. Wagner, H, et al. [The alkaloids of *Uncaria tomentosa* and their phagocytosis-stimulating action]. *Planta Med.* 1985;5:419-423.

400. Wagner, H. Immunostimulants from medicinal plants. *Advances in Chinese Med.* Singapore, 1985.

401. Walker, Morton. M. The anticancer components of Essiac. *Townsend Letter for Doctors & Patients* #173, December, 1997:76-82.

402. Wall, ME, et al. Plant antitumor agents I. The isolation and structure of camptothecin, a novel alkaloidal leukemia and tumor inhibitor from *Camptotheca accuminata. J Am Chem Soc.* 1966;88:3888-3890.

403. Walters, Richard. *Options.* Garden City Park, NY: Avery Publishing Group. 1993.

404. Watson, EM. *Journal of the Royal Society of Western Australia* 1944;30:83.

405. Weed, Susun S. *Wise Woman: Herbal Healing Wise.* Woodstock, NY: Ash Tree Publishing. 1989.

★406. Werbach, Melvyn R and Murray, Michael T. *Botanical Influences on Illness.* Tarzana: Third Line Press. 1994. Reviews major botanical treatments for cancer.

407. Wheelwright, Edith Grey. *Medicinal Plants and Their History.* New York: Dover. 1974 [1935].

408. Wiener, JR, et al. Overexpression of the protein tyrosine phosphatase PTP1B in human breast cancer: association with p185c-erbB-2 protein expression. *J Natl Cancer Inst.* 1994;86:372.

409. Wiener, JR, et al., Overexpression of the tyrosine phosphatase PTP1B is associated with human ovarian carcinomas. *Am J Obstet Gynecol.* 1994;170:1177-1183.

410. Williams, David G. *The skin cancer cure nobody wants you to know about.* Alternatives For the Health Conscious Individual. Kerrville, TX: Mountain Home Publishing. 1995.

411. Willis, A. *The Spread of Tumours in the Human Body.* London: J&A Churchill. 1934.

412. Winston, David. Herbalist & Alchemist: The Art of Alchemy. Broadway, NJ, 1997. *Company catalog.*

★413. Wolff, Jacob. *The Science of Cancerous Disease from the Earliest Time to the Present.* New Delhi: Science History Publications. 1989. [Abridged from Die Lehre von der Krebskrankheit von den ältesten Zeiten bis zur Gegenwart. Jena: Gustav Fischer Verlag. 1907.] A monumental four-volume history of cancer, in which he discussed many unusual treatments. A model of German pre-WWI historical scholarship. This is the one-volume English abridgement.

414. Woodward, Marcus. *Leaves from Gerard's Herbal.* New York: Dover. 1969. A classic of Shakespeare's day.

415. World Health Organization (WHO). Guidelines for the Assessment of Herbal Medicines. *Programme*

on Traditional Medicines, Geneva, 1991.

416. World Health Organization (WHO). *In vitro* screening of traditional medicines for anti-HIV activity: memorandum from a WHO meeting. *Bul. WHO.* (Switzerland), 1989;67:613-618.

417. World Health Organization (WHO). WHO/UNICEF Meeting Report: Primary Health Care; *Report of the International Conference on Primary Health Care.* Geneva, 1978.

417a. Xu, L, et al. [Characteristics and recent trends in endemicity of human parasitic diseases in China.] *Chung Kuo.* 1995;13:214.

418. Yao, XR, et al. Expression of protein tyrosine kinases in the Ig complex of anti-mu-sensitive and anti-mu-resistant B-cell lymphomas: role of the p55blk kinase in signaling growth arrest and apoptosis. *Immunol Rev.* 1993;132:163.

419. Yarden, Y, et al. Growth factor receptor tyrosine kinases. *Annu Rev Biochem.* 1988;57:443-478.

420. Young, James Harvey. *The Medical Messiahs: A Social History of Health Quackery in Twentieth Century America.* Princeton: Princeton University Press. 1967.

421. Zevin, Igor Vilevich. *A Russian Herbal: Traditional Remedies for Health and Healing.* Rochester, VT: Healing Arts Press. 1997.

422. Zhang, L and Tizard, IR. Activation of a mouse macrophage cell line by acemannan: the major carbohydrate fraction from *Aloe vera* gel. *Immunopharmacology.* 1996;35:119-128.

423. Zimmerman, MR. A possible histiocytoma in an Egyptian mummy. *Arch Dermatol.* 1981;117:364.

🌹 Resources

People with cancer, ideally, should be under the care of skilled oncologists who are sympathetic to their use of integrative medicine, including herbs. Finding such an oncologist may be the most important challenge in dealing with cancer.

Patients should also familiarize themselves with the state-of-the-art conventional treatments for their particular diagnoses, as well as the most promising alternatives from around the world. This can be done through reading books and articles (such as those mentioned in the References section), by visiting the most informative Websites (many of which can be accessed through www.ralphmoss.com), or by utilizing a consultation service such as The Moss Reports (see below).

Finding a conventional oncologist is relatively easy, but discovering a talented herbalist can be something of a challenge. Information on herbs is as freely available as dandelions growing in the park. So naturally there is a good supply of well-meaning people claiming expertise in the field. Some are licensed health-care providers, such as medical doctors, osteopaths, chiropractors, naturopaths, acupuncturists, and other professionals. There are also many non-credentialed herbalists, lay practitioners who carry on the thousand-year-old tradition of learning and treating their neighbors with plants.

In the United States, there is no uniform licensure or other requirements for calling oneself an herbalist. There is, however, a goodly number of schools and programs, many of them advertised in the back pages of health magazines. These range from truly enlightening courses taught by outstanding scholars, to total wastes of money and time. That is why it is difficult to know whether a person purporting to be an herbalist can really help you.

Below, I have given the names and addresses of some organizations and publications that can help you find an experienced and ethical herbalist with whom you can work. Often the best recommendation comes by asking around, especially at the local health food store.

Many of the treatments mentioned in this book could be used as part of a self-help program for cancer. But not everything discussed in this book is suitable for self-treatment. Some items must be approached with caution and others should be avoided entirely, except in the context of a clinical trial.

Many herbal treatments are now available through health food stores, mail order companies, or even over the Internet. These include pau d'arco, cat's claw, aloe vera, etc. While most of these products are reliable, on occasion there have been problems with strength and quality. For example, many samples of pau d'arco have been found to lack lapachol, and cat's claw has being marketed with minuscule amounts of Isomer A. In general, I would stick to the larger, most reputable brands, unless you know and trust the herbalist who is preparing the item for you.

CLARK METHOD

Self Health Resource Center
1055 Bay Blvd. #A
Chula Vista, CA 91911
Phone: 619-409-9500
Fax: 619-409-9501

Self Health Resource Centre
14027 63 St. Edmonton, AB
T5A 1R6 Canada
Phone: 403-475-2403
Fax: 403-475-2403

HOXSEY TREATMENT

Bio-Medical Clinic
PO Box 727
General Ferreira #615
Col. Juarez
Tijuana, Mexico
Ph: 011-52-66-84-90-11 or -81
Many other companies and
herbalists have created their own
versions of this famous formula.

ESSIAC TEA and TINCTURE

Trademarked Essiac® is
distributed by Essiac Products
Campbellton, New Brunswick
E3N 2R9 Canada

Flor·Essence is made by:
Flora Manufacturing &
Distributing, Ltd.
7400 Frasier Park Drive
Burnaby, British Columbia
V5J 5B9 Canada
Phone: 604-436-6000

HANSI

Hansi International, Ltd.
2831 Ringling Boulevard, A-102
Sarasota, FL 34237
Phone: 941-953-4863
Fax: 941-366-2023

MISTLETOE (ISCADOR)

Lukas Klinik
CH-4144 Arlesheim
Switzerland
Phone: 011 41 61-701-3333

Physicians Association for
Anthroposophical Medicine
PO Box 269
Kimberton, PA 19442

Mercury Press
241 Hungry Hollow Road
Spring Valley, NY 10977
914-425-9357

Society for Cancer Research
Research Institute Hiscia
CH-4144
Arlesheim, Switzerland
Phone: 011 41 61-701-2323

CURADERM

Masters Marketing Co.
Masters House
5 Sandridge Close
Harrow, Middlesex HA1 1XD
England
Phone: 011-44-181-424-9400
Fax: 011-44-181-427-1994

CoD TEA—N. AMERICA

Institute for Immunostabilization
Research and Information
c/o MDA, Inc.
150 Fifth Avenue #835
New York, NY 10011
Phone: 212-727-0407
Fax: 212-727-0409

CoD TEA—EUROPE

Institut fur
Immunostabilizierungs-
Forschung und Information
Margaretenstrasse 8
A-1040 Vienna, Austria
Phone: 43-1-585-18-05
Fax: 43-1-585-18-05-13

ALZIUM

Chaim Kass
Ced Tech, Ltd.
Phone: 718-871-2856
Fax 718- 871-6493

ANVIRZEL (OLEANDER)

Ozelle Pharmaceuticals
11825 IH 10 West, Suite 213
San Antonio, TX 78230;
Phone: 210-690-0022

CARNIVORA

Helmut Keller, MD
Carnivora-Forschungs-GmbH
Postfach 8, Lobensteiner Strasse 3
D-96365 Nordhalben, Germany
Tel: 49-9267-1662
Fax: 49-9267-1040

ALOE VERA (CARRASYN)

Carrington Laboratories, Inc.
2001 Walnut Hill Lane
Irving, TX 75038
Telephone 214-518-1300
Fax 214-518-1020

HERBAL ORGANIZATIONS

American Botanical Council
PO Box 201660
Austin, TX 78720
Phone: 512-331-8868

American Herb Association
PO Box 1673
Nevada City, CA 95959
Phone: 916-265-9552

American Herbalist Guild
PO Box 1683
Soquel, CA 95073

Herb Research Foundation
1007 Pearl St., Suite 200
Boulder, CO 80302
Phone: 303-449-2265

Medical Herbalism
A Clinical Newsletter
for the Herbal Practitioner
PO Box 33080
Portland, OR 97233

National Herbalists' Association
of Australia
Suite 305 · 3 Smail St.
Broadway
NSW 2007 · Australia

The Herb Quarterly
PO Box 689
San Anselmo, CA 94979
Phone: 800-371-HERB

Robyn's Recommended
Reading
1627 W. Main, Ste. #116
Bozeman, MT 59715

SUPPLIERS OF HERBS

Aphrodisia
264 Bleeker St.
New York, NY 10014
212-989-6440

Caswell Massey Co., Ltd.
100 Enterprise Place
Dover, DE 19901
800-326-0500

East-West Herb Products
Box 1210
New York, NY 10025
800-542-6544

Frontier Herbs
Box 299, Norway, IA
Phone: 800-786-1388
Fax: 319-227-7966
Supplier of bulk herbs to stores
and individuals.

Gaia Herbals
Harvard, MA
Phone: 800-994-9355

Herb Pharm
PO Box 116
Williams, OR 97544
Highly regarded source.

Herbalist & Alchemist
PO Box 63
Franklin Park, NJ 08823.
Has original Scudder and Jones
formulas available, but only to
health professionals.

Blessed Herbs
Phone: 800-489-HERB
Fax 508-882-3755

Indian Meadow Farms
Macomber Mill Road, Box 547
Eastbrook, ME 04634
207-565-3010
High quality herbal farm. All
organic, none wildcrafted
because of ecological concerns.

Mountain Rose Herbs
PO Box 2000
Redway, CA 95560

Phone: 800-879-3337
Fax: 707-923-7867
Has rare and unusual items at
reasonable prices.

Naiman, Dr. Ingrid
Seventh Ray Press
P.O. Box 31007
Santa Fe, NM 87594-1007
Phone: 505-473-5797
Fax: 888-FAX-HEAL
Sells Eli Jones Formula,
Compound Syrup Scrophularia,
Trifolium Compound, "Hoxiac"
(Hoxsey + Essiac),
Red Clover Combination

Penn Herb. Co., Ltd.
603 North Second Street
Philadelphia, PA 19123
Phone: 800-523-9971
Phone: 215-925-3336
Fax: 215-925-7946
One of the largest and
most complete selections,
at excellent prices.

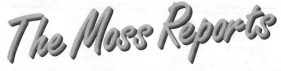

🌹 Index of Plants by Botanical Name

🌹 General Index